THE COMPLETE
NATURAL
HEALTH
CONSULTANT

Michael van Straten

EBURY
PRESS

Published by Ebury Press
an imprint of the Random Century Group
Random Century House,
20 Vauxhall Bridge Road,
London SW1V 2SA

First impression 1987
Second impression 1990

ISBN 0 85223 561 5 (Hardback)
0 85223 454 6 (Paperback)

Edited by Yvonne McFarlane and Vivianne Croot
Designed by Grahame Dudley
Illustrations by Sheila Tizzard and Tessa Land
Cover illustration by Long and Wood Photographic Studios
Additional written material by Anne Charlish and Nancy Duin

Filmset, printed and bound in Great Britain by
Butler & Tanner Ltd, Frome and London

CONTENTS

FOREWORD

A FTER a quarter of a century, my enthusiasm for alternative medicine is still growing, my therapeutic horizons still expanding and my utter faith in the human body's ability to heal itself unshaken.

It may seem contradictory that this book emphasizes the vital importance of the holistic approach to health and disease, and yet contains an A–Z of illnesses and symptoms. However, experience with thousands of patients has taught me not to be dogmatic: if you have a problem, you want to deal with it. I hope this book will not only help you deal with the crises of daily life but also teach you a better way of treating your body, mind and spirit within the environment of the 20th century.

There is no such thing as alternative medicine. There is Good Medicine and Bad Medicine, and Good Medicine is about people. This book is dedicated to the memory of Dr Norman Knox, a country-town GP, who taught me about Good Medicine when I was only seven years old and remained a friend for 40 years.

ACKNOWLEDGEMENTS

This book would never have seen the light of day without the tremendous support, help and bullying—in the nicest possible way—of Yvonne McFarlane, the skill of Anne Charlish and Viv Croot, the endless work by Gillian Haslam, the patience of Beverley and the understanding of my own staff who have suffered. The professional colleagues who also contributed are all busy and eminent and I thank them for their time and knowledge.

INTRODUCTION

In the past decade there has been a consumer-led revolution in attitudes to health care. Millions of people have forsaken orthodox medicine for all but the most serious medical emergencies, and have turned instead to alternative practitioners—osteopaths, naturopaths, acupuncturists, herbalists and others outside the bounds of ordinary medicine.

Why is this?

The reasons are not hard to find: the scandal of tranquillizer over-prescription, surgical errors, the long waiting lists, three-minute consultations, indifference, dehumanization, invasive diagnostic procedures have all contributed to the mass rejection of orthodox methods. Just as important, people are beginning to resent the Olympian mysticism of the medical profession and its ingrained secrecy. They will no longer tolerate being fobbed off with platitudes or patronization when they ask questions, they will not submit to surgery, drug therapy or complex investigations without good reason, and they demand to be involved in decisions which impinge on their own lives. Whose body is it anyway?

People are looking for a new approach. And they are finding it in a medical discipline that does more than just treat the symptoms of a disease: *Holistic medicine*.

The holistic approach
'Holistic' has become a buzz word meaning different things to different people. You can go to an 'holistic' health centre or even have an 'holistic' holiday. Is holistic medicine alternative, complementary or something else altogether?

Imagine a person as a plant which is essentially healthy but has one sick stem. Basically, there are two ways of improving the situation: one way, often the way of orthodox medicine is to treat the sick stem in isolation with fungicides (drug therapy) or to prune it off altogether (surgery); the other method, usually the approach of the alternative therapies, is to encourage the healthy parts and their inherent healing powers by feeding more and better compost (dietary advice) or allowing more sunlight onto the plant (exercise); in this approach, the specific problems of the sick part may be seen as untreatable on their own, or at least not very important. The holistic approach is neither orthodox nor alternative but recognizes and uses the best of both systems. I must emphasize that it is an *approach* rather than a technique. It is not about what you do, but rather how you do it.

An important point to remember is that not all alternative therapies are holistic: sticking needles into someone is no more holistic on its own than prescribing valium. On the other hand, many GPs, even those who deny it vigorously, do use an holistic approach.

What is holistic medicine?
Orthodox (or allopathic) medicine concentrates its efforts on the 'pill for every ill' approach to illness. Alternative medicine focuses on the sick person as a whole, and takes into account all the factors that can contribute to any illness: environment, work, life style, personal relationships, nutrition, and mental state as well as the particular disease. Holistic medicine takes the best from both approaches: it is a person-centred rather than a disease-centred approach; it encourages self responsibility for health, including access to health information and self-help techniques; it advocates the use of a number of different

approaches and sees the health carer more as a guide and educator than a giver of treatment, although the latter role is more suitable to some occasions. How does it work in practical terms?

First, people are seen not just in terms of their bodies, but also of their minds and spirit. Health is seen as the wellbeing of all three parts, not just the absence of disease. Ill health, on the other hand, is seen as the result of damage to this integrated whole.

Secondly, there is an awareness that each one of us has an innate healing power (think how a cut finger heals) and that this can be and needs to be encouraged. Part of this encouragement is to help people become more aware of their own health and to take more responsibility for it on themselves. This implies a shift away from the traditional 'active doctor/therapist and passive patient' relationship to more of an equal partnership, a shift in emphasis from treatment to education.

Thirdly, the health carer themselves need to take greater care of their own health, since it greatly affects their relationships with the people they are trying to help.

Finally, the holistic practitioner uses a wide range of treatment methods which may embrace orthodox systems where these are appropriate. The best complementary practitioners will use or recommend a wide range of therapies, most of which are themselves based on an holistic approach, and self-help techniques.

WHAT IS THE ALTERNATIVE?

To understand the holistic approach you must know something about the alternative therapies. They may be called natural, or alternative or complementary therapies. Natural because they are nearly all based on the idea of the body as a whole, as nature made it, rather than as a series of separate body systems; alternative because that is how their practitioners see them in contrast to orthodox methods; and complementary, that is filling in the gaps (sometimes gaping holes) left by orthodoxy. Of course, they are all three, but in holistic terms, complementary is the

best description, since they are seen as working in tandem with orthodox medicine rather than as a completely separate option.

There is a growing list of complementary therapies, many of which have their origins at the very beginning of medical history. Naturopathy, acupuncture and herbalism are probably the oldest forms of healing we know. Other therapies, such as osteopathy and homeopathy, developed in the late 18th and 19th centuries, while the 20th century has seen many new concepts in psychological approaches to disease such as bioenergetics, autogenics and biofeedback.

But how do they work and what evidence have we of their success?

WHERE IS THE EVIDENCE?

Practitioners of each of the major alternative therapies give some two million consultations a year. The majority of the people who make those consultations derive some benefit from their treatments, quite often after years of unsuccessful conventional treatment. This would appear to be a pretty impressive demonstration of the value of such systems as acupuncture, homeopathy, naturopathy, osteopathy and chiropractic. Even so, there are still many people, not just orthodox doctors, who ask 'where is the evidence?'

In some ways they are right. It is not enough for complementary practitioners to say that they know their treatment works because their grateful patients are walking proof. They are not being totally honest with themselves, or with the public who want clearer guide lines on whom to consult about their health.

One obstacle to objectivity in assessing complementary methods lies in their particular strong point: that they treat the whole person rather than a disease. More attention is given to the individuality of the person, their responses to their environment and the interrelationships of abnormal functions within their body that make up the pattern of illness. This makes some of the methods of conventional medical research inappropriate to many complementary therapies.

Things have not been made easier by the recalcitrant stance of the orthodox medical fraternity who in one breath demand scientific evidence and with the next make assessment very difficult by threatening (until recently) to strike off any of their colleagues who assist in trials or experiments in complementary therapies.

Of course, there are scientific methods which can apply to complementary therapies. Double blind trials can be applied to the testing of nutritional supplements and homeopathic remedies. An interesting point about double blind trials is the interpretation of the placebo effect. Up to 30 per cent of people on placebo treatment in such trials show improvements. Orthodox medicine takes this statistic to indicate that the real drug is not working very well; complementary practitioners regard it as further evidence of the strong self-healing properties of the body, given suitable motivation. The effectiveness of acupuncture or osteopathy can be scientifically tested against a group of people suffering the same complaint but treated conventionally or not at all. Comparative studies of the incidence of certain types of disease among communities with different life styles and eating habits can also provide evidence. For example, communities in rural Africa eating a low fat high-fibre diet have a very low incidence of bowel cancer, diabetes and heart disease compared to a Western urban community. Sceptics will of course try to find other reasons for the differences which must be considered, but such studies give useful pointers to further research.

There is still a long way to go, but more sophisticated instruments will make it possible to measure the subtle variations in body functions which complementary practitioners believe lies at the root of many disorders. We are now entering a new era of exploration, with experts from both orthodox and complementary medicine working together to encourage research into natural therapies and attempts are being made to develop new methods of assessment in which the sick person actively participates rather than being treated as yet another statistical guinea pig.

There are many different points of view and all of them must be aired, but whatever theories abound, and however careful and thorough scientific investigation may be, the final proof of the pudding of complementary medicine will lie in the eating, the outcome of that indefinable and sometimes intuitive exchange between a well-trained practitioner and the person who is involved in his or her own healing process.

HOW THIS BOOK WORKS

The Natural Health Consultant introduces you to the holistic approach to your health. It is divided into three parts:

Part one comprises four essays on nutrition, exercise, stress management, and positive health. In order to maximize the natural healing powers of the human body, it is vital to keep it well nourished, well-exercised and free from unnecessary stress — all of which go to maintain homeostasis, the body's ability to ensure constant physical and chemical conditions within it, regardless of external conditions. This section of the book will help you help yourself to better health.

Part two offers a brief review of all the major complementary therapies—acupuncture, the Alexander technique, healing, herbalism, homeopathy, hypnotherapy, manipulative therapies, massage, naturopathy, relaxation techniques and the main psychotherapies. The more extreme alternative therapies are not included. The holistic approach that informs all these therapies will become apparent, but the section will also help you to find the therapy that you find most compatible.

Part three is the largest section of the book, the A–Z guide to disorders and problems. While there are obvious situations in which orthodox treatment makes the difference between life and death — the inflamed appendix must come out, the broken bone set, the burnt skin grafted, the parasite destroyed — complementary therapies still play a major part in guiding the sufferer towards a better state of general health, which will fortify them in the fight against illness. Other ailments, especially of the digestive organs, respond well to complementary therapies. The A–Z will give you a brief description of the illness or problem, outline the orthodox response, explain what you can do to help yourself and indicate which comp- lementary therapies can help, with specific instructions where relevant.

Hippocrates said, 'the value of any medicine depends more on the faith that the receiver has in the giver that what is given'. This book will help you have faith in yourself as the giver of good health and recovery.

PART I

HELPING
YOURSELF TO
BETTER HEALTH

NUTRITION

Before the fish finger, the food processor and the butter mountain, human beings were hunter gatherers. What we did not find for ourselves we did not eat. With the advent of fire and cooking utensils, we started to include much larger quantities of meat in our diet and so gradually developed into omnivores. As we have managed to survive thousands upon thousands of years in this way, why, you may ask, is there now all the attention being focused on the foods which we eat in our daily lives?

There have been more changes in our eating habits in the past 100 years than in the previous 100,000 years, and in the scale of adaptation and change to suit our changing environment, 100 years is not much more than a blink of the eye. During the last century the change in our population has been dramatic. More and more and more people congregated in the urban conurbations and fewer people lived on the land which was the traditional source of the food which they ate. It therefore became necessary to find ways of transporting vast quantities of food into the cities and of keeping that food fresh and edible for long periods of time. This was the birth of the food processing industry.

In recent years, advances in food technology have spawned a new generation of convenience and junk foods developed to meet the changing needs of our social system. These factors have combined to produce a dramatic rise in the amounts of sugars, refined carbohydrates, salt, animal fats, additives and preservatives which are consumed in the average Western diet.

And what has this done for us? Most Western people today are grossly overfed and at the same time undernourished. While it cannot be denied that enormous advantages result from advances in science and technology, the benefits of civilization are not always positive. The 'over-civilization' of natural body fuel (food) has led to a drastic rise in the incidence of totally avoidable health problems such as obesity, heart disease, high blood pressure, bowel disease and circulatory diseases. For more than 50 years, practitioners of nature cure and other natural therapies have warned against the insidious invasion of the food industry into our daily lives. At last their voices are beginning to be heard.

Food, glorious food

Nutritionists tell us that we need fats, proteins, carbohydrates, vitamins, minerals and trace elements in order to sustain a healthy vital and active body. The only problem with this is that human beings do not like to eat fats, proteins, carbohydrates etc. Humans like food and food should be fun, it should be attractive and above all it must be enjoyable if it is going to do us any good at all. Learn which food belongs to which category, and how to get the balance of fat, carbohydrates and protein right. Healthy eating will follow naturally. First master the basic facts.

Protein

Protein is used to form about 17 per cent of the body — muscle and bone, skin, hair and nails. It is also essential for much hormone and enzyme production that keeps the body working efficiently. Protein is rarely lacking in the average Western diet; in fact, most people eat more than enough. It is found in milk, yoghurt, cheese, meat, poultry, eggs and fish, but also in nuts, seeds, pulses, wholegrains and some vegetables. The trouble with the best known sources of protein is that they are from animal produce and therefore contain saturated fat which can raise chol-

The Affluent Diseases

Below is a list of a wide range of illnesses directly linked to the food we eat. These diseases are virtually unknown in societies that do not live on our Western 'civilized' diet.

Disease	Adverse Dietary Factors
Allergies	*Too much* fat, sugar, salt, cow's milk; *too little* fibre
Breast cancer	*Too much* fat and sugar
Cancer of the large bowel and colon	*Too little* fibre, too much fat
Constipation and piles	*Too little* fibre
Diabetes	*Too much* fat, sugar; *too little* fibre
Diverticular disease	*Too little* fibre
Gall bladder disease	*Too much* fat and sugar
Heart disease	*Too much* fat and salt
High blood pressure	*Too much* fat and salt
Irritable bowel	*Too little* fibre
Mineral deficiencies	*Too much* fat, sugar and salt, *too little* fibre
Overweight and obesity	*Too much* fat, sugar and salt, *too little* fibre
Stroke	*Too much* fat and sugar
Vitamin deficiencies	*Too much* fat, sugar and salt, *too little* fibre

esterol levels in the blood. High concentration of cholesterol is known to be associated with heart disease. Protein is not stored in the body, as are fats and sugars, so it needs to be eaten regularly. Too little protein, a problem in developing countries, can lead to a breakdown of muscle and tissues, too much can put a great strain on the liver and kidneys as well as reducing the mineral balance in the body.

Fats

Fats are an important source of energy. They help to protect the body by maintaining vital organs, cell structure, nerves and body temperature. They also carry the fat-soluble vitamins A, D, E and K into and around the body. Although fat is a necessary part of our diet and contributes to the texture and taste of many foods, most people are now aware that excessive fat intake can lead to heart disease and some forms of cancer.

Fats come in three different mixtures of fatty acids: saturated, animal fats such as butter, cheese, eggs and cream, as well as the fat contained in meat, fish and other animal produce; polyunsaturated fats, from vegetable sources including oils such as wheat germ, safflower, sunflower and corn oil (but not in palm or coconut oil) and in margarines made from these; and nonsaturated fats, such as olive oil.

Although a great deal has been written about the role of the fatty acids in causing heart disease, it is still not exactly clear how they work. Research has shown, however, that people with a high level of cholesterol in their blood are more likely than others to have a heart attack. Saturated fats increase cholesterol, so it makes sense to decrease your intake. However, the debate about fatty acids is far from over. New research has shown that polyunsaturated fat may be linked to premature ageing and cell destruction, although this has yet to be proved beyond doubt. In all, it is sensible advice to reduce fat intake generally.

Carbohydrates

Carbohydrates are the body's main source of energy. They are converted into glucose and glycogen to fuel the muscles, brain and nervous system. The principal sources of carbohydrates in most people's diet are starch and sugars, not in themselves bad things, except when taken in excess and in their refined forms. Refined white sugar, and white flours and breads are high-calorie carbohydrates but have had all their nutrients removed in the processing. They are rapidly absorbed into the bloodstream and provide instant but not prolonged bursts of energy. Taken in excess, refined carbohydrates can lead to blood sugar disorders and obesity.

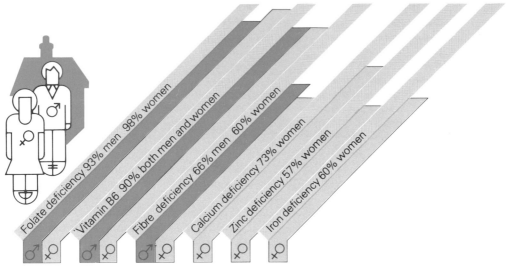

Overfed and undernourished
In spite of our affluence many people suffer important nutritional deficiencies.

It is far better to get your carbohydrates from the starch in proteins, whole grains and pulses (such as beans and lentils) and pastas; also from the natural sugars of fresh fruit and some vegetables. This is because such unrefined carbohydrates are more slowly converted into glucose in the body and are released into the blood in a steadier stream to provide long-term energy.

Dietary fibre

Next to fats and heart disease, fibres and roughage must rank as the great nutritional talking point of our time, yet many people do not fully understand the role of fibre in diet. Fibre is an indigestible substance which occurs naturally in nuts, cereals, beans, fruit and vegetables. Fibre is not actually broken down or digested but passes completely through the intestinal tract. Although it has no nutrients, its importance lies in its capacity to absorb liquid, rather like a sponge, thus helping the efficiency of the bowels by producing large, soft stools which are easier to pass.

Fibre also speeds up the passage of waste products through the bowel and helps to remove toxic matter. Whereas low-fibre foods may take as long as three or four days to pass through the system, high-fibre foods make the journey in less than 24 hours. It has been suggested that

this plays a significant part in reducing the length of time that cancer-causing substances stay in the lower bowel. Fibre may thus help to reduce not only cancer of the colon, but also diverticular disease, gallstones, hiatus hernia and other 'affluent diseases' associated with low-fibre food.

Fibre also appears to affect blood sugar levels and has been known to help some diabetics. By increasing the level of fibre in their diet (under medical supervision) some diabetics have been able to reduce their insulin intake, even discontinue it in some cases.

Sources of fibre

Cereal fibres seem to be the highest in roughage, making waste bulkier and speeding its passage through the body. Whole cereals include whole wheat, brown rice, burghul (bulgar wheat), barley, bran and, of course, their products such as wholemeal bread, pasta and breakfast cereals.

Pulses such as red kidney beans, chick peas, butter beans and lentils and products containing oats, barley or rye are also rich in fibre but work in the intestines in a different way. They form a glue-like substance which is thought to restrict the amount of both fat and sugar absorbed from food eaten. They also seem to lower blood cholesterol levels and may be effective in lowering blood pressure and in dealing with blood sugar problems.

Many fruits and vegetables have significant amounts of fibre and work in the digestive tract in much the same way as pulses and oats. Sweetcorn has a surprisingly high amount of fibre, as do carrots, apples, Brussels sprouts, aubergines (egg plant), blackcurrants, raspberries and dried fruits.

DIFFERENT LIVES, DIFFERENT NEEDS

From the first moments of life until old age we all need food, but how much we need can vary enormously, depending on activity, work, play, sport as well as the age, state of development and general health of the individual. Above all the need is for a balanced intake of essential nutrients together with sufficient calories to enable us to achieve optimum levels of growth and development, and an input of calories to match the output of our physical requirements.

What do expectant mothers need?

What a woman eats during pregnancy affects not just her own health but that of the unborn child. First of all, it is important that a woman is healthy when she conceives a child. There is now a great deal of evidence to suggest that the diet before conception contributes almost as much to a healthy pregnancy as what the mother eats over the nine months. Moreover,

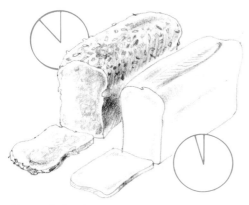

Brown is best
Wholemeal bread contains almost twice as much fibre as white. Four slices a day will provide $\frac{1}{6}$ daily recommended intake.

changes in the woman's body means that she can store more energy and needs more protein than usual during the first four months of pregnancy so eating patterns in these early days are very important.

Basically, the pregnant woman needs a varied, well-balanced diet which contains all the essential nutrients. It is a mistake to eat appreciably more — or less — than normally. Extra weight can cause complications during the later stages of pregnancy and during labour and it is difficult to lose after the birth. Equally dangerous is to restrict food intake to control the mother's weight. The baby's growth and development could be impaired and the mother could find it difficult to breastfeed adequately. A good natural multi-vitamin and mineral supplement, especially one containing folic acid, is always a sensible idea during pregnancy.

During pregnancy a woman also needs more calcium and iron than usual and although these can be taken as supplements along with folic acid, it makes more sense to take them naturally in food. Extra milk, cheese and yogurt will provide calcium, and liver and kidneys along with lots of green vegetables will provide iron. Foods containing vitamin B_6 are said to help with morning sickness but there is no conclusive evidence. Lots of fibre will, of course, prevent the constipation that many pregnant women suffer.

What do babies need?

There is no question that breast feeding is the ideal way to start your baby's life. Breast milk is conveniently packaged, is maintained at the right temperature and need no sterilizing. More importantly, breast milk is ideal for babies' digestive systems and is much less likely to cause digestive problems and allergic reactions.

For a few days after the baby's birth, breast milk also contains colostrum, the source of the mother's antibodies which gives the baby protection against many diseases, especially gastroenteritis. The feeding mother needs a good diet and a high fluid intake, although not large quantities of milk. There is evidence to suggest that the higher the mother's intake

How much is enough?
For a balanced diet, try to divide up the total day's energy intake as follows

Protein
This should make up 11% of the day's calorie intake.

Active adult males	84 g/3½ oz
Sedentary adult male	63 g/2½ oz
15–18 year old male	72 g/3 oz

(US National Academy of Science gives 56 g/2¼ oz for adult males and 54 g/2 oz for 15–18 year old males)

Adult women	54 g/2 oz
15–18 year old girl	53 g/2 oz

(UK NACNE figures)

Fat
Total fats should provide not more than 30% of which not more than 10% should be from hard, unsaturated fat.
This means 90 g/3½ oz, of which 30 g/1¼ oz is saturated fat.

Carbohydrate
This should make up the rest of your calorie intake (that is more than half).
This means 275 g/11 oz a day.
You should also take in **40–60 g/1½– 2½ oz fibre** per day, no more than **25 g/1 oz sugar** and **5–7 g/less than ¼ oz salt**.

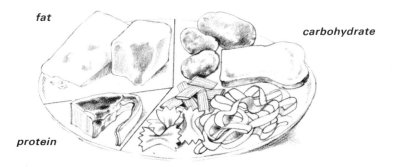

fat

carbohydrate

protein

of cow's milk during breast feeding the more likely it is that the baby can suffer from a number of related problems, specifically skin allergies, eczema, asthma, colic and problems with nasal catarrh. Four to six months is the ideal period for a baby to be exclusively breast fed. Do not add any cereals or other solid foods to bottle feeds until the baby is six months old. Introduce your baby to solid food by puréeing or sieving the food which you eat yourself making sure, of course, that you have not added salt or sugar. Start by offering very small quantities of puréed vegetables, fruit or rice. Introduce new foods gradually, leaving two or three days between each one, so that you can avoid (or pinpoint) any allergies.

What do young children need?
Because of their rapid rate of growth, young children need more protein and other nutrients than adults. Although children go through phases of not eating cer-

tain foods, this is nothing to worry about and certainly should not be fussed over. Children get over such fads very quickly and the important thing is not to bribe them with sweets and biscuits. Remember that your child's future eating habits will be established from early on in their lifetime.

Try to cut out foods containing artificial colourings, preservatives and flavourings, as there is increasing evidence that these can have a profound effect on the behavioural patterns of young children. Avoid foods which have too much salt or sugar. The seeds of future heart disease can very easily be sown during childhood so start your child on the right footing by reducing the amounts of animal fats and using fresh and dried fruits and the root vegetables as healthy sources of sweet foods. Providing that your child shows no sign of adverse reaction, give cow's milk as it is an excellent source of calcium and protein as well as vitamin D.

Children under five years old should be given full milk rather than the skimmed and semi-skimmed varieties recommended for adolescents and adults.

Avoid processed foods, instant packet this and that, takeaways and frozen TV dinners. They are expensive and nutritionally inadequate. Get your children used to home-made soups, beans of all kinds and vegetable casseroles as an occasional alternative to meat.

What do adolescents need?

Teenagers need more of just about every kind of nutrient, because of the rapid growth spurt that occurs during adolescence. (Boys need about 500 more calories per day than girls) Teenagers tend to dislike regular meals and prefer snacks or instant food, most of which is high on additives, salt, sugar or fat and low on protein, vitamins and minerals. Try to make sure young adults have at least a healthy breakfast of, say, a bran cereal, fruit juice, boiled egg and wholemeal toast, and keep the refrigerator and store cupboard well filled with fruits, nuts, homemade hamburgers and pizzas and appetizing and attractive vegetable dishes and fruit desserts.

The adverse effects of food additives are not confined to young children. Alexander Schauss, a leading American criminologist, has shown in his book *Diet, Crime and Delinquency* that food additives and diets high in refined sugars, refined carbohydrates and junk foods can lead to repetitive antisocial and delinquent behaviour in juveniles. It is, therefore, important to make a special effort to ensure that teenagers eat foods they enjoy which are also nutritious.

Remember that this is the age group most afflicted by *anorexia* or *bulimia* (see A–Z section). If you children have been brought up with a healthy regard for food you should avoid this, but keep an eye out for any symptoms.

One piece of good news is the increasing tendency of young people to turn to vegetarianism. Don't discourage your children if they do. A vegetarian diet can be a very healthy basis for living.

Calorie Chart for Children

This chart shows how many calories children and adolescents use up a day. It may be more than you think.

Children	
Age	Cal/Day
1	1,150
2	1,350
3–4	1,550
5–6	1,700
7–8	1,950
9–11	2,200
12–14 Boys	2,650
Girls	2,150
15–17 Boys	2,900
Girls	2,150

Adult nutrition

The same principles apply to the feeding of adults as to children. One of the most important differences is that of calorie requirement which varies from male to female and according to age and amount of normal physical activity (see p. 16).

Healthy eating in later life

The needs of elderly people are often complicated by the fact that they are frequently single, and often living on low or fixed incomes. Many do not enjoy the sociability of eating and tend to snack rather than to eat proper meals. Although the one commodity which they have in abundance is time, they seem to put a great reliance on convenience and frozen and packaged foods. Homemade soups, stews, casseroles, vegetarian dishes all make use of inexpensive ingredients but require more time in their preparation.

Vitamin C and folic acid are both easily destroyed by cooking and by storage. It is important for the elderly especially to pay particular attention to these two essential nutrients. Both these substances are found in green vegetables, citrus fruit, root vegetables, salads, berries, pineapples, wholemeal bread; these all require regular purchasing and this can sometimes be a problem for people suffering from arthritis, rheumatism or other disabling diseases. Loss of teeth can also complicate healthy eating for the elderly. For

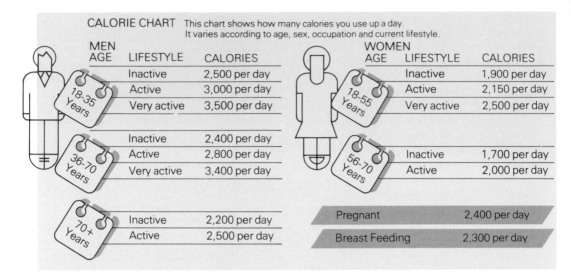

CALORIE CHART This chart shows how many calories you use up a day.
It varies according to age, sex, occupation and current lifestyle.

MEN

AGE	LIFESTYLE	CALORIES
18-35 Years	Inactive	2,500 per day
	Active	3,000 per day
	Very active	3,500 per day
36-70 Years	Inactive	2,400 per day
	Active	2,800 per day
	Very active	3,400 per day
70+ Years	Inactive	2,200 per day
	Active	2,500 per day

WOMEN

AGE	LIFESTYLE	CALORIES
18-55 Years	Inactive	1,900 per day
	Active	2,150 per day
	Very active	2,500 per day
56-70 Years	Inactive	1,700 per day
	Active	2,000 per day
Pregnant		2,400 per day
Breast Feeding		2,300 per day

these reasons, it is a good idea for older people to supplement their diet with vitamins and minerals.

Older people frequently suffer from constipation which can in turn lead to other health problems. This can be avoided by maintaining a high level of dietary fibre in the normal daily food.

What do convalescents need?

People in the recovery phase of illness, or who need a bland diet sometimes risk malnutrition at this crucial time; it is important that their nutritional needs are met, but their carers may not always know how to do this (neither may their medical practitioner).

When you are instructed to feed someone a bland diet, base your menus on the following:
● boiled brown rice and steamed carrots.
● dry wholemeal toast and clear soup.
● lightly cooked vegetables.
● porridge made with water.
● natural yoghurt.
● white fish, steamed or foil baked.

After a week or so (or as advised) the convalescent can be gradually weaned back to their normal diet.

WHAT'S THE ALTERNATIVE?

If the standard Western diet is inadequate, what other ways are there to eat? Many people have turned to alternative kinds of diet. Some, like vegetarianism, are very sound nutritionally; others based on theoretical or philosophical principles rather than knowledge of nutrition, may not be such a good idea to undertake without proper help.

Vegetarianism

Vegetarians eat eggs, milk and cheese as well as all plant products, but refuse meat, fish and poultry.

In UK, the Vegetarian Society estimates that there are now one million true vegetarians and a further million people who eat fish but not meat or poultry. This trend has come about for a number of reasons; the increasing publicity given to factory farming and promoted by the Animal Rights Movements together with growing concern about the long term health effects of meat consumption have made many young people question the traditional eating habits of their parents. There is ample evidence to show that a vegetarian diet is extremely healthy and in the long term far less likely to produce coronary disease, high blood pressure and digestive diseases. Yet there are still doctors who believe that any diet which does not include meat cannot be sufficient for the human need. This is patent nonsense.

Vegetarians get their protein from nuts, pulses, cheese, eggs, milk and milk products. These are excellent sources and providing not too much emphasis is placed on the dairy products, the vegetarian diet will be generally extremely beneficial. The absence of animal fats means that vegetarians have a generally lower calorie intake than meat eaters; few vegetarians who eat properly get fat.

A vegetarian diet is without doubt extremely healthy for any child providing that it is well maintained and balanced. The absence of animal fats from the diet means that it is sometimes difficult to maintain sufficient calorie input for the growing child. However, the equivalent of one pint of milk a day (as cheese or yogurt if you like), will make sure that the child has sufficient calcium and extra protein and the fat soluble vitamins from milk. Try not to use cheese and eggs as the *main* sources of protein, due to the high cholesterol content.

Vegans do not eat any animal products at all and strict vegans avoid honey and even yeast (as well as products made of leather, fur or animal parts of any kind). Nutritionally, the vegan diet is often deficient in vitamin B_{12}, since this is found almost entirely in animal products, and vitamin D, important for the development and growth of strong bones in children, is also frequently lacking. Supplements of these are essential, especially in northern climates or industrial smoggy areas where there is insufficient sunlight for the synthesis of vitamin D in the body.

Bringing up children on a vegan diet needs very special care and attention as it is sometimes difficult to maintain sufficient calorie input for proper rate of growth. Supplementation with the B_{12} and D vitamins is essential.

The Macrobiotic Diet

This form of diet, developed in Japan, is based on the philosophical concept of *yin* and *yang* (see **Acupuncture** pp. 66–9). *Yin* and *yang* represent the two opposing elements of nature, and according to Dr George Oshawa, the diet's popularizer, disease is a result of an imbalance between the *yin* and *yang* foods in the diet.

The macrobiotic diet depends largely on cooked whole grains, cooked vegetables and miso, a paste made from fermented soya beans, brown rice and sea salt which contains enzymes and vitamin B_{12}. The diet contains very little in the way of fresh fruits and salads and almost no animal protein. Occasional periods of 10 days on a brown rice diet are also recommended, and very little fluid. It is an extreme dietary regime and is almost certain to be deficient in vitamins A and C, it is not ideal for children and adolescents, and should be undertaken only with great care and professional guidance.

EATING TO LIVE

So how can you improve your food intake and reduce your chance of disease and increase your positive health factor?

Firstly, follow the **Guidelines to Healthy Eating** (over the page).

Secondly, eat as nature intended. Keep your food whole. Whole foods are those that have undergone minimal processing (or none at all) and contain almost all of their original nutrients. They are also free from additives or preservatives. If possible (and this is increasingly so) they should be grown organically, without chemical pesticides or herbicides. Meat and poultry should come from animals not injected with growth hormones, which are still there when you eat the meat. Eggs should be from free range chickens.

Increasing numbers of nutritionists, and all naturopaths, believe that whole foods may be one way to avoid the affluent diseases. Unfortunately, most doctors and main stream nutritionists have always debunked the naturopathic concept of a whole food diet. Nobody needs food supplements, nobody needs special diets and the majority of people get all they need from their daily food intake. These are the same people who said until very recently that white bread was just as good as wholemeal bead, that there was nothing wrong with animal fats in the diet, that food allergies did not exist. Many of these previously held views have now been changed.

GUIDELINES TO HEALTHY EATING

Healthy eating does not have to turn you into a food faddist. For most people, it means making certain adjustments to their existing dietary habits. Healthy food is not necessarily unappetising, nor an exercise in self-sacrifice, nor expensive.

It means getting the right balance between the various nutrients in your normal everyday foods, and preparing your meals so that they are a pleasure to eat as well as being good for you.

More fresh fruit and vegetables.
They are low in calories but high in vitamins and minerals; use them to provide at least one meatless meal a week; eat at least one salad meal a day.
- Vary your choice as much as possible and stick to seasonal varieties to make sure that foods are at their best and freshest. Better still, grow your own.
- Keep them for as short a time as possible, as they lose nutrients with age. Try to eat them raw and with their skins, if possible.
- Cook them for as short a time as possible and in as little liquid as possible. Steam in preference to boiling to retain more vitamins and minerals. Keep the cooking water to drink or use for stock, sauce or soup (it contains many of the vitamins and minerals from the cooked vegetables.)
- Never add salt or bicarbonate of soda when cooking vegetables.

More fibre
- Eat wholemeal bread, which contains substantial amounts, or a daily breakfast cereal which contains bran.
- Sprinkling bran over food is less effective; take fibre naturally from unpeeled carrots, apples, potatoes or broad beans. All the pulses—lentils, dried peas, soya beans, chickpeas and haricot beans are also high in fibre, as are all unrefined grain foods.
- Increase your fibre intake gradually, over a period of weeks, to avoid a bloated, tight feeling at first.

Less fat
About 40 per cent of our daily intake comes from fat. Quite apart from the relative merits of saturated or polyunsaturated fats, you can probably eat a great deal less fat than you do. Because fat goes unnoticed in many of the ordinary foods we eat daily as sandwiches, takeaway foods or in restaurants and canteens, it is worth keeping a record for several days of what you eat. The fat content could be (and probably is) surprisingly high. Begin a gradual campaign of substitution and within a relatively short time your body will be responding positively to a lower fat intake by declaring some foods formerly favoured as 'too rich' or 'too greasy'.

Follow these simple courses and you need not drastically alter your eating habits.
- Eat lean meat (avoid pork), poultry and more fish.
- Trim all the fat from meat and skin from poultry.
- Grill, roast or casserole fatty meats or fish (such as mackerel or herring).
- Cut down on all meat products— sausages, pies, salamis, pates—all of which contain huge amounts of hidden 'fats'.
- Use low-fat margarines for spreading instead of butter and use non-stick frying pans for cooking. Be sensible about this—a little pure butter is far better than the masses of chemical margarine which has the same number of calories.
- Substitute skimmed milk, low fat yogurt or cheese for conventional dairy products.
- Avoid ice-cream, chocolate cake, fried foods and butter-enriched sauces, as a general rule, and use them only for family treats and special occasions.
- Nuts and seeds, which contain unsaturated natural oils, can be eaten in small amounts. Remember, however, as you nibble them as snacks, that they should be substitutes—not additions—to your natural fat intake from other sources.

Cut out sugar

Refined white sugar, an essential ingredient in so many jams, cakes, puddings, biscuits, canned fruits and soft drinks, has no nutrients at all and in a great number of instances, it is used not to enhance the flavour of the original substance, but to mask it. Once acquired, a 'sweet tooth' is difficult to get rid of, which is why it is important to discourage children from eating sweets in the first place. Because it is a form of addiction, sugar is not easy to give up, hence the profitable trade in artificial sweeteners.

● Monitor your sugar intake in tea and coffee and gradually, slowly, reduce it, so that your taste buds become more sensitive. Use honey to help you, if necessary, since it is a natural sweetener.

● At meal times, serve fresh fruit or cheese instead of a dessert and avoid sweet between-meal snacks.

Less salt

Although some salt is essential, an excess affects potassium levels, causing fluid retention and kidney disorders. The diets of Western civilization contain too much salt. Like sugar, salt is not easy to give up and intake should be reduced gradually, preferably without the aid of salt substitutes.

● Always cook food without salt—it draws out moisture and essential nutrients.

● Add natural flavourings such as herbs and spices to enhance the flavour of food and add a little sea salt, if necessary, to the finished dish.

● Try to eat more foods that contain potassium (fruit, potatoes, dates, wheatgerm).

● Cut down on processed foods which often have a very high salt content.

Sense and Sociability

Working adults have to take the social aspect of eating and drinking into account. Fortunately, a few minor adjustments are all that's needed for you to eat and drink sensibly and sociably without becoming an obsessive, a faddist or a killjoy.

Drink less coffee Coffee and, to a lesser extent, tea, are drugs which stimulate the heart and digestive system. Caffeine, the major stimulant in coffee, can, for example, increase the heart rate, sometimes causing nervousness but more often masking tiredness and fatigue. It also, however, increases stomach acid and makes peptic ulcers more likely. Limit your coffee intake to two cups per day, replacing additional intake with decaffeinated coffee, herbal teas, fruit or vegetable juices and mineral water. All cola drinks contain caffeine.

Drink less alcohol Too much alcohol is damaging and many irreversible liver disorders are linked with a high and persistent intake of alcohol. However, as most people recognize, alcohol does have soothing and relaxing properties and in moderation can contribute to general health and well-being. All drinkers lose vitamin B and C and women drinkers can suffer hormonal imbalances. Limit your drinking to a glass of wine or beer with meals. Drink mineral water or fruit juice at parties and dilute your table wine with mineral water.

Entertaining Elegant, healthy meals can be served to guests and, indeed, the sheer simplicity of such dishes will be welcomed by most people. Fish grilled or cooked *en papillote* (in foil), brochettes of meat or fish served with boiled potatoes tossed in herbs and a salad are a feast for anyone. Start off with a vegetable soup or terrine or a soufflé and finish with a fresh fruit salad or cheese. Or try a Chinese meal which is exotic, quickly cooked and nutritious. If you prepare natural, seasonal products simply and well, there is no need for sauces nor filling pastries or puddings.

Eating out Much the same applies to eating out as for home entertaining, although canteen or pub lunches present something of a difficulty. The sheer problem of catering for large numbers and keeping food warm means that many nutrients are inevitably lost in cooked dishes. Stick to salads or grills as much as possible and avoid dishes made with pastry or refined flour.

OBESITY

Bad nutrition is one thing; to be both undernourished *and* overweight is just adding to your problem. If you are overweight you are at risk. Fat babies become fat adults and fat adults are likely to suffer totally needless health problems throughout their lives. Back problems, arthritis of ankles, knees and hips, heart disease, circulatory problems, high blood pressure, diabetes and respiratory ailments are all infinitely more likely in the obese person. So what can you do about it?

Modern Western society's obsession with slimming has in recent years spawned a host of instant cures for obesity; none of them work. Hundreds of diets aimed at making weight reduction as simple and easy as possible have been devised. Most of these are simply useless, while some are downright dangerous.

Excessive dieting to become thin — encouraged by fashion magazines — can lead to an extremely serious disorder in young women (and increasing numbers of young men), anorexia nervosa, a mental and physical illness caused by compulsive dieting and resulting in metabolic disorder, and if not cured it can be fatal.

Some recent trends in dieting techniques illustrate the dangers of a food intake aimed solely at weight reduction.

Low calorie diet

If you reduce your calorie intake by between 500 and 1,000 calories a day, you will lose weight.

However, the inevitable difficulties of keeping to a diet that is well below 1,000 calories a day produces an off–on effect, whereby after a short time, the dieter finds it impossible to stick to the monotony of raw vegetables, cottage cheese, fruit and low fat yoghurt. Consequently there are recurrent periods of bingeing, when whatever weight has been painfully lost is quickly regained and the dieter becomes cross and depressed and writes off the whole exercise as a dismal failure. This sort of diet does nothing to re-educate your eating habits.

Low carbohydrate diet

This is not a particularly desirable method of losing weight. Instead of counting calories, you simply limit your carbohydrate intake, which should theoretically have the effect of reducing overall calorie intake. Essentially you cut down on all foods that contain sugar and starch such as bread, potatoes, cereals, pulses, honey and jam. The disadvantage of this type of diet is that you can find yourself eating more of other foods, particularly with a high protein and fat content and so lose no weight at all. The other is that you lose out on the vital nutrients and fibre provided by carbohydrates.

High protein diet

The high protein diet involves the consumption of large amounts of animal protein — particularly grilled steaks, fish and meat and very little else, especially carbohydrates.

This form of diet is firstly expensive and secondly deficient in fibre, vitamins and minerals. It is not a balanced food intake and is very difficult to stick to. In addition, high intakes of red meat can lead to the aggravation of existing conditions, such as high blood pressure, arthritis, rheumatism and gout. This is definitely not the way to successful long-term weight loss.

The all fruit diet

These diets, such as the Beverly Hills pineapple diet, the grapefruit diet, the grape diet, all involve the exclusion of virtually all food except a particular form of raw fruit. Apart from the potential damage to the enamel of your teeth, especially true in the pineapple diet, they are a certain recipe for malnutrition and in no way do they train you to eat in a more rational and balanced way.

The high fibre diet

This diet is rather more sensible in its approach, since it does involve a wide range of foodstuffs. Increasing fibre intake and reducing the amount of animal proteins (thus the amount of saturated fats in the diet) is a healthier way of eating and can lead to a substantial weight reduction.

Too, too solid flesh

Discovering (or admitting) that you are overweight, and by how much is not easy. Your ideal weight depends on bone size, body type and height. Ideal Weight Charts are necessarily averages not absolutes. However, you can use them to calculate whether you need to lose weight. If you are 10% above your ideal weight then you are *overweight*. If you are 20% or more, you are *obese* and for your health's sake, if not your appearance, you should do something about it.

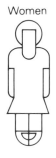

Women WEIGHT (without clothes)	HEIGHT (without shoes)	Men
	1.95m/6.4in	181lb/80.4kg
	1.92m/6.3in	176lb/78.2kg
	1.89m/6.2in	171lb/76kg
	1.87m/6.1in	166lb/73.8kg
152lb/67.6kg	1.84m/6.0in	162lb/72kg
148lb/65.8kg	1.81m/5.11in	158lb/70.2kg
144lb/64.0kg	1.78m/5.10in	153lb/68kg
140lb/62.2kg	1.76m/5.9in	149lb/66.2kg
136lb/60.4kg	1.73m/5.8in	145lb/64.4kg
132lb/58.7kg	1.70m/5.7in	140lb/62.2kg
128lb/56.9kg	1.68m/5.6in	136lb/60.4kg
123lb/54.7kg	1.65m/5.5in	133lb/59.1kg
120lb/53.3kg	1.62m/5.4in	130lb/57.7kg
116lb/52.4kg	1.60m/5.3in	127lb/56.4kg
113lb/50.2kg	1.57m/5.2in	123lb/54.7kg
110lb/49kg	1.55m/5.1in	
107lb/47.6kg	1.52m/5.0in	

It is essential, however, to aim for a very wide spread of food sources to avoid missing out on some of the essential nutrients.

Too much fibre can reduce calcium absorption, which has long term implications especially for woman. So eat calcium-rich foods at separate meals from fibre.

Meal replacements (very low calorie diets)

These are yet another example of short-term success leading to long-term failure and the side effects of prolonged periods of dieting with meal replacements can be measured in terms of bowel disorders and anorexia.

Whether your meal replacement is a biscuit filled with synthetic bulking agents or a drink made from instant powder containing essential nutrients, artificial colourings and flavourings and no fibre, the results are inevitably the same. Many people do lose weight using meal replacements but there is no re-education of food habits nor is there any long-term benefit unless the slimmer continues to substitute one meal a day with one of the meal replacements. Latest research suggests that repeated or prolonged use of VLCOs can lead to muscle wastage, especially of heart muscle.

Positive Action

None of the diets and regimes above will re-educate your appetite. To do that you will have to think in the long term; but there are ways you can help yourself in the short term while gradually changing your life style. Some people find they will have more will-power if they know they are being watched. A slimming club may help them. Exercise will, of course, help everybody.

Slimming clubs

Slimming clubs as pioneered by Weight Watchers have one enormous advantage in that they are supportive of the would-be slimmer. The mere fact of having to weigh-in publicly at weekly meetings is a powerful incentive.

Slimming clubs and especially Weight Watchers have modified their dietary advice over recent years to encompass a greater range of whole foods, high fibre foods and sensible eating patterns. The successful slimming club really does aim at re-educating the slimmer and encouraging him or her to maintain healthy and sensible eating patterns once target weight has been achieved.

EXERCISE

Exercise is a tremendous help in any programme aimed at losing weight consistently. By increasing the amount of exercise you take, it is possible to lose weight without drastically reducing your calorie intake. The type of exercise you take depends on age, physical condition and how overweight you are, and it is most important that you start your exercise programme carefully and sensibly (See **Fit for Life**, p. 29). It is interesting to remember that a simple brisk walk can burn up some 400 calories per hour, so simply by leaving your car in the garage more often, by avoiding the lift and using the stairs or just by riding a bicycle you can speed up your weight loss in a safe and efficient way, while at the same time improving the overall health of your respiratory system and your cardiovascular system.

SLIMMING THE HEALTHY WAY

For successful life-long slimming, you *must* re-educate your appetite and eating habits. No human being, no matter how obese they may be, can live their lives successfully 'on a diet'. The long term answer is to change your way of eating to increase your regular exercise and to end up on a dietary regime which you enjoy, which is nutritious and which will maintain the balance between your energy requirement and your energy input. There is little point

in trying to lose weight to benefit your health if the means of doing it creates other problems which can be just as detrimental to your body.

There is no easy, instant way of losing weight. To do so effectively, you must cut down the amount of food you eat — that is, reduce your calorie intake over a period of time (see Calorie Chart p. 16). To achieve a sensible weight loss, aim to lose about 1 kg/2¼ lb per week, while modifying your normal eating habits so that you can maintain your weight loss. Naturally the more overweight you are the quicker you will lose weight initially but don't forget that as your weight drops the amount of calories you use just moving your body around will become smaller, therefore the rate of weight loss will gradually decline throughout the period of the diet. Dieting is not easy at first, although it becomes less difficult to maintain as you become used to a lower food intake and when you begin to see the results of a slimmer, healthier figure.

While your diet must be well-balanced, containing sufficient nutrients and fibre for healthy living, it must also be as enjoyable as possible. Plan your diet so that it includes low-fat and low-sugar foods that you positively like. Game birds, shellfish and vegetables and fruit such as asparagus and strawberries are not so very expensive as an occasional part of a low-calorie diet and are natural, healthy foods.

Designing your own diet

A certain amount of flexibility is essential in any diet. That is why it is better to devise one that can fit in with your established work pattern or lifestyle. There are, of course, certain diet rules that should be followed and these are listed below.

- **Aim to get your calories** from valuable foods such as wholemeal bread, cereals, lean meat, pulses, fruit and vegetables.
- **Treat yourself** every other day to a little something (not more than 150 calories) as a morale booster.
- **Don't weigh yourself every day.** We all lose weight at a different rate, and

it will only depress you to weigh yourself two or three times a day and see no change.

- **Keep a diet diary.** List everything you eat and drink a week or two *before* you start your diet. You'll be horrified, and it will help to motivate you.
- **Drinks** take plenty of water to cleanse the system—you need about 6–8 glasses, far more than you think you need per day. Limit your tea and coffee intake to no more than two cups a day. Drink fruit and vegetable juices in preference to low-calorie soft drinks which contain all sorts of additives. Drink herbal teas. If you are a milk drinker, switch to skimmed milk. Avoid alcohol or include only as an occasional treat. Drink yeast extracts if you want something hot and savoury.
- **Reduce fat intake** by using low-fat polyunsaturated margarine on breads or crispbreads. Grill, steam or cook in a non-stick pan. Trim all the fat from meat or poultry.
- **Eliminate sugar intake** Substitute a little honey or eat fruit when you have a craving for sweet things.
- **Eat fresh fruit and vegetables,** and plenty of them, choosing low-calorie seasonal varieties that you enjoy eating.
- **Eat at least one salad** of raw vegetables each day.
- **Eat fibre** in a reasonable quantity every day to avoid constipation and to make you feel less hungry.
- **Combine exercise** with your diet, otherwise you will have flabby skin and slack muscles.
- **Don't despair.** If you overeat or drink on one day, do not abandon your diet. Simply cut down the following day and carry on.

Diet suggestions

Think through your daily routine and work out in which parts of the day you need most energy. Balance your calorie intake according to whether you need—or have time for—a sustaining breakfast, lunch or dinner.

FOOD ADDITIVES

Food additives have been in use since the dawn of civilization. Honey and salt were found to have valuable preservative qualities which enabled foods to be eaten out of season. We were our own experimental animals so that the ancient Britons, Greeks and Egyptians knew well not only what was poisonous and what was good to eat but were also aware that foods sometimes had to be prepared in a special way to be safe or, while a little of a food might be good to eat a lot of the same food could be dangerous. To take a modern example, monosodium glutamate, MSG, seems to be fine in small quantities although why you need flavour enhancing is questionable if good ingredients are used. MSG occurs naturally in fermented soya products such as soy sauce but many Chinese restaurants use it in excessive quantities and it can give rise to symptoms including heart palpitations, headaches, dizziness, tightening of the muscles, sickness and weakness of the upper arms with pains in the neck and even a migraine in some people.

Modern Additives

The use of food additives has increased dramatically in the last 30 years. The demand for brightly coloured, easy to prepare, tasty foods that can be stored and cost very little has meant that the manufacturers have had to use colours, preservatives, emulsifiers, stabilizers and antioxidants in quantities so great that estimates indicate that the average consumer in Britain eats more than 6 g of declared additives per day. This figure includes only those substances which have to be declared as additives and omits flavours, nutrients, vitamins and sweeteners. That does not sound much but can be viewed in the perspective of being equivalent to the content of aspirin in 20 tablets.

Some food additives have been tested more or less rigorously, but if the quantities you use are excessive or if the individual has a particular sensitivity then certain additives can have adverse effects. Fortunately consumer legislation in the United States, Australia and New Zealand

and throughout the Common Market means that very many of the additives in use can be identified and a choice made as to whether or not you wish to buy foods containing them.

In the US there are far fewer permitted colours than in most countries and this must be desirable. Europe has the E Code and certain additional numbers without the E which are not used in all the Common Market countries and Australia and New Zealand use the same numerical system without the E and only for those additives permitted in those countries. The UK currently used five colours that are not permitted in the rest of the Common Market which are: **107 Yellow 2G; 128 Red 2G; 154 Brown FK** and **155 Chocolate Brown HT**. These are not used in the USA either, but 107 and 155 are allowed in Australasia.

So you see there is not too much agree-

Additives at a glance

The additives that can affect not only hyperactive children but also can affect some asthmatics and those sensitive to aspirin include the following:

E102	Tartrazine
E104	Quinoline Yellow
107	Yellow 2G
E110	Sunset Yellow FCF
E120	Cochineal
E122	Carmoisine
E123	Amaranth
E124	Ponceau 4R
E127	Erythrosine BS
128	Red 2G
E132	Indigo carmine
E133	Brilliant blue FCF
E150	Caramel
E151	Black PN
154	Brown FK
155	Brown HT
E210	Benzoic acid
E211	Sodium benzoate
E212	Potassium benzoate
E213	Calcium benzoate
E214	Ethyl 4-hydroxybenzoate
E215	Ethyl 4-hydroxybenzoate, sodium salt
E216	Propyl para-hydroxybenzoate
E217	Propyl 4-hydroxybenzoate, sodium salt
E218	Methyl 4-hydroxybenzoate
E219	Methyl 4-hydroxybenzoate, sodium salt
E220	Sulphur dioxide
E250	Sodium nitrite
E251	Sodium nitrate
E310	Propyl gallate
E311	Octyl gallate
E312	Dodecyl gallate
E320	Butylated hydroxyanisole (BHA)
E321	Butylated hydroxytoluene (BHT)
621	Monosodium glutamate (MSG)

622	Monopotassium glutamate
623	Calcium dihydrogen di-L-glutamate
627	Guanosine 5-(disodium phosphate)
631	Inosine 5-(disodium phosphate)
635	Sodium 5-ribonucleotide

Additives are not only implicated in certain adverse reactions but are sometimes there much more for the convenience of the manufacturer than for the consumer, disguising excessive amounts of fat and poor quality raw materials. So another 16 additives can be added to the list above which seem to me to be either unnecesary or can cause bad reactions. These are:

E131	Patent blue V
E142	Green S
E153	Carbon black
E173	Aluminium
E180	Pigment rubine
E221	Sodium sulphite
E222	Sodium hydrogen sulphite
E223	Sodium metabisulphite
E224	Potassium metabilsulphite
E226	Calcium sulphite
E227	Calcium bisulphite
385	Calcium disodium EDTA
E407	Carrageenan
924	Potassium bromate
925	Chlorine
926	Chlorine dioxide

Of these carageenan is possibly the most debatable because some studies and most governments have found it to be perfectly safe and just one group of workers believes that it could precipitate certain gut problems when used in excess. More research is being done.

ment even concerning the question of which colours are safe to use and although the majority of smoked kippers and mackerel in the UK are coloured with brown FK (which stands For Kippers) when they are exported this rather dubious colour is left out and there is a good deal of consumer demand that Britain follows suit.

Additives and hyperactivity

Hyperactivity in children brings the most appalling strain and exhaustion to parents and although some doctors believe this problem to be mostly psychological the fact is that since the publication of Maurice Hanssen's book *E For Additives* literally hundreds of parents have said that by avoiding certain additives and by removing foods containing salicylates from the diet they have seen an improvement in their children's behaviour. Such foods include many soft fruits and pineapple as well as tea, spices, mint, honey, licorice and cucumber, whereas fruits such as custard, apples, pears, bananas, peaches, mangoes and lemons are low in salicylates. Some think that the diet is less important than the additives but the way to find out is to start with a strict diet excluding the potentially troublesome fruits and vegetables and to re-introduce them one at a time.

Additives and you

The message is clear. If you want to be careful about the additives you consume and have an additive-safe diet for you and friends and family, then read the label, find out all you can about additives. Growing public awareness means that there will be ever-increasing numbers of foods not using the one fifth of commonly used additives. Be sure not to fall into the trap thinking that additives are all nasty, because some of them are very useful, completely safe and help bring us better food.

VITAMINS AND MINERALS

Vitamins and minerals have no energy value, but they contribute to good health by regulating the metabolism and assisting the biochemical processes that release energy from the food we digest. They are sometimes called micronutrients.

There are 13 major vitamins: A, C, D, E, K, and the eight vitamins of the B group which work together and are known as the B complex. Vitamins are either water soluble or fat soluble: the water soluble ones are most of the B complex and C, which have to be taken daily in food since they cannot be stored in the body (any surplus is excreted); the fat soluble vitamins A, D, E and K are stored in the body's fatty tissues. Vitamin B_{12} can be stored in the liver.

Vitamins and minerals work together: for instance, vitamin C is needed for iron to be absorbed by the body. Vitamins also assist other vitamins: folic acid (from the vitamin B complex) needs vitamin C to be present to turn into its active form; vitamin E protects vitamin C from oxidation. Vitamins in the correct combination occurs naturally in whole food, and it is much better to eat them this way. Unfortunately, processing, refining and cooking can destroy vitamins (and some minerals) and sometimes a supplement is essential.

The chart below indicates the function, sources and recommended minimum daily intake of the major vitamins and minerals. For more information about deficiency and therapeutic doses and supplements, see Vitamin and Mineral Deficiency in the A–Z section.

Women and vitamins and minerals

Because of menstruation, pregnancy and breast feeding, women have slightly different needs to men for certain micronutrients.

Many need a supplement of vitamin B_6 to bring them up to 25 mg a day for 10 days before the start of menstruation. They also need extra vitamin C, folic acid and vitamin B_{12} and need extra folic acid and vitamins B_{12}, C and E to ensure adequate iron for blood replacement after menstruation.

Pregnant women and nursing mothers need a supplement of all vitamins and minerals (see chart). Women taking the contraceptive pill should also take a supplement of the entire B complex, vitamins C and E and make sure that their zinc intake is adequate.

Vitamin and Mineral Chart

Vitamin	What it does	Where you can find it	How much you need
A (retinol)	essential for normal growth, clear skin, healthy hair and nails, good vision, healthy mucous membranes	eggs, liver, fish liver oils, dairy produce, spinach, broccoli, carrots, apricots, tomatoes	750 μg/2,500 iu

The B vitamins work as a team, and are particularly concerned with the maintenance of the nervous system.

Vitamin	What it does	Where you can find it	How much you need
B_1 (thiamine) (most affected by cooking)	converts carbohydrates into energy; promotes function of heart, muscles and nerves	wholemeal bread, peanuts, wheatgerm, pulses, brewer's yeast, brown rice, bran, beef, liver	1.5 mg
B_2 (riboflavin)	releases energy from foods; essential for growth, healthy skin, hair and eyes	red meat, brewer's yeast, yoghurt, eggs, fish, vegetables, wholegrains, dairy produce	1.7 mg
B_3 (niacin, nicotinic acid)	as B_2; also important on fat metabolism	wholegrains, liver, kidneys, fish, pulses, peanuts, wholemeal bread	19 mg 21 mg during lactation
B_5 (pantothenic acid)	healthy skin and hair; essential for production of anti-stress hormones	wholegrains, liver, fish, eggs, yeast, kidney, pulses, fresh vegetables, royal jelly	10 mg
B_6 (pyridoxine)	growth; metabolism of amino acids (from protein); blood formation; production of vitamin B_3	liver, cereals, pulses, fresh vegetables, bananas, nuts, eggs, milk, yeast	2 mg 10 mg for pregnant women 25 mg for 10 days before menstruation 25–50 mg for women taking contraceptive pill
B_{12}	blood formation; healthy nervous tissue; interdependent with folic acid	dairy products, liver, fish, brewer's yeast	3 μg 4 μg during lactation 5 μg for pregnant women and women taking contraceptive pill
folic acid	formation of blood; interdependent with B_{12}	pulses, raw green leafy vegetables, fruit, liver	400 μg 500 μg during lactation
biotin	converts energy from food; produces fatty acids	liver, kidney, pulses, nuts, yeast extract, cauliflower	300 μg
C (ascorbic acid)	growth, healthy skin, bones, teeth, gums; assists healing, helps body's defences to fight viral and bacterial infections, stress and fatigue	acerola cherries, citrus fruit, fresh vegetables (especially potatoes)	60 mg

Vitamin	What it does	Where you can find it	How much you need
D	maintains calcium and phosphorus levels; building strong, healthy bones	dairy produce, oily fish, eggs, cod liver oil, sunshine	10 µg/400 iu
E (tocopherol)	plays a role in fertility (not yet understood); protects vitamin C against oxidation; protects circulatory system and cell membranes; makes essential fatty acids	vegetable oils, green vegetables, cereals, eggs, wholemeal bread, oily fish, cod liver oil	30 mg
K	controls blood clotting	leafy green vegetables, liver, cabbage, cauliflower, peas, wholegrains, yoghurt, blackstrap molasses	this is usually produced by the intestinal bacteria so there is no recommended daily intake; 500–1000 µg is probably enough

Minerals

Calcium (Ca)	healthy bones, teeth, nails, normal muscle function and nerve function, blood clotting and milk production in nursing mothers	dairy produce, eggs, oily fish, wholemeal bread, watercress cabbage, pulses	1000 mg
Phosphorus (P)	activates the B complex vitamins; forms healthy bones, teeth and nails; depends on vitamin D for activation	cheese, milk, soya flour, brown rice, fish, peanuts, wholemeal bread, yeast extracts, chicken, beef	1000 mg
Sodium (Na)	controls water balance; essential for muscle contraction and healthy nervous system	occurs naturally in whole foods as sodium chloride; also in salt	1200 mg
Potassium (K)	works with sodium to control water balance and muscle contraction and healthy nervous system; also important in enzyme function	potatoes, Brussels sprouts, mushrooms, dates, wheatgerm, meat, fish, poultry, milk, fruit, tea, coffee	3000 mg
Magnesium (Mg)	needed in the body for the use of protein and many vitamins; promotes healthy nervous system and cell structure	seafood, nuts, cereals, green vegetables, wholemeal bread	400 mg
Iron (Fe)	makes haemoglobin (the oxygen carrying component of blood)	liver, black pudding, red meat, wholegrains, fish, eggs, pulses, green leafy vegetables	18 mg
Zinc	growth, healthy skin	offal, meat, fish, green	15 mg

Vitamin	What it does	Where you can find it	How much you need
(Zn)	and hair; promotes healing; works with vitamin B_6 in hormone production; releases vitamin A from liver	leafy vegetables, wholemeal bread	
Iodine (I)	proper thyroid function; produces thyroid hormone; maintains metabolic rate	seafood, water, iodized salt, shellfish	200 μg
Copper (Cu)	makes melanin pigment in the skin; maintains enzyme systems promotes healthy body tissue	fish, shellfish, liver, offal, nuts, raisins, prunes, green vegetables	2 mg
Manganese (Mn)	growth, reproduction, bone formation and development, maintenance of blood sugar levels	cereal grains, pulses, fruit, tea, leafy vegetables	5 mg
Chromium (Cr)	controls use of glucose in muscles, cholesterol synthesis and how fatty acids are used.	brewer's yeast, liver, cheese, wheatgerm, cereals, beef	200 μg
Selenium (Se)	activates vitamin E; helps produce antibodies to fight infection; protects against cell membrane damage	wholegrain cereals, meat, fish, nuts, offal, vegetables, fruit	200 μg
Cobalt (Co)	works with vitamin B_{12}	fresh green leafy vegetables, fish, cereals, dairy produce	1 μg
Sulphur (S)	formation of body tissues; a constituent of all proteins	present in all protein, but eggs, chicken, nuts, pulses, dried fruit, shellfish, mustard, all good sources	800 mg
Molybdenum (Mo)	prevents dental caries; aids iron metabolism and the excretory system; maintains normal male sexual function	buckwheat, wholegrains, offal, eggs, vegetables, fruit, pulses	500 μg

* iu stands for international units; this is an old fashioned method of measuring vitamins, and only three are still measured this way: A, D and E. In the chart, measurements are given in ius (where relevant) and in milligrams (mg) or micrograms (μg).

FIT FOR LIFE

Western civilization has undermined the health of nations—cars, armchairs, supermarkets and the TV have made Western man an obese, sedentary and unhealthy specimen.

The diseases of civilization take a terrible toll. Heart disease, bowel disease, diabetes, circulatory diseases and stress related illness are just a few of the avoidable health problems that fill our hospitals.

Together with a healthy balanced diet (see **Nutrition**, pp. 18–19), a regular programme of exercise and physical activity will bring untold rewards. If you are determined to take a positive approach to your own health care, then start here.

THE CASE FOR EXERCISE

Regular exercise brings about marked physiological changes and improvement in normal body functioning. It increases muscle strength, which can improve posture and prevent or reduce backache; it also has direct effects on the health and efficiency of the heart muscle, lungs and circulation.

As the heart grows stronger and larger, it can pump greater amounts of oxygenated blood to the muscles with fewer beats and less effort. This lowers the strain on cardiovascular muscles. Inactive people in sedentary jobs are more likely to suffer from coronary heart disease than more active people, even taking into account other factors such as obesity, smoking and high blood pressure.

Although exercise does not actually lower cholesterol levels in the blood, it appears to bring down general blood fat levels. It can modify the nature of the fat in your blood, transforming it from large, artery-clogging globules (low density lipoprotein) to smaller, less sticky ones (high-density lipoprotein) which flow more easily round the system.

Exercise involving controlled breathing is also beneficial to sufferers of asthma and bronchitis. Simple stair-climbing and walking exercises have produced significant improvements in bronchitics, while asthmatics who swim on a regular basis find that they suffer attacks less frequently and, in turn, need fewer drugs to control them.

Exercise is also good for the mind. Many people are surprised to find themselves refreshed and invigorated after short bursts of physical activity and it has been shown that exercise can reduce tension, anxiety and in some cases, depression, by promoting the release of hormone-like substances including adrenaline and noradrenaline that affect the emotions. A well-exercised body and the accompanying sense of mental well-being will also help people who have trouble sleeping.

EXERCISING FOR LIFE

Exercise and pregnancy

During pregnancy, it is very important that muscles remain strong and that correct posture is maintained. Pregnancy puts a particular strain on the abdominal muscles, spine and pelvic floor which have to be strong enough to support the weight of the growing baby. Strong leg muscles help good circulation and prevent cramp and varicose veins.

Most ante-natal clinics will recommend a series of exercises especially suitable during pregnancy and these should be practised regularly but without overstraining. Exercise before and during pregnancy will make labour and delivery much easier.

Post-natal exercises are also important to improve posture and shorten and tighten the abdominal muscles. Again, ante-natal clinics will advise suitable exercises which should be carried out for 4–6 weeks after the birth of the baby.

Breathing and relaxing routines frequently help with post-natal depression and the strains involved in looking after a new-born baby. Return to general fitness exercises as soon as possible. They will get your figure back into shape and make you more able to cope physically and mentally with the hard work of parenthood.

Exercise for Children and Teenagers

Generally, children and adolescents get plenty of physical activity at school and naturally engage in sports that suit them. However, it is important to encourage your children's natural sporting abilities and to try to develop an interest in sport and physical exercise in those who show little inclination. If family activities include swimming, cycling, running or other sports from an early age there will be little problem in children accepting fitness as part of their everyday life and this, along with good nutrition, is the best start in life that you can give your children. Most forms of dancing are excellent exercises, great for teenagers, who are sure to enjoy them.

Staying young with exercise

Many people who are physically active and sporting in their youth tend to give up exercise in early middle age, possibly because of less leisure time, more demanding jobs and, for many, various family commitments. This is short-sighted for a number of reasons. This is the time of life when affluent diseases are most likely to strike and when obesity is most prevalent. Exercise can keep the body strong and less vulnerable to a whole host of illnesses, including stress, associated with the onset of middle age. Moreover, it has been shown that exercise can actually delay the ageing process and help retain a youthful appearance by preventing muscles from shrinking, keeping skin healthy, firm and less wrinkled and, of course, removing flab from the body.

Although life-long exercise is desirable if you want to maintain a youthful figure

---

Fat to Fit in easy stages

Yes/No

Before starting any exercise programme you must assess your own fitness. If you are overweight and over 40 and you've hardly moved a muscle since you left school, seek professional advice before you start. To help you decide how you stand, answer the following questions TRUTHFULLY and then add up your score.

Check here: (count your yesses).
0–3   Good: start exercising today
3–6   Just in time; start gently and persevere
6–12 You may not make it to the gym! Get some advice before you start.
NOTE: If you have ever been told that you have high blood pressure or heart disease, you can exercise but you must seek professional advice before you start.

1 Are you over 40?
2 Is it more than 5 years since you took regular exercise?
3 Do you regularly get home and fall asleep in front of the TV?
4 Do you have any joint disease or deformity?
5 Are you more than 7 kg (14 lb) overweight?
6 Do you ever get dizzy or faint?
7 Do you smoke?
8 Do you feel ill if you have had to run for the train?
9 Do you get out of breath easily?
10 Do you have a problem sleeping?
11 Have you ever had a serious back problem?
12 Do you drink more than 3 pints of beer, 3 glasses of wine or 3 'spirits' daily?

and physical well-being into middle-age, you can begin exercise at any age. One interesting Russian experiment carried out some years ago took a group of 60-year olds and put them through a tough physical routine once a week. Ten years later at the age of 70 they were, on all physiological tests, actually younger. This shows how remarkable flexible and responsive the body is.

If you are out of condition, start gradually with gentle regimes. Many women in early middle age, for example, find that yoga not only maintains fitness but provides relaxation from the stresses and strains of family life.

Older people can begin by walking more: gradually increase your pace until you are walking briskly. Do muscle-tightening exercises while sitting down. Use the stairs instead of a lift or escalator, and take up a sport you can do at your own speed such as swimming, tennis, golf, bowls or cycling. Yoga is particularly good for older people. Even for people disinclined to take up aerobic exercises, there is considerable medical evidence on the health benefits to be gained by ordinary exercise in warding off the debilities or age.

Exercise and overweight

In the past, slimming regimes tended to underestimate the role of exercise in weight reduction with the result that the body, though slimmer, was still flabby. Now we know that dieting alone weakens the muscles and causes the loss of valuable muscle tissue which turns to fat as soon as dieting stops. Exercise tones the muscles and as you lose weight your body will become stronger, firmer and leaner. It often takes time for the body to respond to exercise. Persevere and bulges will disappear as you burn up fat and develop firm muscle tissue.

Another reason for exercising when slimming is that research has shown that appetite actually decreases with regular exercise. This is because it prevents a drop on the blood sugar levels which cause hunger. Exercise also speeds up the time it takes food to be processed in the digestive system and it speeds up the metabolic rate in such a way that even when you have stopped exercising the stimulating effect can persist. This means that throughout the rest of the day you are losing more calories than you might expect given your level of exertion.

Take up a regular exercise routine such as the exercises on page 32–37 and/or a sport, If you are on a very low-calorie diet, do not exercise too vigorously or you may feel dizzy and weak. Use caution and common sense. (See the table on p. 42 for how many calories you can use up.)

TYPES OF EXERCISE

These are three different kinds of exercises which serve different functions: *aerobics, anaerobics* and *isotonics*. Ideally, you should include some of each in your physical programme.

Isotonics

These are designed to develop muscular strength and flexibility and include stretching exercises, yoga and weight training. Isotonic exercises are based on exertion of muscles and joints and the aim is to make them more supple and elastic. Although isotonics do not greatly improve overall fitness or strengthen heart/lung functions, as aerobics do, they can make the body supple and graceful and can ease tension out of tired muscles. Stretching exercises are pleasant to do, especially if done to music, and make a good start to a fitness programme for a sedentary person. At first, you will be surprised at how out-of-condition you are! However, aching and stiff muscles will soon disappear as your body becomes toned up and conditioned.

Stretching exercises are also useful in the warm-up routine before you start aerobic activity. They can also help mobility and flexibility in such sports as tennis, skiing and running and, because they develop supple muscles, can also prevent many common sports injuries. Isotonic exercises are especially useful in association with a weight-reducing diet since they can firm up slack muscles, helping the body to assume its natural leaner proportions.

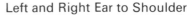

A SIMPLE EXERCISE PROGRAMME

A simple exercise routine
Many of the following exercises are suitable for warm-up and cool-down phases and also for people suffering from back problems. In addition, any combination of the exercises can be used for a routine keep-fit regime.

The first six exercises are for strengthening and relaxing the neck muscles and are useful for loosening and warming up.

Left and Right Ear to Shoulder
Position: Place left hand against left side of head.
Exercise: Try to push your left ear down towards your left shoulder. At the same time pushing with your hand against the side of your head. Hold for 10 seconds. Repeat 5 times, then repeat again with right hand on right side of head.

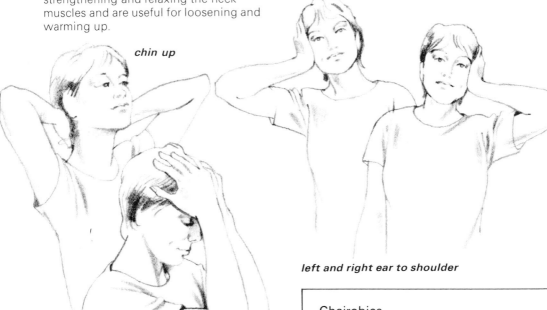

chin up

chin down

left and right ear to shoulder

Chin Up
Position: Clasp fingers of both hands together and place them behind your head.
Exercise: Lift your chin upwards pushing hard against your hands. Maintain the pressure for 10 seconds and repeat 5 times.

Chin Down
Position: Place the palms of both hands firmly against your forehead.
Exercise: Press head against the hands trying to push your chin down towards your chest. Hold for 10 seconds, repeat 5 times.

Chairobics
There is very little movement to the following two exercises and they can be done at work, on the bus and when sitting at home. They are muscle-strengthening and particularly useful for older, relatively inactive people.
Stomach squeeze
Position: Sitting on chair with cushion on lap.
Exercise: Bend knees, raise thighs squeezing cushion against stomach. Hold for 10 seconds and relax gently. Start with 3 times working up to more gradually.
Crossover
Position: Sitting on chair.
Exercise: Grip chair, cross one leg high over thigh and lean towards crossed leg as if pushing chair away. Hold for 6 seconds, then gently relax. Repeat with the other leg. Start with 6 times for each leg working up to more gradually.

shoulder drop

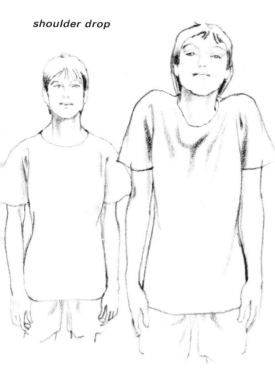

Exercise: Raise the shoulders as high as possible keeping arms by your side. Hold this position for 5 seconds then allow your shoulders to drop with their own weight. Repeat 3 times.

Chest Out
Position: Standing or sitting on stool.
Exercise: Push both shoulders as far back as possible sticking chest out and forcing shoulder blades together. Hold for 5 seconds, relax, repeat 3 times.

chest in   **chest out**

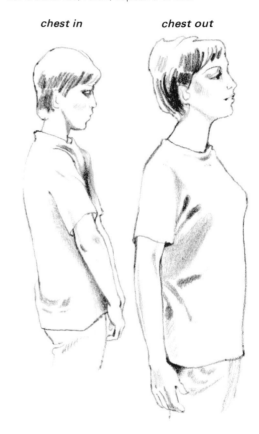

Shoulder Drop
Position: Standing or sitting in a straight chair.

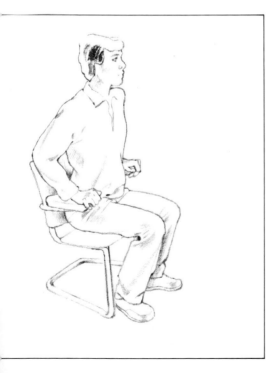

Chest In
Position: Standing or sitting on chair or stool.
Exercise: Push both shoulders as far forward as possible, narrowing the chest and forcing shoulder blades as far apart as they will go, keeping your arms by your sides. Hold for 5 seconds, relax, repeat 3 times.

Body Stretch

This is a useful warm-up exercise which stretches your arms and the sides of your body. (Not illustrated)
Position: Standing with feet just over hip distance apart.
Exercise: Breathe in, raise arms above head. Reach up as far as possible with left arm. Hold for 2 seconds. Breathe out. Repeat with right arm.

Walking on the spot

This is an excellent way of warming up or slowing down if you get breathless or dizzy from more strenuous exercises.
Position: Stand with feet slightly apart.
Exercise: Walk on the spot, rolling on the balls of your feet, as many times as you like, breathing deeply. You can extend this to jogging on the spot, gradually raising your knees, for up to 20 times. (Not illustrated)

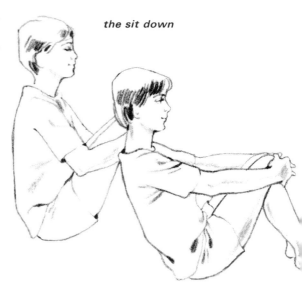

the sit down

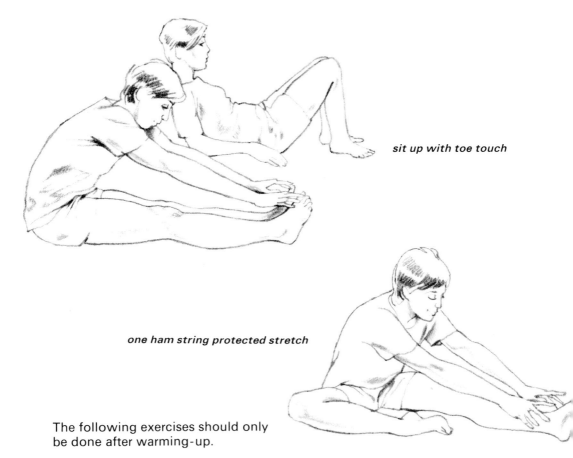

sit up with toe touch

one ham string protected stretch

The following exercises should only be done after warming-up.

Sit Down
Position: Sit on floor, knees bent, arms around knees.
Exercise: Lean slowly backwards using your arms to support the weight of your trunk. Use your arm muscles to pull back into the sitting position. Rest for 5 seconds, repeat 10 times. As your abdominal muscles gain in strength, you can reduce the support of hands and arms until you can perform the exercise 10 times without holding your knees.

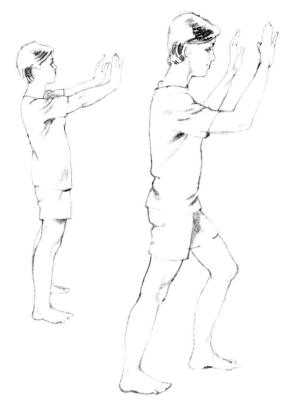

away with achilles heel

Sit Up with Toe Touch
Do not attempt this, until you have mastered the Sit Down.
Position: Flat on back, knees bent, feet flat on floor.
Exercise: Tuck in tail, chin on chest, hands along sides. Roll slowly upright from the neck keeping tail tucked. When upright straighten legs stretching fingers to toes, then roll slowly back to the floor bending knees. Work up to 10 repetitions.

One Ham String Protected Stretch
Many people engaged in sports stretch both ham strings at the same time. The ham strings are large muscles at the back of the thigh and a lot of elasticity in these muscles inhibits lumber flexion and correct spinal movement. Stretching both at once is counter-productive since it can do harm and trigger pain without any real appreciable benefit.

Position: Sitting on floor, bend one knee fully and place foot flat on floor.
Exercise: Allow bent knee to fall outwards and stretch both hands towards the foot of the straight leg as far as comfortable. Now start gentle rhythmic bouncing movement reaching off the foot. Continue for 20 seconds, rest, change legs and repeat.

Away with Achilles Heel:
This stretches shortened Achilles tendons which can impede correct walking and limit the flexion of the knee when bending and lifting.
Exercise: Put arms out in front and lean palms of hands against wall, balanced on both feet. Now place one foot halfway towards the wall, keeping the other leg straight at the knee with heel flat on the floor. Bend the forward knee and both arms slowly and rhythmically. The back heel must be kept on the floor and the tail tucked in at all times. Continue for 20 seconds. Relax, change legs and repeat.

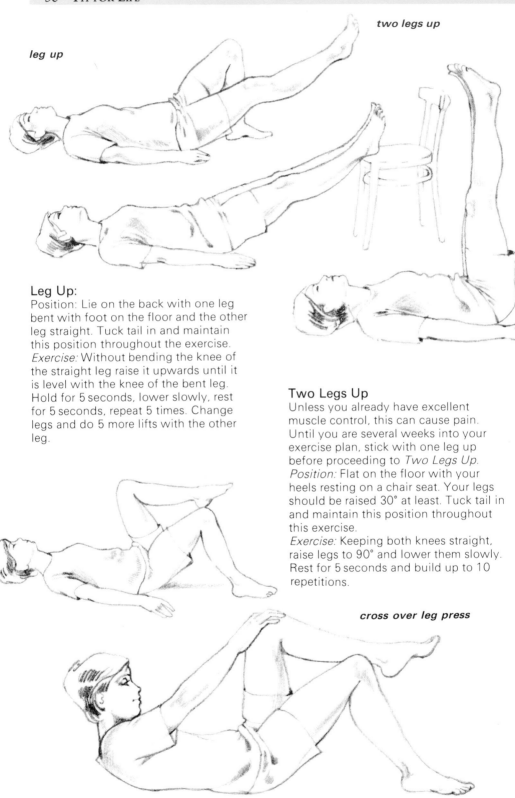

two legs up

leg up

Leg Up:

Position: Lie on the back with one leg bent with foot on the floor and the other leg straight. Tuck tail in and maintain this position throughout the exercise. *Exercise:* Without bending the knee of the straight leg raise it upwards until it is level with the knee of the bent leg. Hold for 5 seconds, lower slowly, rest for 5 seconds, repeat 5 times. Change legs and do 5 more lifts with the other leg.

Two Legs Up

Unless you already have excellent muscle control, this can cause pain. Until you are several weeks into your exercise plan, stick with one leg up before proceeding to *Two Legs Up. Position:* Flat on the floor with your heels resting on a chair seat. Your legs should be raised 30° at least. Tuck tail in and maintain this position throughout this exercise. *Exercise:* Keeping both knees straight, raise legs to 90° and lower them slowly. Rest for 5 seconds and build up to 10 repetitions.

cross over leg press

Cross Over Sit Up

Position: Flat on back, legs straight. Tuck in tail and maintain this position throughout the exercise.

Exercise: Spread the legs apart to 45°, tuck chin into chest and place right arm across body. Now pushing your right shoulder towards your left leg raise your trunk until both shoulder blades are off the floor. Relax and repeat 5 times. Change arms and stretch left shoulder to right leg 5 times.

Skipping

Position: Standing with both feet together and arms out to the sides holding a real (or imaginary) skipping rope. (Not illustrated)

Exercise: Breathe deeply and regularly. Turn the rope and jump just high enough to clear it. Build up the rhythm gradually. Skip forwards to begin with then as you become more practised try skipping backwards.

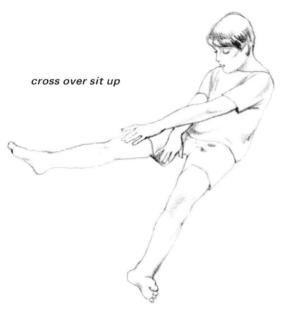

cross over sit up

Jumping

Position: Hands on hips, feet together. (Not illustrated)

Exercise: Breathe deeply and regularly. Jump from side to side, landing flat on both feet. Work this up gradually, then advance to bending your knees as you land and straightening them as you jump. Practise until you can repeat 16 times.

Finish the session with cooling down exercises (as for warming up).

Cross Over Leg Press

This is an isometric exercise which really strengthens the abdominal muscles without movement.

Position: Lie on back, knees bent and feet flat on the floor. Tuck tail in and maintain position throughout the exercise.

Exercise: Raise the right knee until the calf is parallel with the floor. Now place left hand on right knee, keeping your arm straight. Raise head and tuck chin into your chest. Now push hand against knee and knee against hand using the muscle strength of shoulder and arm against knee and hip. This creates powerful action of the abdominal muscles. Hold the pressure for 5 seconds and relax, repeat 5 times. Change over hand and leg and repeat 5 times again.

Weight Training

This is a form of isotonic exercise and should not be confused with heavy weight lifting. Weight training develops your capacity to lift something a little heavier than before or raise a heavy object once or twice more. This lengthens and shortens muscles to build up strength and also helps to burn up excess stores of fat. Many women find 'weighting' good for firming up midriff, bustline and other problem areas. Although not as useful as aerobics, weight training can help the heart and lungs as well, especially if light weights are used in conjunction with a high number of movements and 'repetitions'.

While weight training is frequently carried out at gyms and health centres, barbells and dumb-bells can be bought for home use and you can improvise with everyday items such as heavy books, bags of rice or dried beans and unopened cans. It is advisable for a beginner to go at least once to a sports centre or gym to see the correct weight training style.

Anaerobics

This form of exercise is the opposite of aerobics and relies for its effect on short sudden bursts or energy rather than a sustained rhythmic routine. **Sprinting** and **some gymnastics** fall into this category.

Although this form of exercise does help to develop muscular strength and power, it should really be carried out as a supplement to aerobic exercise in order to make the oxygen in the blood work even more efficiently. Some people are naturally able to summon up great bursts of energy for, say, a sprint but they are usually relatively fit to begin with. Anaerobic exercise is not sufficiently sustained to benefit heart and lungs but if you are fit already and have a natural talent for this kind of activity it can be beneficial.

Aerobics

The word 'aerobic' means 'with oxygen'. Aerobic exercises are sustained, rhythmical exercises that increase the body's ability to deliver oxygenated blood to muscles and organs. They are not simply the series of exercises that can be taken at

fashionable gyms, but include such activities and sports as **long-distance running, cycling, jogging, swimming, rowing, cross-country skiing** or even **brisk or uphill walking** and **skipping.** Apart from sport and exercise, any continuous activity which increases your breathing and heart rates is aerobic; gardening, sawing logs, shovelling snow, all provide your body with aerobic work.

The most aerobically valuable activities are those that produce a high heart rate and a demand for large amounts of oxygen which can be sustained for long periods. When you are aerobically unfit, your cells and muscles cannot supply this oxygen in sufficient quantities, resulting in breathlessness when swimming a couple of lengths or running upstairs. To achieve full aerobic fitness, you must increase your heart rate to a 'training level' and be able to sustain this level for at least 15 minutes, preferably longer.

Training Levels

Most adults have a resting pulse of 60 to 80 beats per minute. Find your pulse rate by pressing your wrist on the thumb side; count the beats for 15 seconds, then multiply by four to find the rate per minute. An aerobic sport or exercise should raise the pulse from its normal beat to well over 100 beats per minute.

Recommended Heart Rates for Best Aerobic Effort

Age	Heart rate per minute
20	138–158
25	137–156
30	135–154
35	134–153
40	132–151
45	131–150
50	129–147
55	127–146
60	126–144
65	125–142
70	123–141
75	122–139
80	120–138
85	119–136

Benefits of aerobic exercises

When you are aerobically fit, your body uses oxygen more efficiently. Breathing

Safety First

Strenuous aerobic exercises or sport should not be undertaken by any person who is not already reasonably fit. This is because the heart, if launched into sudden action, can react abnormally. Many of the movements involved in aerobics can sprain or tear muscles, tendons and ligaments in bodies unused to exercise, so build up to aerobics exercises gently.

- Do not exercise if you have a fever or viral infection. These will not only affect your performance but muscles, joints, heart or respiratory system may become inflamed and your general condition worsen.
- Do not exercise if you feel giddy, faint, out of breath or sick. If symptoms persist, consult a medical practitioner.
- If exercise is really painful, stop. Start again after a day or two with gentle, stretching exercises.
- Train, not strain. Build up gradually to your chosen exercise. Be patient and do not overdo things. It may take several weeks before you feel the benefits of exercise.
- Always warm up and cool down before and after exercise to regulate the heart rate and to stretch and relax muscles, thereby reducing the risk of stiffness and injury.
- After cool down, relax tired muscles in a warm bath or shower.
- Never exercise immediately after eating. In order to avoid stomach-ache and cramps, wait at least 2 hours.
- Never exercise in really hot weather. It is debilitating and you could become dehydrated.

improves, as does the ability to clear out carbon dioxide and other toxic wastes from the lungs. The heart becomes stronger and arteries and veins become more elastic and free from blockages. The American fitness expert, Dr Kenneth Cooper has used aerobics to rehabilitate heart attack victims. He has also shown that people who take regular aerobic exercises generally have lower levels of fats in the blood, lower body fat and fewer heartbeat irregularities than the average. Cooper also believes that aerobics can slow down the ageing process. Oxygen is vital to cell regeneration, and aerobics forces oxygen in every part of the body, including cells and tissue and so makes cell regeneration more efficient.

ON THE FITNESS TRAIL

Long term fitness can be achieved by regular aerobic exercise. That means continuous activity that keeps your heart rate at 75% of the maximal rate for your age. This does NOT mean getting into your leotard and heading for the latest fashionable aerobics class—these are for keeping fit not getting fit. Any exercise which increases the heart rate or the respiration rate is aerobic.

Aim at using 2,000K calories per week. This means three hours of sustained effort which keeps your heart beating at the recommended speed for your age. Choose physical exercises or a sport (preferably both) that will suit you. First of all, you must enjoy what you are doing and not regard your chosen form of exercise as a chore, otherwise you are unlikely to keep it up. Take into account your figure, build, natural ability, temperament and lifestyle in general. Ask yourself these questions. Do I want to take exercise alone or in the company of others? Do competitive sports suit me? How will an exercise programme fit into my daily routine?

HOW OFTEN TO EXERCISE

Ideally, plan your programme so that you set aside a regular time for exercise each week, choosing the time that suits you best. Start off by exercising three times a week, allowing yourself 30 minutes per session with a warm-up and cooling down phase before and after each. If you are taking up exercise for the first time, start with 15 minutes stretching exercises to tone up muscles before you embark on, say, a programme of aerobic exercises. And when you start out, exercise on alternate days at first to give your body a day of rest and a chance to recover.

TIPS FOR BEGINNERS

● You may feel a little stiff at first because your body is unaccustomed to the new unfamiliar movements it has gone through. This will soon pass as you become fitter. If you are in real pain, you have been exercising too strenuously and need to cut back on your training accordingly.
● Always do warm-up exercises *before* you begin the main phase of exercise or sport and cooling-down exercises *afterwards*.
● Always stretch muscles out slowly; short, jerky movement can do damage.
● Take your routine gradually and do not expect instant results. It will take several sessions before you notice any appreciable difference.
● Always take a shower or bath to cool down or relieve tired muscles. Take time and don't rush this. It is most important to relax after exercise.
● If possible, take up your fitness routine with a family member or friend. It is more fun and you are less likely to miss a session.

THE THREE STAGES OF EXERCISE

In order to avoid excessive strain and muscular or joint damage it is vital that each period of aerobic exercise comprises: **a warm-up phase; an endurance phase;** and **a cooling down phase.** Many people often omit the third or cooling down phase and this is the reason that they give up exercise programmes. Without it, waste products are not eliminated from the muscle tissues and consequently you are much more likely to suffer cramp, pain and stiffness in the 48 hours after your exercise.

Warming-up

The warm-up routine improves blood circulation to the muscles, increases the pulse rate and stretches the muscles. This will reduce the risk of injury to muscles or ligaments and get you in the right mood to exercise. The warm-up must last for at least five minutes and it is particularly important if you have taken little or no exercise for years. Choose any combination of the warm-up exercises (p. 28), and vary them from day to day.

Endurance Stage

This should last for between 20 and 30 minutes so that you can push your heart rate up to the appropriate level for your age (see p. 38). DO NOT EXCEED RECOMMENDED FIGURE. Check your pulse rate a few times during the endurance phase. This is best done by stopping and feeling the pulse in your temple with the pad of your third finger. (As above, count the pulse for 15 seconds and multiply by four to get the rate per minute.)

The object is to speed up your breathing and heart rate without gasping for air. As you get fitter, you will have to increase the intensity or the duration of exercise in order to maintain the required heart rate. If, during the early stages of getting yourself fit, you cannot maintain vigorous exercise you should do less intensive workouts but for longer periods of time.

Cooling Off

The cooling-down phase is just as important as the warm-up routine, since it allows your pulse rate to return to normal gradually. (Too abrupt a halt and the sudden lack of oxygen-rich blood in the brain could cause you to faint.)

It should last for at least six minutes and can include any of the stretching warm-up exercises together with brisk walking for four minutes or alternate walking and jogging for two minutes each.

A SPORTING LIFE

Probably the most enjoyable way to take exercise is in sport. Sport is exercise in a social context: it offers goals for the competitive and health-promoting fun for those unconcerned with winning. Ideally, you should combine a sport with a routine keep-fit regime for the best of all possible worlds.

Which sport?

Choose a sport which you are likely to enjoy and which will fit in with your life-style. If time is a deciding factor and it is difficult to travel to or from a swimming pool, tennis court or golf course, choose an activity such as jogging or cycling, that involves minimum time and little bother.

Running and jogging

Running is an excellent form of aerobic exercise which is cheap and can be done any time, anywhere. Not only does it strengthen your cardiovascular system but you will also lose weight (up to 5 kg/10 lbs) if you keep it up for a year. If you are unfit, begin by walking, inter-spersed with a little running. Start with running and walking for just 15 minutes and build up your distance and speed gradually. Don't force yourself to run quickly at first —you could put excessive strain on your muscles—and do invest in a pair of proper running shoes to protect your feet and cushion the body from jolts. The golden rule with running is to train, not strain. As with other routines, allow time for warming up, cooling down and a relaxing shower afterwards.

Cycling

Along with jogging, cycling ranks among the best aerobic exercises. It is also cheap, a practical means of travel and can be easily fitted into the daily routine, for example, by cycling to work or the shops. As with all aerobic exercises, begin gradu-ally by cycling for only 30 minutes, then build up the time to an hour or longer.

Concentrate on the time spent exercis-ing and not on the speed (which, in any case, is not always safe in heavy traffic) and try to keep the pace steady. There are many different styles of bikes to choose from and only you can decide whether you want a 5- or 10-speed gear racing bike or something simpler. In fact, almost any bike will do but it must be the right size so that you can maintain good posture. Well-pumped tyres give an easier ride as do flattish, hard shoes.

Swimming

Swimming is one of the best all-round exercises there is, and it has a high aerobic value. Since the body weight is supported by water, it is particularly suitable for people who are overweight or who have back or joint problems. Unlike many forms of exercise, there is little danger of getting injured as the body is virtually weightless in the water and you do not strain it so much as in, say, running or squash. Fast swimming eats up a considerable number of calories although the buoyant support of the water makes the effort seem less than it is.

Start off gradually with a five-minute session swimming one width of the pool with a walk back to your starting point to complete another. Gradually build up to 15 minutes non-stop swimming, eventu-ally working up to 30 minutes or more. If you are out of condition, begin with backstroke — leg kicking only. Progress to side stroke, breast stroke and, for the really fit, the crawl. Stop for a rest when you begin to feel tired (although this will

Running the Risks

Regular exercise increases the amount of chemicals which your body produces, especially a group called endorphins. These chemicals are the body's own equivalent of morphine-related substances and some runners do get 'hooked' on their own endorphins. This results in obsessional adherence to their running programmes.

DO NOT RUN
- if you have a cold or high temperature
- if you have pains in the chest
- in extremely hot or extremely cold weather
- if you have any persistent joint or muscle pain for which you have not sought professional advice.

While you will need to push yourself in order to maintain any type of regular fitness schedule, you must learn to know where to draw the line between making the effort and going over the top.

become less frequent as your level of fitness improves).

Protect your eyes with anti-chlorine goggles and wear plastic or rubber shoes for walking to and from the poolside to prevent foot infections.

Tennis

Although tennis has only a moderate aerobic value, it is an extremely popular and enjoyable sport which is good for general fitness. It encourages muscular strength and endurance and develops co-ordination and balance.

Tennis can be taken up at any time as long as you are reasonably supple and mobile, although if you have not played since schooldays you may need a brief refresher course on service, footwork and basic strokes. Injuries sometimes occur with beginners because of incorrect play and overstrain, so do get the basics right first before you attempt to build up speed and technique.

Choose a raquet that you can grip comfortably and swing easily, and buy good tennis shoes—they have to absorb the shock of a lot of movement, particularly on a hard court.

Keep up your racket skills in the winter with badminton.

Squash

This is an anaerobically valuable sport which requires speed and skill if played correctly. Like tennis it encourages muscular endurance and co-ordination and can be a way of releasing tension and anxiety. A vigorous game of squash uses up about 600 calories per hour so it is a good way of keeping weight down. Like tennis, a beginner should first be trained in basic play and should build up technique very gradually in order to avoid injury.

Invest in an eye-guard. Squash balls are very hard.

You must be fit to begin with to play squash, so don't make it the first choice if you haven't been exercising recently. It can also be fiercely competitive, so don't let your urge to scramble to the top of the club's ladder impose more stress on you

than that which you are exercising to dissipate.

Leading cardiologists are growing more concerned by the dramatic increase in sudden death on the squash court and within 48 hours of a strenuous game. Apart from the physical exertion, the psychological impact of being shut up in a box with an opponent is reminiscent of the Roman gladiators, and what starts as a game can end, literally, in a fight to the death. If you are over 35 and want to play, then you must play three times a week or not at all.

Burning it Up

If you need extra motivation for exercise, just think how many calories you are burning up. Here is a list so you can compare the rates and adjust your losses.

Sport	Calories burned per hour
Badminton	250
Dancing	300
Skipping	300
Surfing	300
Waterskiing	300
Cycling	350
Tennis	350
Windsurfing	350
Swimming	400
Brisk walking	400
Jogging	500
Squash	600
Skiing	700
Running	800

Golf

Golf is relaxing but is a way of maintaining fitness rather than acquiring it. You would need to play at least five hours a day to get really fit. It is a game where technique counts, so the beginner is wise to take basic lessons and practise frequently at first to develop the co-ordination and balance required to play the game well.

Exercise will keep you fit and enjoying life. It will also help you to deal with the inevitable stress and tension of life in the 1980s.

STRESS AND HOW TO DEAL WITH IT

Stress is rather like human intelligence. Although everybody knows what it is, it is difficult to define and shows itself in many different ways.

Stress is an essential ingredient in our lives, adding spice and motivation. It's important to have a clear view of it and consider its good as well as its bad points.

WHAT IS STRESS?

The original engineering definition describes stress as 'a force which acts on a body, setting up strains within it according to its load-carrying capacity, flexibility, and tolerance'. Or you might compare it to an electric current in a circuit. The circuit is designed to take a certain amount of current and would be functionless without it. It is only when the current becomes too great and the circuit is overloaded that problems arise. The natural capacity of the system is then exceeded and overheating or the blowing of fuses occurs.

Similarly, people whose stress tolerance is exceeded or who handle it in an inappropriate way, not only get hot and bothered but may blow a mental fuse and have a nervous breakdown, blow a cardiac fuse and have a heart attack, or blow up a stomach ulcer.

People vary enormously in their natural tolerance to stress; some people (notably politicans), being 30 amp cooker types, enjoy and thrive on vast amounts of stress, while other people will blow a 3 amp fuse with one evening amongst the bright lights.

The first thing to recognize is how much stress you, as an individual, can tolerate without being affected physically and mentally. Secondly, you need to know what steps to take when stress or tension, however temporary, is getting you down.

AM I SUFFERING FROM STRESS?

How can you tell whether you are suffering from stress? Check with the questions in the panel to see if any apply to you. Stress can manifest itself as lethargy, compulsive eating, inability to concentrate as well as nervous tics, unexplained tearful outbursts or overdependence on cigarettes and alcohol.

Are you stressed?

It's often difficult to take an objective view of yourself to see if how you feel is related to some external stressful factor. Check with these points to see if you could be stressed. Do you:

- feel near to tears most of the time?
- constantly fidget, bite your nails, chew your hair?
- find it hard to concentrate and impossible to decide?
- find it hard to talk to anyone?
- snap and shout at everybody?
- eat when you aren't hungry?
- feel tired all the time?
- no longer laugh at things?
- feel suspicious of other people?
- no longer have any interest in sex?
- sleep badly?
- drink and or smoke to calm your nerves?
- feel you just can't cope?

If you answer yes to more than 4 of these questions, you are stressed. Refer to our other questionnaire and review your life and habits to try and isolate the reasons for your stress. You can't go on like this.

Sometimes stress does not show until the sufferer collapses with a heart attack or other serious malfunction. People who are very busy may think they feel great, whereas in fact they are overloading and about to blow a fuse. In these instances, chemofeedback (a system of measuring stress levels in blood and sweat discussed in **Relaxation Techniques** pp. 96–101) may prove beneficial. This is a system that lends itself to mass screening, and soon may be as automatic a part of life in large companies as mass X ray programmes. It will predict the unpleasant side effects of stress in time to prevent them, and help people to modify their lives to minimize future stress.

HOW THE BODY REACTS TO STRESS

Whatever the cause of stress — and this can range from merely irritating noise, to personal fears and anxiety or to a physically threatening situation like being attacked by a dog — the body's response is the same. The bloodstream is flooded with adrenaline, blood pressure rises, the muscles flex and the whole body feels tense. These are the more obvious symptoms of a wide range of changes that take place in the body and nervous system which are commonly labelled the 'flight or fight' reaction. Primitive man, when face to face with a sabre-toothed tiger probably did just that — fought or fled — but this is rarely possible or indeed appropriate for most people nowadays. Although the body is wound up for action, none takes place and the heightened levels of hormones and chemicals stay in the bloodstream, unused.

When stress occurs repeatedly over a long period without being 'resolved', a chronic state of hypertension is reached when high blood pressure can become permanent, when digestive problems such as ulcers occur and when headaches, aches and pains become common because of muscular tension. These, in turn, can lead to loss of sleep, general underperformance at work or in normal activity, loss of self-confidence and self-esteem and a spiral of declining health.

CAN STRESS BE GOOD FOR YOU?

People cannot, of course, spend their lives avoiding stress and nor should they. Many positively enjoy stress using it to face physical, intellectual or social challenges. Extending yourself in this way keeps you healthy, active and young—as long as you also have the ability to relax. By learning to face each new challenge as it comes along and by switching off before fatigue sets in, you can use stress to make your life more interesting and exciting.

The As and Bs of stress

Dr Ray H. Rosenmann and Dr Meyer Friedmann of California have devised a simple questionnaire which divides people into two categories, Type As and Type Bs. Rosenmann and Friedmann link certain behaviour patterns with susceptibility to coronary heart disease. Type A people, whose lives are full of stressful behaviour, are more likely to succumb than type Bs, who have a more relaxed approach. The characteristics are displayed below: if you identify with half or more of those assigned to type A, you are a type A personality. If you want to avoid overstress or coronary heart disease, try to adjust your style and take in more type B attitudes.

Type A

- Very competitive.
- Bossy, forceful.
- Gets things done quickly (not always well).
- Strives for promotion and high status.
- Eager for fame.
- Easily angered by events or people.
- Reckless when unoccupied.
- Speaks quickly and explosively.
- Moves, walks and eats quickly.
- Will not brook delay.
- Thrives on pressure of doing more than one project at a time.
- Likes to be given (and to beat) deadlines.

Type B

- Uncompetitive.
- Easygoing, reticent.
- Slow, methodical.
- Doesn't care for status or promotion.
- Shuns fame.
- Angers slowly.
- Enjoys creative resting.
- Speaks slowly.
- Does not rush.
- Does not mind delay.
- Likes doing one thing at a time.
- Ignores deadlines.

DEALING WITH STRESS

Once you have established your 'stress threshold', how do you deal with the stress you can't use? Most people work out their own way of dealing with stress. For some, it is a hobby such as gardening or painting; for others it's going to the theatre or cinema; and for many it is a sport or some form of physical exercise. In fact, physical exercise is recommended by many experts as a particularly good form of relaxation since it gets rid of pent-up energy and encourages self-confidence. Studies have shown, for example, that endurance runners who cover long distances in training each week tend to be less anxious and more emotionally stable than their physically inactive contemporaries.

How to de-stress yourself

If you discover that you are unreasonably stressed, here are some tips on breaking out of the vicious circle.
- Work no more than 9 hours a day.
- Take a break of at least half-an-hour in the middle of a working day.
- Take off at least 1½-days per week from your normal work routine.
- Eat regular, healthy meals.
- Get regular exercise through sport, exercise routines or by making everyday activities more 'fitness conscious'.
- Practise relaxation or meditation for 10–15 minutes daily or at least 3 times a week.
- Face up to work or emotional problems and do something practical about solving them.
- Do not use alcohol, cigarettes or drugs to relieve stress; they are only temporarily effective and in the long-term can aggravate and increase symptoms.
- Remember that stressful situations are not always unhappy ones; marriage and promotion at work can both cause stress.
- Learn to recognize your own stress thresholds. Use stress and relaxation positively to take control of your life and channel it in the direction you want to go.

A good diet, high in essential nutrients, vitamins and minerals, can also help combat stress, particularly if it is high in the B-complex vitamins. Vitamin B_{12}, for example, helps protect you against insomnia, depression and fatigue. If you are under temporary stress, it is often worth taking supplements of vitamin B to help you cope with the crisis.

If you feel you need to take more positive steps towards relaxation, there are a number of techniques and therapies from which to choose. Turn to the **Relaxation Techniques** chapter (p. 96) for more information on autogenics, biofeedback, meditation and yoga as well as some relaxation exercises. You may also find the chapter on **Massage** (p. 86) and **Hypnotherapy** (p. 80) helpful. Some other alternative therapies will also exert a beneficial effect on your stress levels, although this is not their primary function. These include **Acupuncture** (p. 66), the **Alexander Technique** (p. 69) and **Herbalism** (p. 74).

LOSING SLEEP

One of the most common symptoms of anxiety and stress is sleep disturbance. This can take many forms:
- inability to get to sleep.
- fitful and disturbed sleep.
- early waking with anxiety preventing further sleep.
- lack of proper sleep produces fatigue and even more stress and tension and so a vicious circle is set up until the sufferer, defeated and exhausted, more often than not resorts to sleeping pills.

Types of sleep

Central to mental and physical health and probably to life itself, there are two kinds of sleep, equally essential. Slow-wave, orthodox sleep restores and replenishes the body. Rapid-eye movement (REM) sleep (dreaming sleep) maintains our emotional and mental stability. During the night, you alternate between periods of orthodox and REM sleep, beginning with a period of orthodox sleep when the body relaxes, blood pressure drops and heart and breathing rates slow down. This is followed by a lighter, dreaming phase

(REM sleep) when the closed eyes move rapidly and fingers and toes often twitch. Predictably, your brainwaves become irregular, temperature and blood pressure rise, the heartbeat increases and your breathing gets faster. The whole cycle from dropping off to sleep to the end of the first dreaming phase takes less than 2 hours and REM sleep probably lasts only from 10–20 minutes before you resume normal orthodox sleep. Thereafter, it recurs about every $1\frac{1}{2}$ hours throughout the night, ending in a longer 30 minute session in the morning before you wake up.

The importance of dreaming
REM sleep is especially important for mental health. It is believed that it helps to sort out and code new information and to slot it into the brain's memory bank and also removes tension and resolves inner conflicts. Experiments have shown that if you are deprived of REM sleep, even for relatively short periods of time you become tense and depressed and some people become psychologically disturbed. Poor sleepers spend less time in REM sleep. Alcohol and sleeping pills, frequently taken to help sleep, can also repress REM dreaming phases, causing you to wake up feeling tired, irritable and depressed.

What to do about it
The first thing is not to worry about it; all that does is increase your stress levels and aggravate the problem. If you find it hard to sleep, don't. Put the light on (if this is possible), read a favourite book, have a warm milky drink. If it's the first time, it may be just a temporary matter and should not be escalated into a problem.

Regular exercise and a good diet should automatically predicate good healthy sleep. It is possible that some sleep problems are diet-related and are caused by deficiencies of zinc, calcium or vitamin E. Make sleeping pills and tranquillizers your very last resort. There are other ways to a good night's sleep.

Do
- Try relaxing exercises to calm the mind and release tension from the body.
- Take a hot milky drink or soothing herbal tea before bedtime.
- Take a warm relaxing bath before going to bed.

Don't
- Drink strong coffee or tea or lots of alcohol.
- Exercise strenuously before going to bed.
- Take sleeping pills.
- Worry about it.

See *also* **Insomnia** in the A–Z Section.

A check in time
Don't pile on the stress by worrying about your health — that can be a disease in itself. Make sure you have regular checks, and then forget about it.

Since hypertension shows no symptoms until the damage is done, you should have your blood pressure checked whenever you see your GP or practitioner.

Tests	When to have them
blood pressure	under 40s: every 2 years
	over 40s: yearly
heart function	ditto
respiratory function	ditto
urine	ditto
optical	yearly
dental	every year

Women under 35 should have a cervical smear test every two years, women over 35 once a year. All women should have an annual breast examination.

POSITIVE HEALTH:

A BODY MAINTENANCE PROGRAMME

Positive health means taking a positive attitude to your body and its functions; taking your life in your hands, in fact. It is *not* about firefighting and spectacular emergency action when your body breaks down. It *is* about a continuous process of doing all the things that are good for mind, body and spirit: eating well, taking regular and enjoyable exercise, getting enough sleep, making time to relax properly— and avoiding things that are bad for you: excess alcohol, smoking, drugs of all sorts, junk food and sloppy postural habits which can make you tired and irritable.

The body maintenance programme in this chapter will show you how to look after your body from top to toe, how to monitor and control your drinking, how to be kind to your back, how to recognize the signs of drug taking and what to do about it, and how to make sure your children enjoy positive health as well as you.

TOP TO TOE

Looking after the outside of your body is just as important as making sure it us functioning properly within. Signs of ill-health often manifest themselves first in the eyes, in the hair or on the skin; equally, everyday hygiene has an important part to play, too.

Skin

The very best treatment for a healthy skin is fresh air and sunlight; keeping it clean comes a close second. It is best to avoid any perfumed soap; medicated soaps should never be used as they kill off the body's natural bacteria and dry out the mucous membranes. For the same reasons, disinfectant and antiseptic should never be added to the bath, and nor should foaming detergents (bubble baths or bath crystals). Use good quality natural soaps and natural oils, free of synthetic ingredients. These are available from good chemists and health food shops. Oatmeal soaps are particularly good for the skin.

If you can, it is better to shower than bath. It is cleaner, and cheaper as it uses less hot water. Those women who are prone to thrush and cystitis, especially, should shower rather than bath and, if they have to bath, they should not soak in hot soapy water as this destroys the bacteria that keep the level of fungus down.

● **Bidets** should not be used for douching. Those in which the water fills up from a tap are perfectly all right, but those that produce water in a spray up into the vagina are not recommended, as they can drive local bacteria up into the womb.

● **Spa baths** The question you should ask yourself is 'How would you like getting into your morning bath knowing that 40 other people had got into it before you?' Unless whirlpool baths are properly maintained, you are at grave risk of contracting all sorts of infectious diseases, some of which can be serious, such as Legionnaire's disease. Less serious hazards include boils, rashes, sore throats, thrush and cystitis. If you use a spa bath, make sure that it is checked several times a day and regularly maintained for bacteria levels, the filter cleaned and the water changed regularly. You should always shower both before and after using one.

● **Swimming pools** These are usually better maintained than whirlpool baths, but there are nevertheless hygiene precautions to be observed. Always wear a swimming cap, particularly if you have long hair; wear goggles to prevent eye infections; and wear rubber shoes in the changing rooms to prevent the possibility of picking up athlete's foot.

Hair

Wash your hair as often as your skin can take it; if you wash it too often, you may dry out the scalp and strip off lubricating oil.

If you do wash it every day, choose a mild shampoo, preferably plant-based, and shampoo only once. Pay special attention to rinsing thoroughly. Don't spend a fortune on miracle conditioners: really healthy hair is the direct result of healthy eating and plenty of exercise to stimulate the circulation. Regard conditioner as a back up to help make hair more manageable and look shinier (it's the light bouncing off the fine film of oil that imparts the gloss). Again, choose a plant-based product to suit your hair type.

Take care with hair colouring products. Many people are allergic to them, so always patch test first. There is some evidence that some permanent hair dyes may be carcinogenic. If you want to colour your hair, go for hennas or other plant-based products.

Eyes

Our eyesight almost inevitably deteriorates to some extent as we become older. A system of eye exercises to reduce eyesight deterioration as a result of ageing was formulated at the beginning of this century by Dr William H Bates (1881–1931), an American opthalmologist. Naturopaths believe that these exercises, combined with a good diet, (plenty of green and yellow vegetables for vitamin A, the fundamental vitamin for eyes) can do much to preserve eyesight which is failing only as a result of age.

Eyestrain

Eyes have to be rested just like any other part of the body. You should not expect to carry out close work for many hours on end and not have pink and possibly swollen and itchy eyes as a result. If you are doing close work, look up and into the distance frequently so that the eyes have to refocus.

If you wear glasses, be sure to have regular eye tests and to make sure that your glasses fit correctly. If they are falling down your nose, you will not be looking through the optical centres and this can result in eyestrain.

Damage to the eyes

Take care to avoid burns to the cornea from aerosol sprays containing oven cleaner, hair spray, garden pesticides; take care with bleach, caustic soda, plaster lime and cement and with car battery liquid. If you get any of these things in your eyes, flush them out immediately with water and then go to your local medical practitioner. Radiation also causes retinal burns so:

- never look directly at the sun or through a telescope or binoculars at it.
- never look at an eclipse of the sun.

Of lice and men

Lice can live on our bodies and hair. They are unpleasant but easy to get rid of. See Lice in the A–Z for how to deal with the various kinds that affect humans. Meanwhile, here are the facts:

The truth about lice

- Head lice prefer clean scalps to dirty ones.
- You cannot catch head lice from other people's hats or combs or from swimming pools, mats in gymnasiums or upholstered aeroplane, railway or bus seats.
- Head lice find it easier to get at a scalp covered with thin or closely cropped hair than to one covered with longer, thick hair.
- Body lice die if they cannot feed regularly and/or are not kept in a warm temperature, so second-hand clothes are very unlikely to be infested.
- Body lice can carry certain diseases, including typhus.
- Pubic lice do not carry sexually transmitted diseases, but they can be associated with them.

● if you work with lasers, never point them at the eyes.
● wear optical quality sunglasses in the snow, when skiing, for example, to avoid damage by reflected sun.
● never look at sunlamps—*always* wear goggles.

Sunlamps are especially hazardous for the eyes. You should always close your eyes and wear goggles, even if you have your back to the lamp because of the reflected light. UVA lamps are particularly dangerous, since they cause internal damage with a delayed pain response: so by the time you're feeling pain, the damage has been done. Always wear swimming goggles to avoid the possibility of conjunctivitis which is easily contracted in swimming pools. Finally, remember that smoking, which is bad for every part of the body may also cause defective eyesight as nicotine affects the arteries in the eyes.

Medically induced eye problems
I recently met Donald Pitts, Professor of Visual Science at the University of Houston, Texas and adviser to NASA. His research shows that many commonly prescribed drugs often used for long term therapy, increase the sensitivity of both skin and eyes to UV light. That doesn't just come from sunlight but also, albeit in very small amounts, from fluorescent light sources and computer screens. More younger people are getting cataracts and the overall incidence of malignant melanoma (a type of skin cancer) has increased dramatically in recent years.

The commonest drugs which have this effect are:
● **oral contraceptives** (all kinds)
● **tetracyclins** (commonly used long term against chronic chest infections)
● **phenothiazines** (major tranquillizers such as largactil)
● **benzodiazepines** (tranquillizers) all minor tranquillizers (valium, librium)
● **chloraphiozides** (diuretics)
● **sulphonamides** (often used against chronic urinary infections such as cystitis)

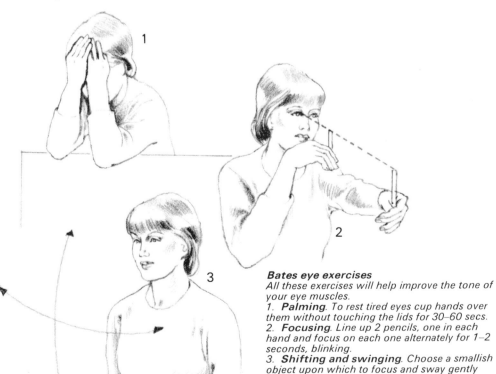

Bates eye exercises
All these exercises will help improve the tone of your eye muscles.
*1. **Palming**. To rest tired eyes cup hands over them without touching the lids for 30–60 secs.*
*2. **Focusing**. Line up 2 pencils, one in each hand and focus on each one alternately for 1–2 seconds, blinking.*
*3. **Shifting and swinging**. Choose a smallish object upon which to focus and sway gently from side to side, blinking, without taking you eye off the object.*

- **sulphonyluveas** (oral diabetic drugs)
- **griseofulvins** (anti fungals used for skin and nail infections often for a year at a time)
- **psoralens** (for psoriasis; also found in some sun tan lotions and in Earl Grey tea as essence of Bergamot)

Taking any of these drugs long term, means extra care in the sun. Use high protection factor sun screens (*without* psoralens), avoid excessive exposure to extreme sunlight, don't use sunbeds and wear high quality sun glasses or goggles when skiing or at the seaside. Look out for glasses or contact lenses made from *permaflex*, a material which absorbs UV light.

Teeth

Good dental hygiene is essential if you are to avoid tooth decay, gum disease and bad breath.

Decay occurs when the bacteria in your mouth, fuelled by the sugar you eat in food, manufacture an acid which attacks the tooth enamel, eventually getting through to form caries. Normally, saliva bathes away this acid, and the trouble occurs when food particles lodge in the crevices and fissures of your teeth and cannot be flushed out. It is therefore important to clean your teeth regularly (morning and night, and after every meal if possible) with a toothbrush and dental floss. Some dental hygienists recommend you clean before eating as well, as this gets rid of the bacteria temporarily so they cannot thrive on the food you are eating, but this seems hardly practicable. Better to avoid sugar as much as possible at meal times and in between. Remember that sugar comes in drinks as well.

Sugary, starchy foods also encourage the formation of dental plaque. This is serious, as plaque can lead to gum disease. Plaque is a thin veil of bacteria and saliva, which collects round the bottom of the teeth, where they fit into the gums. It takes 36 hours to form, so should be routinely removed by brushing, provided you brush regularly, paying special attention to the tooth/gum border. If not removed, it will go hard, and the bacteria trapped behind

---

Eyes and VDUs

If you work with a VDU, do not work in front of the screen for longer than 2 hours without a break. The ideal is 2 hours on, 1 hour off. This is not always possible of course; aim for 15 minute break every 45 minutes or at least 10–15 minutes every 1½ to 2 hours. Make sure that the line of sight is correct and that the background lighting is comfortable. Have your eyes tested at any sign of strain, such as sore eyes or persistent headache.

VDUs are not *per se* harmful to the eyes, but will aggravate any defect already present. Contact lens wearers may find problems with VDUs simply because they concentrate for too long without blinking or without looking up or away: the tear liquid dries up and the lenses then irritate the eyes.

Normal sight line

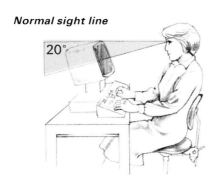

Pay attention to line of sight and posture.

The Fluoride Question

As fluoridation is now a *fait accompli* in the UK, a discussion of the pro's and cons is irrelevant, even though the matter is still controversial.

Find out if your water supply has been treated by contacting your Water Authority. If it is, you are getting quite enough. Indeed some people — those whose work makes them sweat a lot and consequently take in more water than the average — may be getting more than they need.

Cleaning your teeth

Before you clean your teeth with a brush, remove food particles from between them with dental floss. Break off a long piece of floss and slide it between each tooth as shown. Never use a wooden toothpick as it may splinter or break off.

Unbelievably, many commercial toothpastes contain sugar (!) so make sure you buy a sugar-free version from a health shop. Otherwise salt or bicarbonate of soda work just as well.

It is not necessary to clean your teeth in any particular way (up and down, side to side etc) as long as you do it *long enough*. Three minutes (use an eggtimer) is what it takes.

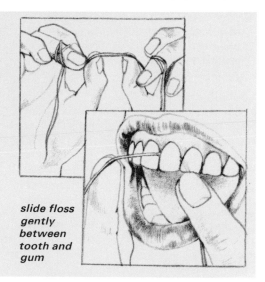

slide floss gently between tooth and gum

it will eat their way into your teeth. Hard plaque also irritates the gums which may become infected. Shock yourself by using a disclosing tablet to see just how much plaque (it's colourless) there is on your teeth.

There have recently been questions raised about the possible risk of mercury amalgam fillings and the toxic and allergic reactions which reputedly occur when the fillings start to break down. Generalized symptoms of fatigue, loss of muscle strength and neuritis (inflammation of the nerves) have all been attributed to this problem. In some cases these symptoms have disappeared after the removal of the mercury fillings.

Feet

Comfortable shoes and attention to hygiene are the best ways of ensuring healthy feet. Uncomfortable, poorly fitting shoes can cause foot problems such as bunions and corns (see A–Z) and will also adversely affect posture, leaving you fatigued and with the evidence of discomfort showing upon your face.

What to wear:
- wool or cotton socks; cotton, wool or silk stockings or tights. Avoid synthetics as they cause the feet to sweat, thus increasing the likelihood of **fungal infections** and athlete's foot.
- shoes with properly constructed innards and preferably flat or with a low heel.
- nothing at all, whenever you can, especially around the house. This allows your feet to breathe and the muscles to work to the full.

What not to wear:
- high heels as a matter of habit, as they cause the weight to be thrown forward. The lumbar lordosis consequently becomes exaggerated (see A–Z). High heels also cause the toes to be compressed because your weight is thrown down to the front of the shoe. Additionally, they cause the muscles and tendons at the back of the ankle to contract, which reduces the mobility of the ankle.
- Fashion trainers; they are the worst innovation in the context of foot care that one could imagine. They cause the feet to sweat profusely and they offer no arch support, which means the arches will eventually drop. Normally, the arches act as a shock absorber, taking the weight of the body as the foot touches the ground, but once the arches are dropped, the back takes the full impact. Good sports shoes are excellent for the purpose for which they were designed, but there is no such thing as a general purpose sports shoe.

● pop socks and hold-up stockings as they hamper the circulation and lead to aching feet and legs. They also can lead to varicose veins and oedema (see A–Z for both).

Looking after your feet.
Wash your feet at least once a day with warm water and mild, not medicated or perfumed soap. Dry carefully between the toes to avoid athlete's foot. If you have the common problem of sweaty feet, wash them morning and evening and use foot powder. Remove rough skin with a pumice stone and massage in a foot cream if you have dry skin.

Keep your toenails short, cutting them straight across with nail clippers, not scissors. Do not clip down the sides of the nail as this causes ingrowing toenails. Keep the clippers clean by wiping with disinfectant and drying after use. Wipe with disinfectant again before use.

If you wear proper shoes and look after your feet, you should not be bothered by corns or bunions. However, do not hesitate to consult a chiropodist if you have painful feet or ingrowing toenails, as these can often cause you to alter your posture which may lead to back pain.

Happy Feet

These simple exercises will help keep your feet in trim. Take shoes and socks/tights off and:
● pick up pencils with your toes (you can do this while reading or sewing).
● put feet out in front of you and loop a wide elastic band across both big toes. Start with feet together, then gradually turn them to a 10 to 2 position, stretching the elastic band. Do this about 20–30 times. This exercises the big toe joint to prevent the onset of bunions (see A–Z).
● take an old fashioned waisted glass bottle (cola bottle is ideal) and lay it at right angles to your foot. (Do this exercise on a rug or towel, never a slippery floor). Lean on the back of an upright chair, put your toes on the bottle and your heel on the ground. Roll your foot across the bottle so your toes are on the ground and your heel on the bottle. Roll back and forth 10 times. This exercises the longitudinal arch of the foot.

Now turn the bottle parallel with your foot. Place your whole foot on the bottle and roll it from side to side. This exercises the lateral foot muscles and ankle joint.

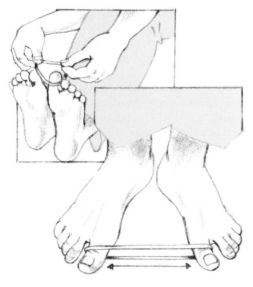

elastic band exercise

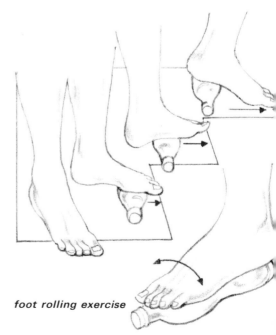

foot rolling exercise

THE BACK PACK
A back maintenance programme

The human back was originally designed to enable us to walk on all fours, and for that purpose it is admirably constructed. However, since we adopted an upright posture many thousands of years ago, we have been having problems with our backs. We have a combination of normal curves in the spine, to increase its supportive strength, flexibility and mobility. When these curves become exaggerated, as a result of poor posture, backpain results.

Backache and back injuries account for more days off work than any other cause. Backache may be psychological, in response to emotional stress, but more frequently it is the result of poor postural habits and the failure to treat our backs with respect when bending to pick up something, lifting, carrying or doing the gardening, housework and decorating.

Putting your back into it

Much of this back trouble is totally avoidable, and you can do a great deal to help yourself avoid it. Follow the five guidelines to healthy back maintenance below and the backbuilding exercises illustrated, and you may never know the misery and inconvenience of an aching back.

How the back works

The spine, running from the base of the skull to the pelvis, is made up of 24 small bones or vertebrae which are separated by spongy discs to allow free movement and to absorb shock as the weight of our bodies comes into contact with something — such as the ground, when walking, for example. As the spinal cord gives rise to many individual nerves, which connect the brain with other parts of the body, a healthy back and spine are essential for the efficient functioning of the body's nervous system.

The spine is a column of 24 bones (*vertebrae*) stacked one on top of the other, and it is divided into three main sections. The *cervical* spine consists of the seven vertebrae that support the head. The *dorsal*, or *thoracic*, spine makes up the middle section of the back and contains 12 vertebrae. The *lumbar* spine, or lower back, contains the largest and strongest vertebrae, of which there are five. The whole column is supported on the *sacrum*, a large triangular bone: attached to the sacrum is the *coccyx*, which is all that remains of your tail.

Sandwiched between each pair of vertebrae is the intervertebral disc. The spinal cord passes through a central opening in each of the vertebrae. Between each pair of these is a small opening, or foramen, through which pass the spinal nerves, supplying the rest of the body. The whole structure is supported by ligaments and muscles.

Standing Tall

Posture is a subconscious concept. We do not think about the muscles we use to maintain it or what they are doing from minute to minute. Why don't you fall over when you raise one arm to the side? Why don't you pitch face down in the dirt when you bend to weed your garden? How can you stand on one leg? All these are made possible by the 'synergistic' contraction and relaxation of your postural muscles— you do not know a thing about it.

Unfortunately we develop bad postural habits very quickly and easily. They are more difficult to eradicate than to acquire. The best way to stand tall is the old-fashioned deportment trick: practise standing and walking with a book on your head (and a solid, heavy one at that). Pushing up against a heavy balanced weight realigns the body and helps to flatten out exaggerated curves in the neck as well as the lower back.

Correct posture makes you look better, which will make you feel better. It can also help considerably with most minor aches and pains in the back. Check your current position with the pointers below.

Head: keep this lifted upwards as if you were suspended on a string.

Chin: hold at right angles to your throat.

Ribs: lift upwards, pulling in the stomach and opening the chest to breathe freely.

Pelvis: keep centred and balanced; avoid tilting the pelvis down in front, poking

GUIDELINES FOR HEALTHY BACK MAINTENANCE

1 **Make good posture** second nature to you, whatever you are doing: standing, sitting, lying down or walking.

2 **Learn (and use) the correct techniques** for:
—bending
—stretching
—lifting
—performing regular household tasks such as (bedmaking, bath cleaning)
—moving furniture
—using tools develop a proper rhythm; it should be smooth and flowing, not jerky with staccato movements)
—decorating
—gardening
—driving
—unloading and loading a car

3 **Use well-designed furniture** to support your back. This means:
● avoiding squashy sofas and soft beds, neither of which can support your back. Be sure to take as much trouble and time selecting your child's bed as your own.
● making sure that work surfaces are at the correct height. These include tables, desks, kitchen surfaces, ironing boards; your child's desk at school; and your office desk or work station.
● asking hotels for a bedboard in advance of your stay, to be sure of proper support.

4 **Plan jobs** so that you do not work at any one thing, such as decorating or weeding the garden, for example, that places unaccustomed stress upon your back for too long a period. When you are gardening, do 15 minutes weeding, 15 minutes pruning and 15 minutes digging. If you dig for one hour, you will probably end the day with backache and the osteopath.

5 **Wear correctly fitting shoes** that are properly constructed and see that your children do as well.

Postural Chairs
Multi-positional postural seating should be standard furniture in every workplace. This type of seating maintains ideal posture and adjusts to suit different functions.

the abdomen forward—a common fault in many women and in men with a paunch.

Knees: keep relaxed and not stiff.

Neck: lengthen the back of the neck. This will happen naturally if you hold your chin and shoulders correctly.

Shoulders: keep them balanced directly above the hips and pull them down from the ears. Slouched shoulders are a very common postural fault, producing a rounded spine and inhibiting breathing. Another common fault is to pull shoulders too far back, making the chin jut out and producing tension in the upper back.

Arms: let them hang loosely and naturally at your sides.

Spine: stretch the whole of the spine upwards. If you hold your pelvis and shoulders correctly, this should happen naturally.

Feet: keep your weight balanced evenly between the heels and balls of the feet.

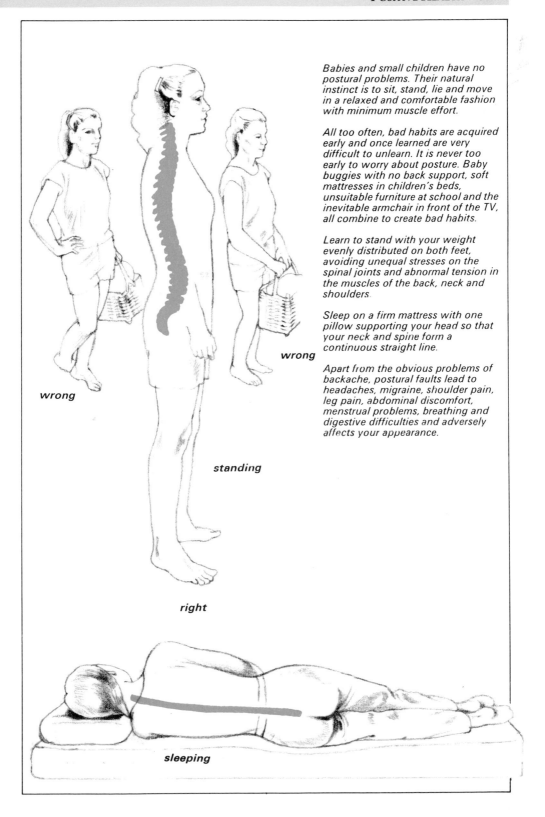

wrong

wrong

standing

right

sleeping

Babies and small children have no postural problems. Their natural instinct is to sit, stand, lie and move in a relaxed and comfortable fashion with minimum muscle effort.

All too often, bad habits are acquired early and once learned are very difficult to unlearn. It is never too early to worry about posture. Baby buggies with no back support, soft mattresses in children's beds, unsuitable furniture at school and the inevitable armchair in front of the TV, all combine to create bad habits.

Learn to stand with your weight evenly distributed on both feet, avoiding unequal stresses on the spinal joints and abnormal tension in the muscles of the back, neck and shoulders.

Sleep on a firm mattress with one pillow supporting your head so that your neck and spine form a continuous straight line.

Apart from the obvious problems of backache, postural faults lead to headaches, migraine, shoulder pain, leg pain, abdominal discomfort, menstrual problems, breathing and digestive difficulties and adversely affects your appearance.

All natural daily activities involve using the spine. Apart from gradual damage as a result of misuse, most people suffering acute attacks of back pain got them as a result of simple everyday activities such as making the bed, cleaning the bath, doing the ironing. Those simple tasks, if performed incorrectly, continue bending and twisting movements which place enormous stress in the lower spinal joints. Train yourself to protect you back at all times as illustrated on these pages.

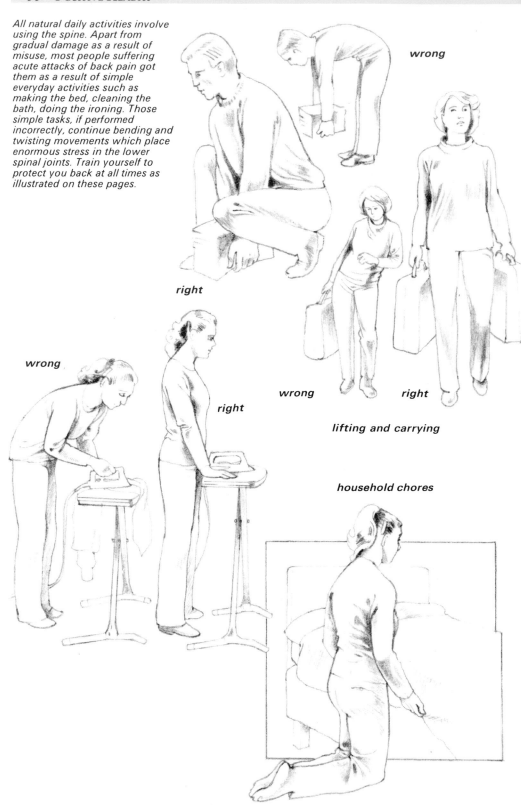

wrong

right

wrong

right

wrong

right

lifting and carrying

household chores

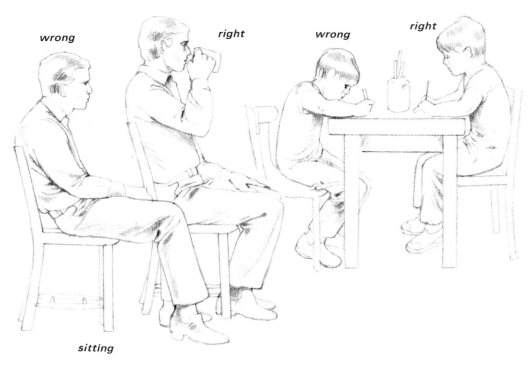

wrong   right   wrong   right

sitting

Children learn most things by imitation, including posture. The best way to teach good posture is by example. If you slouch at the table and slump in your armchair, so will your children.

Back seat driving

The price of your car does not always reflect the quality of its seats. In the excitement of choosing a gleaming new machine most people think about the colour, the power, the economy, the sunroof, but seldom take sufficient care when trying the driving seat. This is not so important if the car's main use is a twice weekly trip to the supermarket, but for those whose driving forms a large part of their working life, the seat is the most important factor. It must adjust to suit your body shape and height. It must support your back in a comfortable and safe driving position It must support your thighs. It must give lateral support and the head restraint must have forward and backward movement as well as up and down.

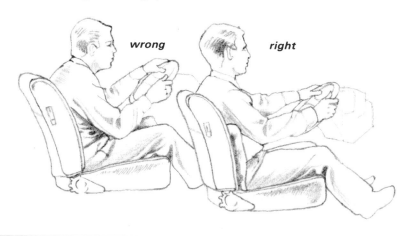

wrong   right

Basic Back Building

These four exercises will help to develop a strength and mobility in your back. They are also useful for getting muscles working before starting an exercise routine or taking up a sport. Sufferers from severe back pain will find that these exercises can help relieve the pain of acute episodes.

lumbar flexion

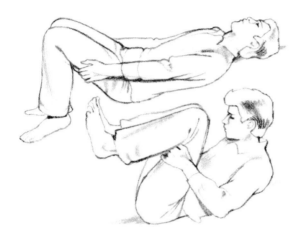

Low Back Stretch

The following stretching exercises are designed to lengthen both muscles and ligaments, thereby breaking into the cycle and changing the established behavioural patterns of the tissues. Before starting the exercises, you may find that the application of ice packs (frozen peas are ideal), gentle heat or the alternate use of both will induce relaxation of the tissues. This usually makes the movements much easier and relieves acute pain.

Lumbar Flexion This uses the legs as a lever to flex the lower part of the back. This exercise should be done on the floor or a really firm surface.

Lie flat on your back with a small cushion under your head, knees bent and feet flat on the floor. Place your hands behind the thigh just below the knees; using your arm muscles, pull your knees up to your chest and raise your head. Your pelvis must be raised off the floor. When you reach the limit of movement and comfort hold the position for 15 seconds, then try to increase flexion gently. Do this in progressive steps for 1 minute.

After the exercise it is essential to lower

pelvic tilt

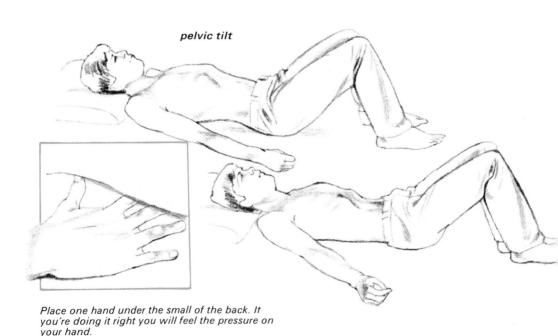

Place one hand under the small of the back. If you're doing it right you will feel the pressure on your hand.

one leg at a time slowly in order to maintain the gain in flexion and avoid the possibility of pain.

Side Bending Stand with feet 45 cm/18 in apart. With slow, deliberate easy movement, bend to the left 5 times, sliding your arm down your thigh. Hold each bend for 5 seconds. Follow by 5 bends to the right.

As you find the bends easier, bend the knee on the side to which you are moving. This increases the stretch imposed on the spinal muscles. Do not allow your trunk to bend either forward or backward.

Tuck your Tail In

Buttocks that stick out cause an excessive lumbar curve that distorts the entire spinal posture; it creates pressure on the rear part of the lower spinal joints squeezing the discs and nerves and encouraging permanent changes in the muscle and ligament tension of the whole back structure.

Learning to tuck in your tail means constant repetition of the exercises and concentration on your posture during all your waking hours.

The Pelvic Tilt: This is suitable for all types of back pain, even acute disc pressure. Lie flat on your back with both knees bent and feet flat on the floor. Place a small pillow under your head. Press the small of your back down to the floor, flattening the curve of your lumbar spine. Practise by placing one hand on the floor under your back and then feeling the downward pressure on the hand as you contract your abdominal and buttock muscles at the same time. If you get it right you will feel a squeezing sensation in the hips and thighs.

Flatten your back, raise the pelvis, hold for 10 seconds; relax the pelvis but keep the back flat; rest for 5 seconds; raise the pelvis and hold for 10 seconds. Repeat 10 times.

Once you have mastered the knack of flattening your back, move on to raising your buttocks from the floor. Do not lift your back from the ground; use your abdominal and thigh muscles in this movement.

When you have stages one and two under control, start gradually straight-

standing tail tuck

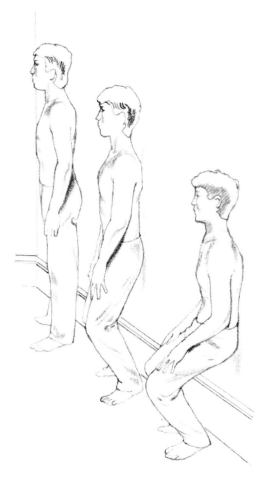

As well as helping to retrain your posture this exercise develops the thigh muscles and is a favourite with skiers.

ening your legs until you can perform the exercise easily with both legs straight out in front of you. This prepares you for the next exercise.

Standing Tail Tuck: Stand with your feet 15–22 cm/6–9 in away from a wall. Press the small of your back against the wall. Slowly move your buttocks off the wall, keeping your lower back in constant contact with it. Now practise slow knee bends, keeping your low back firmly pressed to the wall and your tail tucked in.

THE HEALTHY CHILD

As long as your child is well nourished, well exercised and well loved, you should not hover constantly over them expecting illness. Acquaint yourself with what is normal behaviour and achievements for their age group to avoid any unnecessary worry.

Children vary greatly in what are known as the neurological milestones (movement, understanding, speech), but there are nevertheless identifiable stages of development which should be noted at the time that they occur. The sequence of development is the same in all children but the rate may be different. If you have any worries about your child's development, you should ask your GP to refer you to a pediatrician.

The patterns of growth in children, both weight and height, vary perhaps even more than the neurological milestones: not only do they vary from boys to girls but individual variation is great as well. Girls generally grow quicker and attain maturation more quickly. The child's weight and height growth patterns are a useful guide to the child's general state of health and, although variation is the norm, it is nevertheless true that certain diseases affect growth. If you have any worries about your child's physical development, you should insist that your local medical practitioner refer you to a specialist. Although growth rates vary, there is both an upper and a lower limit beyond which growth is abnormal. The sooner any growth problems are detected, the more effective any treatment is likely to be.

Do not be fobbed off with platitudes from your local practitioner. Specialists would rather see 20 children who are normal than see one with abnormal growth, too late to be helped.

For more information on individual children's diseases, see the A–Z section; for healthy nutrition in childhood, see **Nutrition** pp. 14–15.

DRUGS, SMOKING AND ALCOHOL
DRUG TAKING AND ADDICTION

The consumption of illegal drugs appears to be on the increase and the age at which these drugs are taken is getting earlier. It is no good thinking that it couldn't happen to you or your child or a member of your family. Learn all you can about the signs and behaviour patterns of a person taking drugs and don't hesitate to get help as soon as you think you see such signs. Remember, it's not just illegal drugs that can cause problems.

What are the signs of drug-taking?

It's difficult to tell when someone is using drugs only occasionally—unless they are caught in the act, or when intoxicated (like being drunk). But here are some of the things you may notice:

- Sudden changes of mood from cheerful and alert to sullen and moody.
- Unexpected irritability or aggression, combined with secrecy about movements.
- Lost appetite.
- Losing interest in hobbies, sport, schoolwork or friends.
- Bouts of drowsiness or sleeplessness.
- Telling lies or behaving furtively.

Of course, in an adolescent these could just be signs of normal growing pains—particularly those higher up on the list. So don't jump to conclusions. The following are more serious indications:

- Money or belongings disappearing.
- Unusual smells, stains or marks on the body or clothes, or around the house.
- Unusual powders, tablets, capsules, scorched tinfoil or (more rarely nowadays) needles or syringes.
- A chemical smell on the breath or unexplained traces of glue or other solvents found either on the body or on clothes.
- A sudden unexplained interest in glue, nail varnish or other solvent-based products.
- Unusual soreness or redness around the mouth, nose or eyes.
- Persistent, irritable cough.
- Slurred speech.

● A sudden and uncharacteristic decline in school performance possibly combined with the start of truancy.

What if drugs are taken?

Don't over-react and take it out on your son or daughter before you know all the facts — or you could make a small problem bigger.

First, take time to talk to your husband or wife, or perhaps your family doctor, other parents or teachers. Try to find out if your youngster has any other worries or problems.

Above all, show them that you care and will give them all the support and help you can — even if they are in trouble with the law. See **Addictions** in A–Z section for more information.

SMOKING

Unlike an occasional glass of wine or half a pint of beer, even the occasional cigarette is bad for you. Every time you smoke one cigarette, you shorten your life' by five minutes. In Britain alone smoking accounts for the death of 100,000 people every year. Lung cancer is an extremely unpleasant and painful way to die and chronic bronchitis does not just mean a persistent cough: you'll be on oxygen supply at home to help you breathe, you'll be very ill every winter, you'll need help to cope with daily life and you'll probably hardly ever leave the house.

Lung cancer, heart disease, chronic bronchitis and emphysema (see A–Z) are the chief smoking-related diseases but smoking is responsible for a lot more, such as:

● cancer of the mouth and throat, gum disease.
● ulcers.
● diarrhoea.
● cancer of the bowel from excreted carcinogens.
● angina.

What's in a cigarette?

Tobacco smoke contains nicotine, carbon monoxide, carcinogens and irritant substances, and traces of other gases with unknown effects. Nicotine in small doses stimulates but in large doses, as in regular and heavy smokers, it acts as a depressant. Carbon monoxide combines with up to 15 per cent of the body's haemoglobin (converting it to carboxyhaemoglobin) and so prevents it from transporting oxygen around the body. This increases the risk of heart attack. Carbon monoxide also leads to the development of cholesterol deposits in artery walls, which, in turn, causes heart attacks and strokes. One of the chemicals that smoke contains is hydrogen cyanide which inflames the lining of the bronchi and thus puts smokers at risk from bronchitis.

Three facts that smokers do not want to know:
● smokers lose 10 to 15 years of their lives on average.
● forty per cent of heavy smokers die before they reach retirement (only 15 per cent of non-smokers die this young).
● ninety per cent of all those who die from lung cancer and chronic bronchitis are smokers.

Tobacco kills four times as many people as the total killed by drink, drugs, murder, suicide, road accidents, rail accidents, air accidents, poisoning, drowning, fires, falls, snake bites, lightning and every other cause of accidental death all put together.

Because nicotine makes the heart pump faster, it has to work harder, thus increasing the likelihood of heart disease. Additionally, nicotine can cause palpitations and a generalized feeling of anxiety, despite the fact that smokers claim it allays anxiety. The positive effects, which are almost immediate but rapidly decline, that makes smokers want to continue smoking are the stimulant effect and the fact that smoking aids concentration. However, since it increases anxiety, any gain in stimulation and increased concentration is immediately lost. Additionally, the fact that any positive effect declines rapidly makes the smoker want to smoke all the more, thus creating an addiction.

SO WHO SMOKES?

The British government's figure for smokers in Britain is now 18 million. One in four of all adolescents have started to smoke by the time they leave school. Children of parents who smoke are much more likely to become smokers themselves. In one survey, 22 per cent of children who smoked said that they had their first cigarette with their parents. More men than women smoke, but many more men are giving up than women. Some pregnant women still smoke, even though they know that their babies may have low birthweights, that their babies will have a one-third greater perinatal mortality rate in the first month of life than those of non-smokers and that, provided the baby does survive, it will have a greater chance of respiratory and lung problems than that of the non-smoker.

Passive smoking

Although you may be a non-smoker yourself, you may still be at risk. A cigarette produces two sorts of smoke:
- mainstream smoke, which is filtered by the cigarette and inhaled by the smoker.
- sidestream smoke, which goes directly into the air. This is not filtered and therefore contains high concentrations of many of the substances that make smoking harmful.

If you are regularly exposed to sidestream smoke you may have a decreased lung function as severe as that found in light smokers. You may also have indications of small airways obstructions. Your blood carboxyhaemoglobin levels may rise and you will be at increased risk of lung cancer.

Children are also affected by sidestream smoke. Children who live in smoking households have decreased lung function and small airways obstruction. They are more likely to have serious chest illnesses such as pneumonia and bronchitis and to be susceptible to general upper respiratory tract infections and middle ear infections.

'I DON'T SMOKE, THANKS'

If you are well and truly addicted to smoking, this is the hardest thing to say. 'I don't smoke' has to become an attitude of mind: there is no shortcut to giving up smoking and the most powerful weapon in your armoury is your own willpower. Once you have decided that it's dirty, unhealthy, inconsiderate, anti-social and outmoded, you'll be some of the way there.

Britain's Health Education Council recognizes four stages in giving up:
1. Thinking about your reasons for stopping
2. Preparing to stop
3. Stopping
4. Staying stopped

The reasons for stopping are now well-known and described above.

Preparing to stop means getting rid of any secret stores of cigarettes and your lighter, washing the ashtrays and giving them away. Then arrange to do things, particularly in the first few weeks, which prevent you from smoking — take up swimming and other sports, see non-smoking friends, go to the theatre, open a deposit account into which you pay the money that you would have spent on smoking. Get friends and family to sponsor you. Make an agreement with another smoker to stop smoking. Decide on the day.

Above all, practise: start cutting down. Reduce the number of cigarettes you smoke every day. Start smoking later each day: there is evidence to show that the earlier in the day you smoke, the greater the *frequency* of smoking will be during that day. Gradually ban the rooms in which you allow yourself to smoke, starting with the bathroom, kitchen, bedroom. Practise giving up by not smoking at all for a few hours when you are out with friends. Allow yourself to run out of cigarettes now and again. Don't ever buy more than one pack at a time.

Stopping On the day you stop, arrange to do lots of things that you enjoy. Drink fruit juice for breakfast — the taste is fresh and the acidity will help get rid of the nicotine. Plan treats for yourself. Don't just sit there wanting a cigarette: get up and do something, even if it's only the washing-up. Take up something for which you'll need your hands all the time, such as knitting, gardening, carpentry, re-decorating.

Staying stopped is difficult, particularly if you have been a heavy smoker. You'll be used to a regular supply of nicotine — from 100 to 400 puffs every day — and your body will demand its regular drug. You may feel depressed, irritable, impatient and anxious. You may get sto-mach cramps, headache, an unpleasant taste in your mouth (but you had that anyway) and an increased tendency to cough with more phlegm being produced (but that's a good sign — before, you were congested). Some people do not experience these withdrawal symptoms from the drug at all, but if you do, they will last only a few weeks in any case.

'I can't imagine giving up'
If you really want to give up, you will. You may find it helpful, however, to use some form of support, such as:
- acupuncture.
- hypnotherapy.
- a stop smoking group, based on the same principles as Weight Watchers and Alcoholics' Anonymous (ask your doctor or naturopath if there is one in your area).
- aversion therapy (in which you might be forced to smoke 60 cigarettes, non-stop, and be shown X ray pictures of lungs diseased by cancer and blackened by tar).
- substitutes, such as nicotine chewing gum. Don't, however, turn to chewing tobacco, an alternative now being promoted in the United States, as it is a serious cause of mouth cancer and just as difficult to give up.

Whether you try any or all of these, wanting to is your strongest ally. In the end, if your motivation is high enough, you'll succeed in beating the addiction to nicotine, rather than letting it beat you.

DRINKING AND ALCOHOLISM
A little of what you fancy.... There is some evidence that moderate drinking (a daily glass of wine or the equivalent) does indeed do you good, warding off high blood pressure and heart disease (alcohol combats cholesterol in the blood). All too often, unfortunately, the limit is exceeded and what was a pleasure becomes a pain for you and your family and friends.

Who drinks?
Nine out of ten people drink to some extent. Men on average drink the equi-valent of $1\frac{1}{2}$ pints of beer or 3 glasses of wine each day, while women drink about $\frac{1}{2}$ pint of beer or 1 glass of wine a day— on average. Less than 1 in 20 of us con-sistently exceeds what is regarded medi-cally as 'safe'.

Young adults drink 40 to 50 per cent above the average adult population and about one-third of children between 13 and 16 drink at least once a week.

Knowing your Limit
Heavy drinking is defined as 5–7 pints of beer a day or 10 to 14 glasses of wine (2 standard bottles) a day for men and $3\frac{1}{2}$ to 5 pints of beer or 7–10 glasses of wine (1 litre bottle) for women.

There is no need to cut out alcohol totally (unless on doctor's advice). The sensible limit is 2 to 3 pints of beer or 4 to 6 glasses of wine for men and 1–$1\frac{1}{2}$ pints of beer or 2–3 glasses of wine for women two or three times a week.

That may not sound much, but alcohol is dangerous in large quantities.

Are you drinking too much?
You probably know already if you or someone close to you is drinking too much. Your emotional reactions may become exaggerated and erratic. Your physical reactions will probably by clumsy and slow. You probably won't be able

to think clearly. Hangovers will become commonplace and you may feel more or less depressed all the time. Regular long term heavy drinking increases the drinker's chance of suffering lasting impairment of physical and mental functioning, including liver disease, ulcers, heart and circulatory disorders and brain damage. Accidents and cirrhosis of the liver are particular hazards for the alcoholic. Impaired memory is one of the obvious signs of brain damage and this is irreversible: your chances of holding down your job are slight if you have no memory capability. You won't be able to remember what you *have* done, what you're *meant* to do, nor the reasons for decisions.

Know your own strength
- Extra strength lagers (where all the sugar turns to alcohol) are almost three times as strong as ordinary beer.
- A glass of wine is as strong as a single whisky.
- A pint of beer is as strong as a double whisky.

Why can men drink more than women?
Between 55 and 65 per cent of a man's body weight is made up of water, but, only 45 to 55 per cent in women. Alcohol is distributed around the body through the body's fluids, so in men the alcohol is more diluted. Also, women absorb or take up the alcohol more 'efficiently' and therefore their liver is more likely to suffer alcohol damage than a man's.

Can you ever drink and drive?
If you intend to drive you should not drink alcohol at all. It takes the body one hour to work off the alcohol from one standard drink (glass of wine, half pint of beer, measure of spirits). And the legal limit is 80 milligrams of alcohol to 100 millilitres of blood. Drinking and driving should be regarded as mutually exclusive activities. However, if absolutely necessary, most men can manage if they have drunk one pint of beer (or two glasses of wine) and most women on half that amount.

Cutting Down
If you have checked with the CAGE questions you may think you need to cut down. Another factor to remember is that alcohol delivers lots of calories; those watching their weight can cut 180 calories off their intake for every pint of beer they refuse. Pregnant women should avoid all alcohol if possible.

Getting out of the CAGE
Doctors use a set of four questions in taking a medical history to detect those why may have a significant drinking problem:
- Have you ever felt you ought to *cut* down on your drinking?
- Have people *annoyed* you by criticising your drinking?
- Have you ever felt bad or *guilty* about your drinking?
- Have you ever had a drink first thing in the morning to steady your nerves or get rid of a hangover (an *eye-opener*)? The questions can be remembered by the mnemonic CAGE from the first letters of **C**ut, **A**nnoyed, **G**uilty, **E**ye-opener. Anyone who answers yes to two or more questions is likely to have a significant drinking problem.

If you are a heavy drinker or think you have a problem and want to cut down, or even out, consult your medical practitioner, to discuss the idea of joining a self help group, such as Alcoholics Anonymous.

There are other methods of self help.
- Don't keep drink in the house.
- Don't go out more than once or twice a week until your drinking is under control.
- Push back the time you start drinking by one hour every week.
- Keep a drinker's diary to see how well you are doing.
- Do something else instead—take up an exercise or sport to fill the times when you would be drinking (you'll be surprised how revitalized you feel)
- Give yourself rewards — new record, new shoes, extra hour in bed.
- Don't succumb to pressure; 'one more for the road' may be your downfall. Remember, you're in charge.

PART II

THE MAJOR NATURAL THERAPIES

Not so long ago all unorthodox treatments were thought of as fringe medicine. The purpose of this book is to introduce to the uninitiated reader a selection of those natural therapies that are more widely accepted by orthodox medicine and to give to those who already have an interest a more detailed knowledge of the therapies and how they can be used, both by practitioners and by people themselves.

There are many other therapies of value but these are still considered 'beyond the fringe' in most scientific circles.

Modern trends, happily, are moving towards closer cooperation and it is with practitioners of the therapies in this book that the medical profession is building bridges. It cannot be long before these bridges are completed, allowing greater collaboration between the disciplines.

ACUPUNCTURE

Something like half the world's population is treated by acupuncture—in China, Vietnam, Japan, the Philippines, Korea, Singapore, Malaya and Sri Lanka. In China, all doctors who study western medicine are required to study traditional medicine before they are allowed to start practising. The traditional Chinese system has been used for thousands of years; it is based principally on acupuncture but also uses herbal remedies, good nutrition, exercise (in the forms of T'ai Chi and the martial arts), specialized forms of massage, manipulation and moxibustion (see below).

In traditional Chinese medicine, it is believed an energy called *Chi* flows through our bodies. No-one can deny that we all have energy: without it we would not be living. Chinese traditionalists believe that *Chi* enters the body in at least three ways:

● into the developing foetus as inherited energy derived from the father's sperm and the mother's ovum
● after birth, from food
● from air taken in by the lungs

Chi flows through the body in a series of vertical pathways, known as meridians, each of which passes through a major organ which gives the meridian its name. The meridians are not related to the body's nervous system. They comprise an independent autonomous system which has no identifiable link with the central nervous system. Tributaries and cross channels link the meridians to each other so that all organs and tissues have access to *Chi*. The acupuncturist locates certain key points on the body, at which he or she can insert small, sterile needles which will have direct access to the required meridian. The acupuncture points are located not always on the organ or part of the body which requires treating, but on the meridian with

which it connects. That is why it is perfectly normal to treat a liver complaint, for example, with needles inserted in the foot.

The traditional Chinese doctor or acupuncturist will make a diagnosis, firmly based on the holistic approach, in four stages:

● **Observing** the colour and texture of skin and the tongue; noting blemishes such as pimples, warts or moles, and any swellings or other irregularities.
● **Listening** to the patient's breathing, any creaking of joints, and the quality of the patient's voice which can reveal much about their emotional frame of mind as well as their physical state.
● **Asking** the patient how their

Meridians
Acupuncture points are distributed over the body surface along precise lines known as meridians, each of which relate to a specific organ or function.

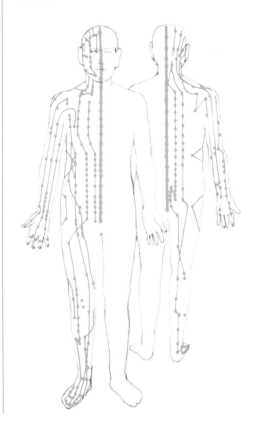

complaint relates to events in their life: shock, stress, climate, time of day, month or year and even phases of the moon.

● **Palpating,** examining by touch as orthodox western doctors do. The traditional Chinese doctor also takes a total of 12 pulses, six at each wrist. Ten of these pulses relate to major organs of the body, the remaining two to functions.

Six of the pulses relate to Yin organs and six to Yang organs.

Traditionally, the surface of the body is yin or yang as shown here. The ancient symbol for yin and yang reflects the true nature of Chinese philosophy which aims at balance — a little positive in the negative, a little male in the female, a little dark in the light, a little light in the dark.

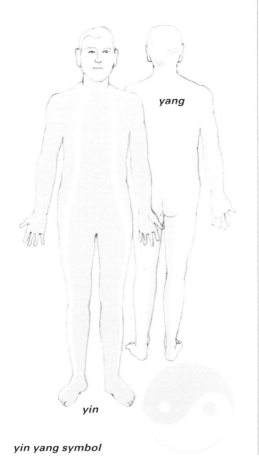

yang

yin

yin yang symbol

YIN AND YANG

Yin and Yang are regarded as the body's life forces, between which there is a constant movement of energy. This movement is the activating force behind *Chi* or energy. Yin and Yang can be thought of, roughly, as opposites, male and female or positive and negative; they are each complex entities, however, with their own set of characteristics.

When Yin and Yang are in perfect balance, the body is healthy. When either one or the other is disrupted, the balance is upset and diseases and ailments result. The traditional Chinese doctor or acupuncturist seeks to determine the state of their patient's Yin and Yang and their balance in relation to one another. The flow of *Chi* can be obstructed by a number of factors in the patient's lifestyle, almost all of which can be easily remedied once observed:

● poor nutrition
● lack of exercise
● bad posture
● shallow breathing
● pollution
● insufficient rest and sleep
● extremes of climate
● poor response to stress and pressure
● inability to cope with the negative emotions of grief, anger and fear
● mechanical obstructions such as tumours, scar tissue

RESTRICTING THE FLOW

Health is regarded as a measure of the freedom of flow of *Chi* and the balance of Yin and Yang. Ill health is seen as a reflection of the fact that *Chi* is prevented from circulating freely and therefore unable to nourish and protect the body. The flow of *Chi* is seen to be disturbed in three different general ways:

● **When it is insufficient** and cannot flow freely. This may manifest itself as chronic fatigue or deep depression, or in a physical complaint such as oedema (fluid retention, notably around the ankle joints).
● **When there is a deviation** in the flow, so that there is a deficiency in one pathway or meridian, or area of the body, with a corresponding excess in

another. Many common ailments fall in this category, from frozen shoulder and sciatica to constipation and painful menstruation.

● **When an excess** of *Chi* builds up and assumes an explosive character. This is what is believed to occur in hypertension, migraine and acute arthritis, for example

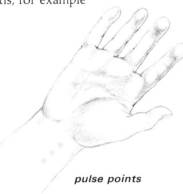

pulse points

Chinese pulses
In each wrist there are 3 superficial and 3 deep pulses. Each of these 12 pulses relates to a meridian.

RESTORING THE FLOW

The touchstone of traditional Chinese medicine is concerned with restoring the flow of *Chi* and thus the balance of Yin and Yang. The flow of *Chi* is thought to be restored either by instilling energy into the body in the form of heat (to tonify) or by dispersing pent-up energy (to sedate):

Moxibustion

This method of instilling energy into the body to correct deficiencies of the flow of *Chi* is used as an adjunct to acupuncture. The needles are inserted at the appropriate acupuncture points in the normal way and the heads of the needles are then heated by wrapping dried moxa (the mugwort herb, *Artemisia vulgaris*) around the head of the needle and burning it. The burning moxa generates a moderate heat which is taken down the needle into the acupuncture point. Cones of smouldering moxa may also be used directly over the skin at the acupuncture points and removed when the heat becomes uncomfortable.

this is done by inserting sterile needles at the intersections of the relevant pathways or meridians. Sometimes the needles just penetrate the skin; in other cases they are inserted to a depth of several centimetres. The energy is drawn into the body by the acupuncturist rotating the needle rapidly between finger and thumb. The process is virtually always painless and the most that may be felt is a slight sensation, as if a pin just touched the surface of the skin, and possibly a sensation (described variously by those who experience it) when the needle reaches the energy.

Sessions usually take from half an hour to an hour and a course of sessions is usually recommended. Only the very lucky experience the spectacular success of a cure in just one treatment.

HOW CAN IT HELP?

It has long been established in China and other parts of the Far East that acupuncture is an effective anaesthetic—or, more correctly, an analgesic (pain reliever) which allows it to be used during surgery or childbirth. It has been shown that stimulating the specific acupuncture points for analgesia releases chemicals in the brain known as endorphins (closely related to morphine), which are the body's own natural painkillers.

Acupuncture is particularly helpful in relieving pain, and treating any disease or ailment that can be reversed. (Cancer, for example, cannot be treated if it has already been recognized as irreversible.) It is commonly used to treat asthma, eczema, tension headache, arthritis and to correct the action of organs that are functioning sluggishly, the liver, for example. In 1979, the World Health Organisation listed some 40 diseases that could be successfully treated with acupuncture, including breathing problems, digestive problems (such as stomach cramps and ulcers), disorders of the nervous system (such as tinnitus and migraine) and painful menstruation. It is also effective when used in combination with another treatment: back pain, for example, can be treated by an osteopath to manipulate and realign and an acupuncturist to relieve pain.

ACUPUNCTURE AND ADDICTIONS

There is no magic short cut to giving up smoking or alcohol, getting off any of the illegal drugs, or eliminating dependence on prescribed drugs such as tranquillizers and sleeping tablets. It is hard work. However, acupuncture can relieve some of the symptoms experienced in nicotine withdrawal, for example, such as stomach cramps and poor concentration. Acupuncture treatment reduces the level of withdrawal symptoms from any drug by interfering with the transfer of messages from the subconscious mind. Of all the addictions, smoking is felt to be the most manageable. The acupuncturist can monitor the success rate because it is easy to tell if someone has been smoking or not. Treating alcoholics and drug addicts is considerably more difficult. The key to curing any addiction is high motivation on the part of the sufferer.

ACUPUNCTURE AND THE RISK OF AIDS AND INFECTIOUS HEPATITIS

As with all skin piercing treatment (ear-piercing, tattooing etc) great care must be taken to avoid these serious diseases. Many acupuncturists now uses pre-sterilized disposable needles. Before accepting any acupuncture treatment, ask to see the needles, and make sure they are still in sealed packs. If your acupuncturist does not use these, he should have a proper autoclave (sterilizing machine). Boiling

water, hot ovens and glass bead sterilizers do not provide a sufficient degree of sterilization.

THE ALEXANDER TECHNIQUE

The Alexander Technique is a process of physical re-training that has far-reaching positive effects on both mental and physical health.

The human body is a complex, delicately balanced piece of engineering. Muscles and bones are designed to interact harmoniously in such a way as to enable us to walk and move with maximum ease and minimum strain. All of us are born with a natural ability to use our bodies the way they were intended: but from a very young age most people start to misuse them, developing mannerisms that throw the whole body out of true: slouching at the desk at school; stiffening unnaturally straight for gym. Constant repetition makes these bad physical habits feel 'right' and we lose our inborn instinct to return to correct, healthy posture. The result of misuse is a malfunctioning of our whole system. The Alexander Technique aims to help you relearn the correct way to use your body by substituting a set of positive habits for the bad ones, so that gradually you become aware of your body's misuse and are able to correct it by returning to a better use of self.

HOW IT WORKS

The Alexander teacher conveys the technique by gently realigning and manipulating the student's body. As he or she works they will repeat certain key phrases, such as 'neck free, to allow the head forward and up, back to lengthen and widen'. Through repetition the student comes to recognize the feeling of correct use, and connects this with the corresponding phrases, or 'directions'. In everyday life

Acupressure

Traditionally, every Chinese father knew the secrets of acupuncture first aid or acupressure. This is the application of pressure to certain acupuncture points for the relief of minor health problems such as headache, stomach ache, nosebleed, fainting. Pressure is applied with the finger or, in the case of children, a small blunt-ended instrument such as the cap of a ballpoint pen. It is distinguished from acupuncture by the fact that no needles or other equipment are used. The A–Z section contains guidelines for do-it-yourself acupressure for the relief of certain conditions.

they will soon be able to feel when they are slipping into bad use, and 'come back to their directions'. The key is the relationship between the head, neck and back. The head is very heavy, so needs to be properly balanced. Thrown back or tipped too far forward—the two most common misuses—the muscles of the neck strain to hold this heavy object, creating tension, and limiting the 'free' movement of the head. The spine, too, is often contracted or thrown out of shape by misuse which means it is impossible to use the rest of the body correctly.

The Alexander teacher also concentrates on correcting *endgaining*—the common habit of striving too hard to do something so that you tense your muscles at the very thought of what you have to do. You might, for example, grip a pen too tightly. It is comparable with the energy and force you expend when you pick up an empty suitcase, thinking it is full. Learning to inhibit this instinctive reaction allows you correct control.

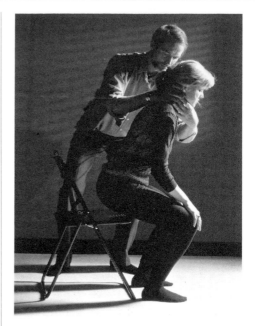

Everybody sits down and stands up many times each day. Learning to do this with the minimum of effort saves wasted energy.

ALEXANDER LESSONS

Alexander lessons are given on a one-to-one basis. Because your own ingrained habits have come to feel so comfortable, it is impossible to correct them yourself: the theory is not enough to convey the technique. The teacher shows by gentle manipulation and the explanatory 'directions' how proper use should feel. The adjustments are small and subtle. There is no wrenching or forceful realigning. As some wrongly used muscles must learn to lengthen, and other under-used muscles must start to work, the technique coaxes rather than pushes to allow the body to come into a more balanced position.

Teachers apply the technique in their own ways. But each teacher's method hardly varies from lesson to lesson. The student is shown correct use in the basic positions of sitting, standing and lying down. The technique of getting in and out of a chair is included in each lesson, because it is something we do many times each day—and it demonstrates our misuse in movement. The repetition of exactly the same movements and positions in each lesson serve to create the necessary new habits and awareness.

The hardest thing for a student to learn initially is not to interfere, 'non-doing'. When the teacher lifts your arm or guides you into a sitting position, it is automatic to give some help with your own muscular effort. Learning to inhibit these unconscious muscular movements is an important first step towards correct conscious control. But all students report an extraordinary feeling once the teacher has moved them into the perfect balanced position. There is a general feeling of wellbeing, a lightness and an exhilaration.

Each lesson lasts for half to three-quarters of an hour. It is usually recommended that new students have lessons three times a week for the first few weeks; after that, once a week is enough. An average of 30 lessons is considered sufficient to re-educate yourself to the point where you can carry it on into daily life, though some people choose to continue for many years, returning periodically for reminders.

DOING IT YOURSELF

Although you cannot learn the technique without a teacher/student relationship, the

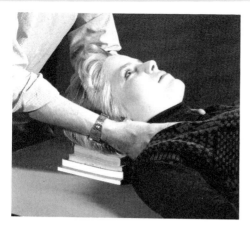

The head, neck, trunk relationship is the key to good posture.

HEALING

Healing by 'the laying on of hands' has been practised for centuries with or without the support of the Church or the approval of the orthodox medical establishment. Until as recently as 1977 doctors in Britain who cooperated with healers risked being struck off. In the USA, despite the fact that it is here that the greatest professional application of healing has been initiated, healing remains technically illegal in most states unless the healer is a church minister. Many American practitioners therefore have to purchase a certificate conferring upon them this status.

whole aim of the teaching is to enable you to carry out the technique in your everyday life. Some teachers recommend that you practise the 'lying down' as you have been taught, for 15 minutes or so a day. This position, following your directions, with your head slightly raised by a book, and your knees bent, puts your spine in its correct, lengthened position.

How Can It Help?
The Alexander Technique has a beneficial effect on any number of physical problems, including hypertension, asthma, peptic ulcers, spastic colon, ulcerated colitis, rheumatoid arthritis, tension headaches and low back pain. The positive health benefits in improved performance are recognized by athletes and major drama and music colleges, which have resident Alexander teachers. (Alexander was himself an actor.)

The technique has a positive effect on the general functioning of the body especially the circulation of the blood and breathing. It is enormously beneficial in dealing with stress. Muscle tension is fed back to the brain as feelings of stress and panic. Relaxation techniques usually only help for the period that they are being used, whereas the Alexander awareness will enable you to recognize whenever a muscle in any part of your body tenses up, and therefore to release it and prevent stress build-up.

The Therapeutic Touch
'In the United States of America healing remains technically illegal in most states, unless you are a church minister. Dr Dolores Krieger, a Professor of Nursing at New York University until her recent retirement, presented a course for nurses as a part of their formal training. Entitled "The Therapeutic Touch", it was essentially a euphemism for the outlawed practice of healing. She had discovered that healing not only helped patients mentally and physically but that it could also be scientifically quantified. Tests showed that nurses trained in this simple "laying on of hands" brought about improvements in haemoglobin levels in their patients, which did not occur in patients who had not received healing.

Professor Normal Shealy, Clinical Associate of Neurosurgery at the Universities of Wisconsin and Minnesota, has been using healers and psychics at his Pain Rehabilitation Centre. In a four-year period over 1,000 patients were treated at his clinic: 90 per cent were off drugs when they left, while 80 per cent had some 50 to 100 per cent pain relief at the end of his programme. It would be good for medical students to participate in healing conferences where they can see the laying-on-of-hands.'

The Church appears to feel that it has a monopoly on healing, and that all healers should be Christian. It disapproves of healing outside the Church environment.

Some healers do believe that their power comes directly from God and that they are simply the medium. These are known as faith healers, spirit healers, spiritual healers or spiritualist healers. Secular healers believe that their energy comes from within themselves and that, motivated by a profound and powerful desire to heal they are able to communicate this restorative energy to the patient. These are known simply as healers or hand healers.

All healers work by laying their hands, sometimes over the affected area, sometimes not. They often experience a sensation of heat and so, too, does the patient. All healers believe that they are transferring into the patient an energy in the form of heat. This energy is believed to correct the disharmony in the patient's body that their disability reflects.

That some sort of transference between healer and patient does appear to take place was demonstrated by Maxwell Cade (see **Biofeedback,** p. 97) in London in the 1970s. Using an electroencephalographic brainwave monitor, he found that the brainwave patterns of both healer and patient altered simultaneously as the healer started to concentrate.

Matthew Manning, an internationally respected healer, demonstrated, in scientifically controlled laboratory conditions, between 1977 and 1982 that he could 'heal' cervical cancer cells which had been grown in plastic flasks. The conditions of their culture made it easy to measure the number of dead or injured cells. After healing the number of injured or dead cells increased by anything from 200 to 1200 per cent. The experiment was repeated 30 times in the United States and subsequently over several successful trials at the University of London.

Matthew Manning describes his beliefs about healing and his work.
'Healing has for countless decades been inextricably entwined with religious ceremony. Yet healing remains the most natural therapy in the world. Take the small child who trips and stumbles over a kerb and grazes a knee. As the child cries, a caring mother will gently place her hands on the painfully scraped wound.

"I'm going to count to ten, and the pain will be gone." And it has. The mother is also a healer. That is how simple it is. For years healing has been handicapped with its familiar prefix of "faith". For a long time healing remained within the domain of the Church and it was always believed that if it was unsuccessful it was because the recipient did not have sufficient faith in God. It has been thought, too, that the patient needs faith for the healing to work and so the image of healing has been inextricably associated with religious ceremony.'

'The "faith" healing label is misleading for two reasons. Firstly, you don't actually need any faith! I treat people who come to me believing that I am the only person who will be able to help them. What better act of faith in a healer could one ask for? Yet, sadly, I cannot always help them. Surely, if my results were based on faith alone, all would respond? Secondly, I also treat patients with little or no faith in me at all: they probably seek me out when all else has failed.'

'I expect my patients to be prepared to help themselves rather than relying solely on me. When prospective patients learn this, about 40 per cent do not want to know any more, which prompts me to believe that a large proportion of the public still view my role as that of a miracle-worker. Whereas previously the healer closed his eyes and placed his hands on the patient, many healers now encourage patients to take some initiative rather than completely abdicate responsibility to others, as we normally do when treated by a medical practitioner. Neither a doctor nor I can magically remove a patient from a stressful job, relationship or environment any of which may lead to migraine, angina, high blood pressure, back pain or ulcers for example. The medical solution has been to prescribe tranquillizers or sedatives, which mask the symptoms efficiently but fail to deal with the cause.'

'As a first step I make my patients familiar with a variety of relaxation methods: these include breathing exercises, yoga, mental imagery and even laughter. Relaxation does not mean sitting in front of the television or sleeping. It is a positive skill which has to be learnt and practised regularly to achieve its effect upon mind and body. A short period of relaxation has been shown to lower blood pressure, slow down the heart rate, overcome fatigue and improve concentration, as well as relieving a variety of common symptoms which may be due to tension, such as backache and headache.'

'I encourage my patients to investigate the element of emotional contribution to their illness. I find, for example, that many of my adult cancer patients have experienced the loss of a stabilizing influence in their life six to 18 months before their disease was noticed. This loss can be that of a spouse, due to death, divorce or separation, of a job or even moving from one area of the country to another. I would not suggest that everyone who experiences such a loss becomes ill, but rather that we have a choice as to how we adapt to the situation in which we find ourselves. The person who responds to such a loss with feelings of complete and utter despair is most at risk.'

'Finally, I teach my patients to use what I call visualization or mental imagery. Typically, I ask them to visualize their white blood cells, the body's defence system, being active and powerful as they overcome the disease. Some patients find it helpful merely to talk to their body and "instruct" or "order" it to get better. One young patient who had tumours on various nerve endings throughout her body imagined the tumours as slices of cheese and her white blood cells as white mice that several times each day devoured the cheese.'

'Such ideas certainly seem alien to some of the people I treat when they first seek my help, and orthodoxy has for a long time been sceptical. I suspect that eventually these ideas will become absorbed into mainstream medicine as with the teaching of relaxation now.'

'When I work, I start by placing my hands upon the patient's shoulders which helps me to gain an "attunement", after which I experience considerable heat and tingling in my hands which is often also felt by the patient. Research, in which I have participated as a subject, suggests that this sense of "attunement" to which healers refer is not entirely subjective: the brainwave patterns between myself and my patient have been found to become synchronized to within one tenth of a second. Where I place my hands may superficially have little or nothing to do with the precise location of the problem but, like an acupuncturist, I feel that I work more on some form of "energy grid" throughout the patient's body.'

'As with some of the other complementary therapies, healing can sometimes cause an adverse reaction before any appreciable benefit is noticed. Occasionally cancer patients with whom I have been working experience nausea, vomiting, bouts of diarrhoea, or profuse sweating within 48 hours of my treatment. This usually lasts for just a few hours and is followed by feelings of well-being and a reduction in pain levels. Since about 30 per cent of the body's toxins are excreted through the skin, it seems logical that feverish sweating may be experienced. Typically, however, there are four possible responses to healing.'

'The first is that I cannot effect an improvement. If after two or three sessions there is still no improvement, I advise the patient to seek the help of another healer as I know that I often get results where another healer has not and vice versa.'

'The second possibility is that an improvement occurs but the problem to some degree remains. An arthritic joint may be free of pain and inflammation but movement is still restricted.'

'The third possibility usually occurs with patients suffering from diseases which affect the nervous system, for example, multiple sclerosis. The patient gets no better but gets no worse either. This at least is preferable to a continuing degeneration.'

'Finally, there is the hope that healing will be completely effective in eliminating the problem. This, however, is dependent on three crucial factors: the awareness that healing is rarely miraculous but rather a slower process; the understanding that the patient must also make some contribution with their own self-healing efforts, where necessary or possible; and, lastly, the attitude of the patient for this is where all healing starts. Healing, probably like any other therapy, tends not to be very successful with people who do not possess some *inner desire to get better. In the end, attitude is most important which is why much of my work is devoted to teaching self-help.'*

There is no governing body to which all healers belong or are trained. The closest we get is the National Federation of Spiritual Healers, set up by the great healer Harry Edwards (1893–1976), who was almost single-handedly responsible for gaining medical and perhaps legal respectability for healing. However, although many healing practitioners have been trained to a certain level of proficiency and professionalism by the NFSH, a good many have not. Paradoxically, most of the better known healers are not NFSH members. The best way to find a responsible and helpful healer is first by recommendation and, secondly, by their possible NFSH membership. The disadvantage to the patient with our present legal status is the number of unscrupulous practitioners who do immense damage by suggesting that the patient give up other therapies, relinquish essential drugs or surgery, or who make phony "diagnoses" and then claim they alone can help the patient.

HERBALISM

It may surprise you to discover that the origins of modern medicine, with its heavy reliance on drug prescription to treat specific diseases, lie in herbalism. Just as the medical herbalist has at his or her disposal a large number of drugs from plant and plant material, so has today's conventional allopathic doctor. A surprising proportion of the drugs that today's doctors prescribe are little different from those handed out in the 19th century, and some of the best modern drugs are purified products of herbs.

PLANT POWER
Some very well-known drugs have been refined from plants and are in worldwide use: digitoxin from the foxglove (*Digitalis purpurea*) and digoxin from the closely related *D. lanata* are both used as a cardiotonic and to treat heart failure; atropine from deadly nightshade (*Atropa belladonna*) is used to dilate the pupil (in eye surgery, for example); morphine from the opium poppy (*Papaver somniferum*) as a powerful painkiller; quinine from *Cinchona officinalis* to treat malaria; and perhaps best known of all, aspirin. Aspirin was originally synthesized from the salicylic acid of the white willow (*salix alba*). It should be added in this context that some of the more dangerous modern drugs are not derived from herbs or plants but are manufactured synthetics, such as Valium and sleeping tablets, for example, and it is these that tend to cause the most side-effects.

HOW SAFE ARE PLANTS?
Herbal treatments have been in use for thousands of years. Herbal remedies have been passed down the generations, first by word of mouth and then in illustrated herbals: their drug trials, therefore, have been carried out on previous populations. With today's drugs, new products have to be used in trials first on animals, then on human volunteers, and finally on the market. It is not all that rare for a so-called wonder drug to be withdrawn comparatively quickly after its release because of unsuspected side-effects. Certainly, there are plants which are poisonous or which cause undesirable side-effects, but the herbalist has very extensive trials and records at his or her disposal enabling them to prescribe safely. So, while herbalists are able to prescribe drugs with no harmful side-effects, it may be that their drugs are not as powerful as those of the allopathic doctor.

THE WHOLE STORY
The crucial differences between medical herbalists and today's orthodox doctor is, firstly, that the herbalist looks at the patient as a whole, while conventional doctors look for symptoms which enable them to diagnose and treat diseases. They

see the patient as a disease carrier, whereas the herbalist regards them as a diseased person, requiring a holistic treatment.

Secondly, the medical herbalist is using whole plants or plant products containing active constituents, while doctors use these constituents in refined and isolated forms or synthetics.

Herbal medicine involves use of the whole plant, the combination of all its constituents, which work together in natural harmony to exert specific therapeutic effects on the body. Any plant contains a number of constituents which may contain alkaloids, glycosides, tannins, gums, resins, trace minerals, essential oils, antibiotic substances and hormone precursors. Each of these has a function and may reinforce, support or control the action of the others. Herbal practitioners are strongly opposed to the principle of isolating one constituent, knowing from experience that the gentle action of their remedies is effective, safe and in harmony with the body's therapeutic needs.

PLANT INTERACTION

One constituent of the same plant may either negate a potential undesirable side-effect of another of that plant's constituents or can potentiate the effect of a third constituent (a process known as *synergism*). This makes it desirable, herbalists believe, to use whole plants rather than only the active substances. Furthermore, and this is what is essentially the skill of medical herbalism, plants can interact with *each other* to produce either a different, better or worse remedy.

Several different plant extracts may be contained in one preparation with the intention that each will produce its specific effect to accomplish a beneficial combined effect. Herbal combination therapy, which is clearly complex, is the rule rather than the exception for medical herbalists and that is why you should seek a reputable practitioner.

HERBAL RENASCENCE

The resurgence of interest in herbalism today has taken place partly in response to an increasing demand for natural foods, natural remedies and a growing distrust of synthetics in all fields, and partly as a result of the increased scientific research in plants themselves. There are an estimated 750,000 species in the world, and while only a small percentage has been evaluated so far, this area of research is continuing. The World Health Organisation, in its quest to provide adequate medical care for all by the year 2000, is investigating and supporting traditional herbal medicines in third world countries. Studies are being carried out into the traditional herbs used in these countries and people are being encouraged to share knowledge and to undertake training. China is also directing further research into herbal medicine.

NATURAL REMEDIES

The regular use of herb teas and tisanes to replace coffee, tea and other social drinks, in cooking, and in the early stages of illness, do much to promote good health. A simple infusion of elderflower (*Sambucus nigra*) and peppermint (*Mentha x piperita*) taken hot in the first hours of a cold or influenza has been found to disperse the infection quickly. If combined with garlic capsules taken each night during the winter, recurrent colds and catarrh, with their potential complications—such as bronchitis—become something of the past.

Modern stresses of life are responsible for a tremendous increase in nervous problems, such as depression, anxiety and insomnia—and a resultant dependence on tranquillizers and sleeping tablets. There are many herbal nervines which have a gentle sedative action on the nervous system, such as scullcap (*Scutellaria lateriflora*), valerian (*Valeriana officinalis*), vervain (*Verbena officinalis*) and balm (*Melissa officinalis*). These can be taken regularly or occasionally without the hazard of withdrawal symptoms. Stress-related disorders can also be treated with Bach remedies, created by Dr Edward Bach who practised from the 1910s until his death in 1936. These are plant tinctures given in homeopathic dosages (see *Homeopathy* p. 76) to treat negative moods and states of mind.

Hypertension and angina, both often stress-related, can respond to herbal treatments. Neither are suitable conditions for self-treatment, but it does help to take tisanes of lime blossom (*Tilia cordata*) or chamomile flowers (*Chamaemelum nobile*) in place of coffee and tea, which are both stimulants. They will also reinforce hypotensive remedies intended to help lower the blood pressure.

An extensive range of herbs is available to treat migraine, but the causes should be assessed before specific remedies are taken. The herbal remedy which has gained the most popular renown recently is feverfew (*Chrysanthemum parthenium*), recommended over 400 years ago for vertigo and used today for certain types of migraine and for various other conditions.

HOW DOES THE HERBALIST WORK?
A medical herbalist initially takes a careful history from the patient, using orthodox methods of diagnosis. The practitioner will investigate the patient's diet and lifestyle, assessing the integrity of the body's systems, looking for any imbalance and disharmony, seeking always the cause of illness, and regarding the patient as a whole person and treating him or her accordingly. Treatment will consist of an individual prescription of herbal remedies, and will include guidance on nutrition.

Practitioners with the letters FNIMH or MNIMH are members of the National Institute of Medical Herbalists, and have had to reach a high standard of knowledge and training to pass the entrance examination. Founded in 1864, the NIMH is the oldest organization of its kind in the world, and endeavours to maintain the highest professional standards. Members of its research department contributed to producing the *British Herbal Pharmacopoea*, a definitive work on the medicinal plants used in Britain.

Students of the School of Herbal Medicine and Phytotherapy undergo an intensive course of training, at the end of which the successful student may sit the examination set by the NIMH for membership.

The Herbalist's Vocabulary
Many of the descriptions of herbal treatments are the same as those used by conventional doctors: for example, antispasmodic, expectorant, diuretic, emetic, stimulant. Some, however, are used only rarely by other types of practitioners:

- **carminative**—relieves flatulence and colic
- **cholagogue**—helps or stimulates the release of bile from the gallbladder
- **demulcent**—soothing substance for the skin
- **emmenagogue**—stimulates menstruation
- **emollient**—used internally to soothe membranes or on the skin to soften
- **nervine**—calming
- **vulnerary**—used to treat and heal wounds

Alternative names for herbalism that you may come across are eclectic medicine, plant healing, physiomedicalism, medical herbalism, botanic medicine and phytotherapy.

HOMEOPATHY

Homeopathy means, literally, 'like disease'. It is a system of medicine in which the sufferer is treated with a very small dose of medication that would bring on the symptoms of the disease if taken by a healthy person. This is by no means a new-fangled notion. The foundations of homeopathy were probably known since the time of Hippocrates, and the 16th-century physician Paracelsus selected his remedies on a similar basis. However, homeopathy as we know it today dates from the late 18th century and the work of German physician Samuel Hahnemann (1755–1843).

THE HOMEOPATHIC PRINCIPLE
It was in the late 1780s when Samuel Hahnemann gave up his medical career in

disgust at the practices of his profession, such as bleeding and purging, which just weakened the patient. He turned to translation for a living; while working on a herbal textbook by Cullen of Edinburgh, he came across the statement that quinine was good for malaria because it was a powerful astringent. Realizing that this was not the whole story, as stronger astringents than quinine were available, Hahnemann determined to find out why quinine was better by trying it ('proving' it) on himself.

For several days Hahnemann took a dose of quinine producing some of the symptoms of malaria in himself (although there were obviously no bugs). When he stopped taking quinine, the symptoms disappeared. Hahnemann formulated the theory that the symptoms of malaria were not, in fact, those of the disease but those of the body's *resistance* to malaria. The symptoms, therefore, would best be encouraged rather than suppressed, in order to help the body fight the disease. Hahnemann reasoned that quinine was good for malaria precisely because it was capable of producing in a healthy person similar symptoms to those produced in a patient suffering from malaria: in other words, quinine could imitate and thus supplement the body's fighting mechanism for malaria.

To test his theory, Hahnemann experimented on his family and friends and then tried further drugs and poisons of plant and mineral origin for other conditions. He came to the conclusion that like will cure like—*similia similibus curantur*.

POTENTIZATION

When Hahnemann began treating people with his new system of medicine, he quickly found that they often got worse before they got better. He attributed this to the sudden switching on of the Vital Force or healing power in the body, a bit like the dust which flies up in a long deserted room when it is first cleaned by a broom. In an attempt to overcome this, Hahnemann started to dilute his remedies more and more until there was very little of the original substance left. He then

found that their effect was too reduced to be beneficial. To correct this, Hahnemann shook each successive dilution of the remedy vigorously (a technique known as *succussion*). This process of dilution and succusion he called *potentization* for, to his surprise, the less there was the quicker and better the remedy worked.

Hahnemann had discovered a way of maximizing the potential of a remedy to its fullest effect, not by increasing its strength but by appreciating its optimum potency. He believed that this potentization made the remedies capable of working on the subtle, energetic level in the body where true healing comes from, rather than working on the physical body. One of the scales that Hahnemann used to express the potency of a remedy was a scale of 1 in 100 (the centessimal scale): a 1c potency would mean that the solution contained one part of the remedy and 99 parts diluent (usually alcohol).

THE MATERIA MEDICA

Hahnemann built up his pictures of the effects of substances on the human body from toxicology (the orthodox study of poisons of plant and mineral) and from his provings. In 1811, 21 years after his discovery of the nature of the true benefit of quinine in cases of malaria, Hahnemann published the *Homeopathic Materia Medica*, from which several fundamental principles emerged:

- homeopathic treatment stimulates the body's own auto-immune system into action to provide a cure
- that cure can be effected only by the body, not the substance
- if the body is sensitive to the particular substance that is being used as a treatment then only small dosages are required
- the appropriate remedy is the one that produces in a healthy person the symptoms of the disease.

The pictures Hahnemann recorded have been added to by later homeopaths to give us the modern *materia medica* (the remedy pictures) and the repertoires in which the remedies are listed by symptoms, so that the homeopath can treat patients with any disorder, as doctors do, rather than a limited range as some of the alternative therapies do.

HOMEOPATHY V. ALLOPATHY

The medical profession has been at pains to protect its territory from encroachment by homeopaths despite the existence of sound scientific evidence to show that homeopathy treatment can be effective. Doctors and other scientists maintain that the remedies are so far diluted that they cannot possibly have any effect: however work carried out in the late 1970s, in the Glasgow Homeopathic Hospital substantiated the claims for homeopathic treatment, and the tests were carried out on stringently scientific lines with double-blind trials (in which patients are split into two groups with one group being given the treatment and the other placebo medication, with neither patients nor medical supervisors being allowed to know which group is which until the trials are complete).

Despite the cynicism shown by the medical establishment for homeopathy since its inception, one aspect of it has been accepted and taken up by conventional medicine and that is immunology. It has long been accepted that a healthy person injected with a certain virus (or bacteria)—such as that for measles (or tetanus), for example—will develop, with the help of the body's auto-immune system, the antibodies to effect an immunity to the disease. This is the basis for all vaccination and inoculation; and it is very close to the basis of homeopathy, except that homeopathy uses *similar* not *identical* substances to effect a cure.

HOW DOES THE HOMEOPATH WORK?

What can you expect when you consult a homeopathic physician? In addition to the usual examinations and questions any doctor might ask regarding your problem, you will be asked in detail about the factors that you may have already noticed which make your problem better or worse, including the time of day, the seasons, the

weather, and a hot or cold atmosphere. You will also be asked general questions about yourself such as the sort of weather you feel best in, which foods you enjoy or dislike, how you feel generally.

From your answers the homeopath will build up a picture (the symptoms or disease picture) and will match this against the picture of the remedies (the drug picture) and prescribe the remedy whose *total* picture most closely matches the picture of your problem. High potency remedies (200c and above) are usually given when the picture is very clear, or the problem is acute, or if it is felt that the problem is of a general nature rather than local; low potencies (30c and below) are given when the problem appears to be of a local nature with little general disturbance to the body.

CHOOSING A HOMEOPATH

Most homeopaths are doctors who have trained in orthodox medicine and then undergone a further training in homeopathy. In recent years, however, some homeopaths have trained only in homeopathy.

The best way to find a good homeopathic doctor is either by personal recommendation or through a professional association; in Britain, for example, the **British Homeopathic Association.**

HOMEOPATHIC REMEDIES

Homeopathic remedies can be bought from homeopathic and some orthodox chemists and from many health food shops, but 30c potencies and above are more difficult to obtain.

The remedies are available in a variety of forms from tablets, powders and granules to tinctures and ointments. Their potency is commonly graded to a centessimal scale and the usual potencies found in shops are 6c or 30c. 1c signifies 1 part potency to 99 parts dilutent (usually alcohol). A 2c potency is obtained by diluting 1 drop of a 1c dilution with 99 parts of alcohol and then succussing. A 6c potency, therefore, is that process repeated six times, the solution being succussed at each stage.

Dosage is indicated in 'doses' which can mean any of the following:

- 1 or 2 pilules
- 1 tablet
- 1 powder
- enough granules to cover the bottom of the cap of a 7 gm bottle
- 5 drops of liquid

Biochemic Tissue Salts

Homeopaths, as well as naturopaths, herbalists and other practitioners in holistic medicine, prescribe tissue salts when they believe that minerals or 'tissue salts' are not being formed in the body in sufficient quantity for health.

The 12 biochemic tissue salts were introduced by Dr Wilhelm Schuessler of Germany in the late 19th century. He believed that disease processes were always due to the deficiency of certain inorganic substances and that if these were replaced in a minute form, the body would heal the disease by itself.

We now know that Schuessler's dosages were far too small to be effective, but it has been proved that the tissue salts are very beneficial both in acute and in chronic cases. They may act not so much as a nutritional supplement but rather on the controlling mechanisms that govern how much of a substance is taken into the body or excreted from the body or the way in which it is distributed through the body. If someone is iron-deficient, for example, the bowel will absorb *more* iron than it would otherwise: evidently, there is a mechanism that stimulates the bowel to absorb more iron. The tissue salts may work in the same way: giving a message to the body to absorb more of a certain substance or to get rid of it if there is an excess. The main tissue salts and their functions are listed below.

1 CALC. FLUOR Calcium Fluoride
Maintains tissue elasticity.
Over-relaxed tissue, deficient enamel of teeth.

2 CALC. PHOS. Calcium Phosphate
Constituent of bones and teeth.
Indigestion, teething problems, chilblains.

3 CALC. SULPH. Calcium Sulphate
Blood constituent.
Pimples during adolescence, skin slow to heal, sore lips.

4 FERR. PHOS. Iron Phosphate
Minor respiratory disorders, blood stream oxygenation.
Coughs, cold symptoms, chills, feverishness, chestiness, in alternation with Kali Mur.

5 KALI MUR. Potassium Chloride
Minor respiratory disorders.
Coughs, cold symptoms, wheeziness and chestiness, in alternation with Ferr. Phos. Children's feverish colds.

6 KALI PHOS. Potassium Phosphate
Nerve soother.
Temporary nerviness, nervous headache or nervous indigestion due to worry or excitement.

7 KALI SULPH. Potassium Sulphate
Maintains skin condition.
Minor skin eruptions with scaling or sticky exudation. Brittle nails. Catarrh.

8 MAG. PHOS. Magnesium Phosphate
Soft tissue. Salt.
Cramp, flatulence, occasional minor pains.

9 NAT. MUR. Sodium Chloride
Distribution in body water.
Watery colds with flow of tears and runny nose, loss of smell or taste.

10 NAT. PHOS. Sodium Phosphate
Acid neutraliser.
Gastric indigestion, heartburn, rheumatic pain tendency.

11 NAT. SULPH. Sodium Sulphate
Body water balance.
Queasiness, digestive upsets, flu symptoms

12 SILICA Silicon Dioxide
Conditioner, cleanser.
Pimples or spots, brittle nails in alternation with Kali Sulph.

If the remedy you choose has not worked after the number of doses indicated, you should consult a homeopathic physician.

In acute situations the most appropriate remedy is given, up to every 15 minutes, in a 30c (if possible) potency for up to 6 doses. In less acute situations a 6c potency is given every 4 hours for up to 6 doses. In chronic cases a 6c potency is given three times daily for up to five days. Where the problem is mainly emotional or mental, the 30c is used.

The remedies are very delicate and should never be touched with the fingertips. Unless they are for external use, remedies must always be put on or under the tongue either 15 minutes before or 30 minutes after food, drink, or strong smelling substances. They should be sucked and not swallowed for at least two minutes. They do not interfere with any drugs your own doctor may wish to give you, and they do not have any side-effects providing you follow the above schedules, but they may sometimes aggravate symptoms. This aggravation rarely lasts longer than 24 to 48 hours.

Keep the remedies in a cool, dark place, in an airtight container away from strong smelling substances, such as mothballs, for instance. Don't drink coffee, real or decaffeinated, during homeopathic treatment.

HYPNOTHERAPY

Many of us talk and act as if our conscious mind were the most important part of us, running everything in our mind and body, making decisions and permitting us to do things. By contrast, the unconscious mind is often regarded as something fairly peripheral, doing rather vague things of which we are not aware. A moment's thought begins to make it clear that the opposite is true: the unconscious mind is constantly working, monitoring all the physical and psychological functions of the mind and the body, from blood pressure and hormone levels to states of hunger and fatigue, even when we are asleep. The conscious mind, on the other hand, only deals with the 'here and now', and indeed turns off when we are asleep.

The unconscious mind also copes with much of our memory of what has happened, remembering a very large proportion of our experiences—far more than we could remember consciously. Hypnosis is a method whereby the practitioner can speak to the unconscious mind directly, and can therefore communicate with that part of the mind that controls everything, from perception to memory. It is, essentially, a complex process of attentive retentive *concentration* with diminished awareness of surroundings.

Hypnosis is not really normal sleep: it is better to regard it as 'turning down the volume' of the conscious mind, so as to be able to gain direct access to the unconscious mind. With this sort of direct access, 'reality testing' is disconnected, and the distinction between the imaginary and the real disappears, so that the mind reacts to the imaginary (in other words, whatever is suggested to it) as if it were real. It can therefore be an extremely valuable tool in a programme of treatment, but it cannot be regarded as an end in itself.

HOW IT WORKS
Imagery produces responses in us in everyday life, and can affect our behaviour: and this is what the hypnosis practitioner uses, while making the imagery more powerful, more specific and more 'real' to the person being hypnotized. Adequate preparation is important, and the practitioner will spend some time discussing the problem that has driven the patient to seek help. He or she will then explain what will happen in hypnosis and take the patient into the first trance.

In the first stage of the trance, a rapport is established, with the patient becoming receptive to the practitioner's signals, such as concentrating upon an object or upon a spot on the ceiling, for example, to enter the full trance. (This sort of visual fixation tires the eyes and the conscious mind very quickly.)

The practitioner indicates the likely

mental and physical phenomena, such as drowsiness, that will be experienced. Provided that the patient is receptive, he or she starts to experience the mind and body effects predicted by the practitioner. The next stage of trance can be called the plunge, in which the patient more or less relinquishes their critical faculties and gives themself up to the practitioner.

Once in the trance, then things may be suggested to the patient that his conscious mind will remember. He can be taught quicker methods of going into a trance, so it is much easier in future sessions, and the level of trance can be made progressively deeper.

The patient may experience sensory changes such as paraesthesia (the sensation of pins and needles), analgesia, anaesthesia, partial amnesia and, after the treatment is over, compliance with simple signals that the practitioner will have arranged during the period of hypnosis, while the connection between reality and imagery is broken.

How Can It Help

Once this connection is broken, changes may be suggested to the patient. These can be things that will affect **behaviour,** such as: feeling more relaxed in stressful situations; losing the desire to eat excessively (or, for those with anorexia nervosa, encouraging a positive feeling towards eating more); or losing the need to smoke. Alternatively, they can be things which are **internal,** such as stopping pain, curing insomnia, soothing the discomfort of eczema, easing the stress of childbirth, or alleviating asthma and allergic conditions.

Hypnotherapy can also be used to modify the individual's **reactions** to the world, as in the treatment of depression, anxiety, fears or phobias. Indeed, some practitioners go so far as to say it can enhance significantly your performance in things like learning or sport. Certainly the effects are profound and real; even hypnotic anaesthesia is possible in highly hypnotizable patients, and operations and dental extractions have been carried out in this way.

One of the most positive features of

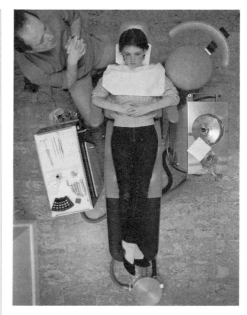

Many people cannot tolerate anaesthesia. Hypnosis provides an alternative and is widely used in dentistry.

hypnosis is that it is something done together; the practitioner cannot 'do it to you' without your full co-operation; indeed, it has been said that all hypnosis is in fact self-hypnosis, and the practitioner is really only a guide. Some people are more susceptible to hypnosis than others: those of a rigid or suspicious frame of mind will only succumb slowly, as the practitioner searches for appropriate techniques, while for those who cooperate, the process will naturally prove more swift and easy.

The Advantages of Hypnosis

The value of hypnotherapy lies in its ability to cut through the patient's verbal evasions or discussions, in which it could take hours to resolve a single issue, as it penetrates the unconscious and releases information which might otherwise be withheld.

The true hypnotherapist will not promote the instant cure—the stage hypnotist's domain—as they work, usually over four to five sessions, by altering ingrained patterns of thought and behaviour. A compulsive eater, therefore, is treated so that he or she not only eats less but deals with the fundamental issues that gave rise to overeating in the first place.

It is important that the therapist takes time with the patient, with the goal of altering these deeply ingrained patterns of thought: the smoker who enjoys smoking but who is addicted to the nicotine and would prefer to give up may be treated successfully and quickly. The smoker who uses the habit as an outlet for some deep-seated anxiety will probably need longer to deal not only with the habit itself but to confront the psychological component of the problem. If that problem is not dealt with, the patient could inadvertently discover a different outlet.

It has already been said that the unconscious remembers a great deal of our life experiences—possibly everything. Under hypnosis, we can find these memories, learning of experiences that have affected us in the past, and working through memories which may be repressed but which may yet still give us pain.

Lastly, hypnosis is a very pleasant experience; and it will teach you things about relaxation and coping with the world which will almost certainly be of wider application than the problem that originally made you seek treatment.

MANIPULATIVE THERAPIES

OSTEOPATHY

Osteopathy is a system of healing primarily concerned with the structure and correct alignment of the body and thus the body's function. The bones, joints, ligaments, tendons, muscles and general connective tissue, and, most importantly, their interrelationship, comprise the body's musculo-skeletal system. Many osteopaths believe that the body will keep healthy provided there are no structural defects, such as a displaced bone or vertebra, which can be corrected by manipulation. These musculo-skeletal

defects are thought to affect local nerves and, therefore, because the nervous system functions as a whole, defects will adversely affect the organs of the body, all of which are controlled by the nervous system. Once the defects are corrected, one can reasonably expect the benefits to be transmitted throughout the nervous system and thus to the organs of the body.

'It is necessary to know the spine and what it's natural purposes are, for such a knowledge will be requisite for many diseases.'

Hippocrates

WHAT IS OSTEOPATHY?

The term osteopathy was first used by its founder, Dr Andrew Taylor Still (1828–1912) of Missouri, in 1874. He believed that the human body was self healing and that an uninterrupted nerve and blood supply to all the tissues of the body was indispensable to their normal function. If any structural problems, such as curvature of the spine, interfered with this nerve and blood flow, the self-healing power was disrupted and disease would result. With this in mind, Still worked out a system of manipulation intended to realign any structural deviations or abnormalities.

Manipulation of the musculoskeletal structure has a long history. Until Still's time however, spinal manipulation was used solely to treat conditions of the back at least in western orthodox medicine. Still extended the use of manipulation to cover the treatment of the whole body, adopting many of those techniques that were valuable and rejecting those that were of no use or possibly even dangerous, to create a complete and practical therapy in which structure and function of the body are seen to be completely dependent on one another. In 1892, Still founded the first school of osteopathy, in Missouri. One of his students, John Martin Littlejohn, who had earlier studied physiology for three years at Glasgow, founded the British School of Osteopathy in 1917 a few years after his return from the United States.

How CAN IT HELP?

Most people who consult an osteopath

for the first time are usually suffering from back problems or pain and discomfort in other joints and muscles. It is not unusual, however, to find that after treatment for the main complaint, patients also report improvements in other conditions which they did not think suitable for osteopathic treatment. For example, the patient suffering from neck and shoulder pain and stiffness may find that manipulation of the vertebrae in the neck has also relieved dizziness or headache.

Modern research in American osteopathic hospitals has shown how abnormalities of the spinal column can affect organs such as the lungs, heart, stomach, intestines, bladder and uterus. It can also be demonstrated that these organs can affect the spine. Manipulation, therefore, can be shown to be of great value in the treatment of many conditions, especially migraine, asthma, constipation, menstrual pains, heart disease and digestive disorders.

Osteopaths do not consider the spine to be the only factor in the cause of disease; illness can be caused by genetic factors, dietary, environmental, psychological and bacterial influences. While osteopathic treatment may relieve some of the symptoms of these problems, it cannot claim to cure diseases of this nature.

How Does the Osteopath Work?

The osteopath examines the patient from the moment he/she enters the consulting room:

- How do they walk?
- How is their posture?
- How are their movements?
- Are they stiff and rigid?
- Are they bent at the waist?
- Is their back out of alignment?
- How do they sit in the chair?

All these things are vital clues to the origin of the patient's problem. Before an osteopath treats a patient for the first time, he or she takes a detailed medical history. This is followed by a complete physical examination in which the osteopath will examine posture and the way in which the patient moves, and will observe restrictions or exaggerations of movement in any area of the spine. Then a detailed examination of the spinal column follows, testing the movement of each vertebra, looking for tenderness, stiffness or displacement. Further tests, such as X-rays or blood or urine analysis may be recommended to help reach an accurate diagnosis.

Assuming that osteopathic treatment is appropriate to the condition and that there are no contra-indications to manipulative treatment, the osteopath sets out to improve the mobility of impaired joints, restoring function to those which are not working properly and relieving areas of pressure (which may be affecting those nerves supplying very distant parts of the body) by manipulating the patient's back, limbs, or other joints.

The osteopath may use techniques of manipulation, deep neuromuscular massage along the nerve routes, relaxation and postural re-education, all with the object of relieving the cause of the patient's condition. It is not uncommon for patients to suffer some form of reaction, such as the aggravation of existing symptoms or discomfort in the treated area, after the first one or two osteopathic treatments since the manipulative thrust which is used to readjust the spinal joint can sometimes irritate the surrounding tissues.

Patients often expect the osteopath not to be in favour of the use of drugs or surgery for the treatment of back problems and this in broad principle is true. There are situations, however, when anti-inflammatory drugs, preferably non-steroidal, or painkillers should be recommended for brief periods at times of acute pain. There are a few situations in which spinal surgery is inevitable but osteopaths believe that many people submit to it before exploring all the alternative possibilities of manipulative treatment. More and more orthopedic surgeons are recommending their patients to try osteopathic treatment, where other orthodox forms have failed, before resorting to it. This complementary use of the skills of the orthodox orthopedic surgeon and the osteopath is undoubtedly in the best interest of the patient and produces results which in some instances neither practitioner could achieve alone.

BACK MATTERS

It is the holistic approach taken by the osteopath that accounts for the high success rate in the treatment of back problems. Many patients who have suffered back problems for years have never had a thorough spinal examination. The visit to the osteopath is often the first time the back sufferer has been asked to take his clothes off. Yet it is quite impossible to arrive at any diagnosis of a back problem without examining the patient standing, sitting, lying and moving without clothes on, feeling the skin and muscle tone and establishing an understanding of the integrity of the underlying structures.

An osteopath looks at the patient as a whole entity. Although back pain may be the symptom with which the patient presents himself in the osteopath's surgery, the root cause of that pain can be far removed from the back itself. Simple problems with the feet, ankles, knees or hips can frequently result in back pain. Changing the height of the chair in which the patient works, altering the height of the bench in the factory or workshop or merely changing the type of shoes he wears can dramatically improve long-standing and chronic back problems.

Cranial Osteopathy

Cranial osteopathy is a specialized technique described as 'indirect' as no manipulative thrust is applied to any spinal joint. The cranial osteopath believes that the fine joints, or sutures, of the bones that form the skull allow tiny movements to occur between them. By stimulating this movement, the circulation of cerebro-spinal fluid is encouraged which may relieve local symptoms and also affect other organs such as the pituitary gland. This technique can be especially helpful in the treatment of children with learning difficulties and those with some forms of brain damage. Gentle, rhythmic pressure is applied to the head in order to encourage movement of the skull sutures.

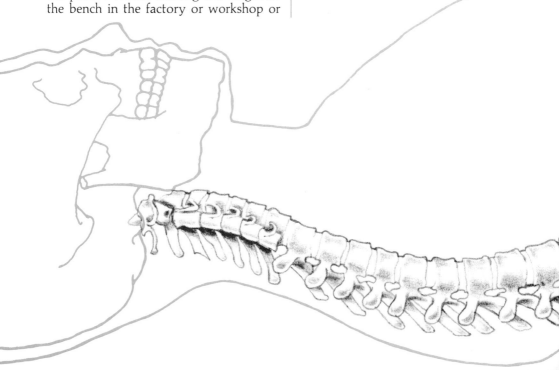

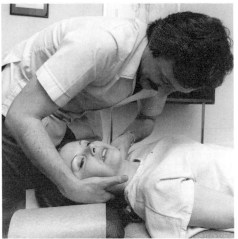

The section of the spine between the shoulder-blades is often treated manipulatively for the relief of respiratory diseases.

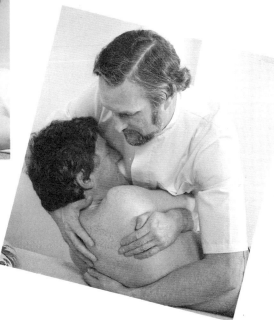

Manipulative treatment to the neck region, above, is of great benefit in the treatment of headaches, migraine, neck, shoulder and arm pain. It is frequently used in the relief of severe stress and tension and in the hands of the qualified osteopath or chiropractor, is a safe, painless technique.

When your osteopath puts his hands on your back this is what he sees in his mind's eye. He is able to build a complex image of this remarkable structure. His sensitive fingers enable his to detect restrictions of movement, abnormal patterns of muscle and ligament tensions and to identify areas of malfunction.

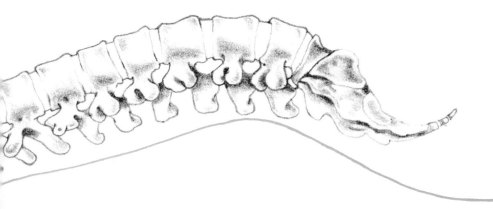

CHOOSING AN OSTEOPATH

It is essential to be treated only by a trained osteopath as osteopathy in the wrong hands can be dangerous.

Little more than a thousand of the many so-called osteopaths in Britain belong to the organized and responsible professional bodies whose requisites for membership are a completion of a four-year fulltime course of training. Osteopaths in the USA are registered medical practitioners, who will have carried out their training at osteopathic medical colleges, where they are trained in medicine with an osteopathic bias. The situation in Australia is less easy to define as regulations and practice vary from state to state.

CHIROPRACTIC

This is a form of manipulative treatment closely aligned to osteopathy. The concept of chiropractic (it means treatment by the hands, or manipulation) was developed by David Daniel Palmer (1845–1913) in 1895 in Iowa. He believed, like Still, that displacements of the structure of the spine cause pressure on the nerves which in turn cause symptoms in other parts of the body. The main differences between chiropractic and osteopathy are mostly historical since both forms of manipulative therapy now subscribe to the modern concepts of anatomy and physiology, although they both use manipulative treatment for the relief of a wide range of disorders rather than just disorders of the spine. Like the osteopath, the chiropractor considers the patient as a whole, with the emphasis on the body's structure, in relation to the patient's specific problem.

The chiropractor tends to place a greater reliance on X-rays in the diagnosis of spinal problems than the osteopath and the techniques of manipulation are slightly different to those of the osteopath. The chiropractor tends to use less leverage and more direct thrust against the specific vertebrae. Chiropractic treatment can achieve excellent results in the treatment of back pain, other musculo-skeletal disorders and certain systemic diseases, such as asthma, migraine, digestive and menstrual disorders.

In Australia and the USA, the chiropractor has the same status as osteopaths do in Great Britain since they remain outside the realms of orthodox medicine. Like the British osteopaths, there are many British practitioners calling themselves chiropractors but far fewer who belong to the established chiropractic association. There are more osteopaths than chiropractors in the United Kingdom, although the establishment of the excellent Anglo-European College of Chiropractic has led to a growing number of highly qualified practitioners. In Australia there are more chiropractors than osteopaths. The regulations and practice varies from state to state both for chiropractors and osteopaths. (See Appendix for details of professional bodies and colleges for all three countries.)

MASSAGE

The ancient art of massage is both luxurious and relaxing and, in the context of natural health, the most innocuous of all the therapies. A good massage can soothe headache, relieve tension and stress in the body, help insomnia, relax taut muscles, lower the blood pressure and, above all, induce a feeling of calm, suppleness and wellbeing. It is well worth taking massage as a regular basis for relaxation and as a preventative treatment for stress.

HOW IT WORKS

Massage concentrates on the soft tissues of the body, the muscles and ligaments, in order to stimulate the circulation of the blood and the functioning of the nervous system. At the same time, the blood pressure is lowered as a consequence of the soothing movements.

Footballers, athletes and dancers find massage particularly beneficial as it negates the unpleasant side-effects of hard exercise and prevents the muscles becoming too taut. During exercise, waste products are released into the muscles and these wastes are later drained away by the lymphatic system. This process can take up to several days, and the accumulation of waste products is what causes stiffness after exercise. Massage speeds up the draining process by stimulating the lymphatic system and the circulation of the blood. Massage is also a useful adjunct to physiotherapy and manipulative therapies.

TYPES OF MASSAGE

There are two principal systems of massage: **Swedish massage,** which is the system used chiefly in the West, and **Shiatsu massage,** from Japan, which combines massage with acupressure on the body's meridian system and acupuncture points (see **Acupuncture** p. 66).

Swedish massage relies on the four basic techniques of *effleurage, pétrissage, pressure* and *percussion* carried out in turn on the back, arms and hands, abdomen, feet and legs, head and face. The most important point to remember in mastering the techniques is that contact with the body should not be broken. The ideal is to create a rhythmic and continual movement, with the techniques producing an alternating soothing and stimulating effect.

EFFLEURAGE

This is a rhythmic stroking movement with open, relaxed hands, designed to soothe and relax the body and to maintain a rhythm throughout the massage so that one movement flows into another. Effleurage movements are always directed *towards* the heart, while stroking can take any direction.

PÉTRISSAGE

This is an intermittent deep movement of lifting, rolling, pressing or squeezing, not unlike kneading bread. It is designed to stimulate the muscles and areas of fatty tissue. It stretches those muscles that have seized up and become shortened and relaxes contracted muscles.

PRESSURE

The third technique is designed to set up friction in order to stimulate the body's superficial tissues. Small circular movements are made with the thumbs, finger-

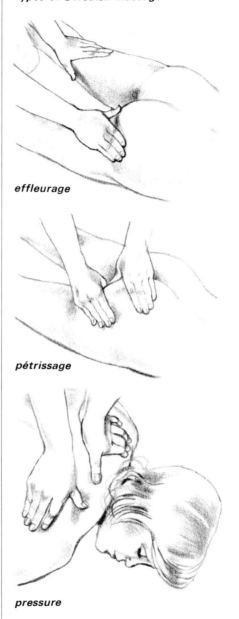

Types of Swedish massage

effleurage

pétrissage

pressure

tips or heel of the hand. Pressure is exerted before each circular movement and, during the movement, the skin moves under pressure from the fingertips against the underlying body structure. It is designed to relieve specific areas of tension, such as around the neck, shoulders and buttocks.

PERCUSSION

Percussive movements are the most difficult for the non-professional to perfect: they are brief, brisk, rhythmic, springy movements applied in series with alternate hands. They consist of cupping, hacking, flicking, pummelling and clapping movements in order to stimulate the skin and, in turn, the blood circulation. These are followed with effleurage in order to soothe and to maintain a rhythmic contact with the body.

Although massage is for the most part beneficial, remember that you must not have a massage if you are suffering from any of the following:

- any infectious, erupting skin complaint
- large bruises
- varicose veins
- temperature/fever
- inflamed joints or are at the acute stage of arthritis
- thrombosis or phlebitis, as a blood clot could be disturbed

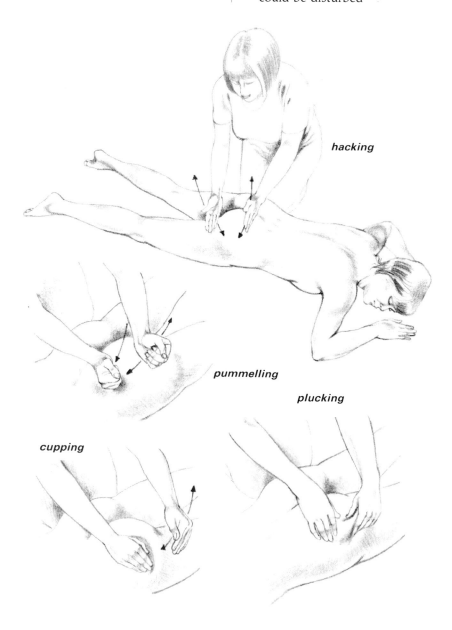

hacking

pummelling

plucking

cupping

AROMATHERAPY

'The way to health is to have an aromatic bath and scented massage every day ...' declared Hippocrates many centuries ago. Certainly, the use of aromatic oils greatly enhances a massage treatment, turning it into a positively pampering experience. Using essential oils during massage to treat specific disorders is known as aromatherapy, a technique based partly on the fact that different smells produce different emotional reactions and partly on the individual properties of essential oils which may exert a therapeutic effect on the body. Recent research at Kneipp Institute in Germany has demonstrated that the essential oils are absorbed by the skin, enter the bloodstream and can be measured in the exhaled breath, having done their therapeutic job on the way.

Concentrated essential oils can cause stinging and allergic reactions, so just one or two drops of essential oil to every 5 ml (1 teaspoon) of 'carrier' vegetable oil is sufficient. The masseur applies a little of the oil to his/her palms and applies it to the body in one long stroke.

Types of oils

The essential oils are used either singly or as a mixture. In perfumery, scents fall into three categories, depending on their rate of evaporation: top, middle or base notes. The top note makes the initial impact, the middle note provides the mellow note and the base note is long lasting.

NATUROPATHY

Naturopathy essentially comprises a commonsense attitude to health based on the body's own healing capabilities. The principal elements of naturopathy are fresh air and sunlight, exercise, rest, good nutrition, hygiene, relaxation and hydrotherapy (water therapy). The naturopathic way of life means people taking responsibility for their own health and its very simplicity makes this easily possible.

WHAT IS NATUROPATHY?

Naturopaths believe that what orthodox doctors regard as symptoms of disease are frequently indications of the body's attempts to reject disease and to throw off the toxic accumulations — the poisoning — that an unhealthy way of life has produced. They further believe that the body has the power to heal itself provided that it is properly treated and maintained. Naturopaths attempt to remove obstacles to the normal functioning of the body, such as stress, poor posture and bad diet,

Taking the Waters

Spas, saunas and whirlpools are all commonplace these days and they are an essential part of hydrotherapy. Other forms include:

- balneotherapy (therapy with different sorts of bath, such as Epsom salts baths, oatmeal baths, and mud baths, for skin conditions)
- sitz baths (a form of hip bath in which the pelvic area is immersed alternately in hot and cold water with the feet in water of contrasting temperature— known as contrast bathing) to stimulate the pelvis and abdominal area for gynaecological, digestive and rectal problems
- hot and cold fomentations (a moist compress which is usually a towel wrung out in water and applied moist, either hot or cold) to promote circulation and stimulate skin reflexes by application to those areas that have reflex connections with the internal organs, such as, for example, the upper back to the lungs
- sprays to stimulate skin function
- friction rubs, such as with sea salt packs (ice packs and warm packs)
- thalassotherapy (therapeutic use of sea water, and sea air, which has a higher proportion of negative ions than that of urban areas and contains more ozone)

and apply treatments which will stimulate or promote natural functioning. In essence, therefore, naturopathy is the promotion of health or the practice of preventative medicine rather than the treating of disease.

VITALISM

Fundamental to all natural therapies is the concept known as vitalism: living things are made up of a sum of the structural, the biochemic and the emotional. As naturopaths believe that disease is not an external invasion of bacteria or viruses but an expression of the body's healing properties at work, so they claim that this process should not be suppressed (with drugs) but should be supported in its efforts at all three levels to resolve the crisis, provided the body has the inherent vitality to cope (very young children and old people are exceptions).

In the treatment of chronic disorders, signifying a deeper level of dysfunction, naturopaths try to stimulate the more active phase of disease and this is why naturopathic treatment at first sometimes seems to aggravate the condition before it cures it.

RESTORING NORMALITY

Naturopaths attempt to restore normality to the body at three interrelated levels:

● **The structural level** Naturopaths work closely with osteopaths (some naturopaths are themselves osteopaths). At this first level of healing, they seek to correct the alignment of the body, looking at the musculoskeletal system, in particular the spine, and to remove the physical causes of pain. Spinal misalignment can lead to an interference in the functioning of the nervous system, which may adversely affect organs such as the heart, lungs and digestive system, and the rest of the musculoskeletal system. Muscular tensions, strained ligaments, stiff joints and poor posture all reduce the body's efficiency.

● **The biochemic level** The chemistry of the body fluids can be upset either by dietary deficiency or excess or by the retention of waste products as a result of inefficient functioning of the lungs, kidneys and bowels. The body is dependent on adequate nourishment for health and vitality. If the nourishment it receives is inappropriate (in the form of harmful substances that are either excessive such as caffeine, nicotine, alcohol and certain food additives, or in the form of too highly refined foods) then the body will work less efficiently and vitality will decrease.

Extensively processed foods containing preservatives, colourings and other chemical additives increase the accumulation of waste products in the body by speeding up oxidation in the body's cells. Naturopaths believe that metabolic waste products lay the foundation for disease: and nowhere has this been more clearly supported by doctors in the western world than in the relationship of highly processed, high fat food to heart disease.

Naturopaths advocate eating foods that are as near as possible to their natural state, because that way they contain a high proportion of essential nutrients, such as minerals and vitamins and enzymes. Fresh and raw foods are the most valuable to us. Any preparation of food will cause a reduction in quality, and boiling vegetables is a good example of this: much of the goodness escapes into the water.

Apart from the food we eat and the chemical additives that some of it contains, naturopaths and many experts believe that chemical pollutants, such as crop sprays, lead and other heavy metals in the atmosphere, also contribute to ill health.

● **The emotional level** Emotions play a significant part in the structural integrity of the body and in our biochemical functions. Function of the body can be impaired by stress which may be due to worry either at home or at work. If we are undergoing emotional strain, we often reflect this in muscular tension and our posture: we may be bowed down and getting a pain in the neck if we live with one, for example. It has been established that people with undue emotional stress in their lives involuntarily depress their immune system and consequently become vulnerable to disease. The body may be strong enough to survive but does not have enough energy left for the efficient working of the immune system.

When the body is under stress, it produces lots of adrenaline, the hormone which would give it the extra power needed for 'fight or flight'. However, it often happens in stressful situations that neither fight nor flight are available options and so the adrenaline cannot discharge. The resultant build-up creates physical tensions.

As the body's chemicals affect the emotions, if it lacks either sufficient nutrients or the right type of nutrients to produce adrenaline, for example, the brain and the nervous system will suffer. The individual suffers lack of concentration, irritability and depression. Not only is energy depleted, but the muscles and tissues also decline in function. So, by extension, nutrition is just as important to our emotional wellbeing as to a healthy, pain-free back, for example.

How Does the Naturopath Work?

The naturopath first takes a **medical history**, in the same way that orthodox doctors do, and also investigates the patient's lifestyle, social conditions, the possibility of emotional strains and dietary habits. He or she will assess the patient's nutritional intake in order to consider the possibility of an unsuitable diet or food sensitivities, either of which could be responsible for the symptoms presented.

The next stage is **examination**, in which the heart, lungs, blood pressure and the blood itself are tested and X-rays taken. Whereas orthodox doctors use the results of this sort of examination to conclude their diagnosis and initiate treatment, the naturopath interprets them as a total pattern of dysfunction, rather than trying to identify a particular disease.

Some naturopaths may also use **hair analysis** and **iridology** to give them further information about the patient's gen-

eral health. Analysis of hair is carried out in a sophisticated process based on a comparison of energy frequencies, known as spectroscopy. From this it is possible to determine the levels of some essential minerals such as zinc, copper and selenium and also levels of toxic minerals such as lead, mercury and aluminium.

Iridology means, literally, the study of the iris; it is based on the fact that the eye, especially the iris, has zones that reflect the condition of the whole body. It is possible to observe changes in these zones which might indicate the level of skin function, the tone of the nervous system, the state of the intestines and of the lymphatic glands. When used in conjunction with clinical assessments, it is an invaluable guide to the main areas of the body that are causing trouble and therefore a pointer to the appropriate treatment.

Natural Treatment

The naturopath will decide from the diagnosis whether the treatment should be **catabolic** (breaking down) for those whose bodies are in a congested, toxic state, or **anabolic** (building up) for those weak patients who need supplements of minerals and vitamins, for example. Those who require catabolic treatment may be advised to fast for two to three days in order to cleanse their bodies completely, or to follow a light diet programme.

Although fasting for a period as long as three days does not sound attractive, many people can happily undergo longer fasts under supervision. Fasting revitalizes the system in a quite unexpected way. (Losing the appetite is regarded as a completely normal occurence in illness and may happen in order to allow the escape of toxic accumulations and because the digestive organs are too weak to function.) The unfortunate but shortlived accompaniments to fasting can include halitosis and headache.

The patient will then be given a programme which will include guidelines on constructive nutrition, hydrotherapy, breathing, exercises and the herbs to encourage cleansing and renourishing

Fast Work

A short fast will rest the body physiology and detoxify the tissues.

It will revitalize you, undertaken occasionally, or when you have minor ailments such as a cold, skin rash or digestive upset. Before you start, however:

● advise your doctor or naturopath of your intention
● not do so for more than two to three days without the supervision of a practitioner
● not attempt to drive on the second or third day
● be prepared for headaches, halitosis, diarrhoea, constipation, or a coated tongue in the first or second day
● drink three pints of fruit juice and water each day, taken at intervals (more if wanted)
● not take any vitamins or minerals during the fast (they will activate the digestive system)
● take small vitamin and mineral supplements *after* the fast

after fasting. Psychotherapy may also be advised.

The essential simplicity of naturopathy is such that most people can carry out the treatments in their own homes, incorporating them into their lifestyle — and this is how naturopathic treatment should be regarded. What may start as a professional treatment can then be extended through life for the maintenance of good health.

How Can It Help?

Recurrent conditions, such as allergies and undiagnosed ailments, that do not fit in with the orthodox categories of medicine, but which nevertheless cause patients considerable distress, can be treated naturopathically. Such conditions are considered by the naturopath more as a pattern of dysfunction rather than disease, and may include irritability, headache, migraine and skin conditions.

Degenerative disorders such as arthritis and heart disease can be treated according to the naturopath's principle of building up the body, increasing its ability to cope and affording it relief.

Children can be treated for skin complaints, such as eczema, as well as asthma and catarrh. Naturopaths can also treat for digestive, gastro-intestinal and gynaecological disorders. PMT is treated in menstruating women while, in menopausal women, the naturopath looks at the nutritional and structural aspects of the body to assist the smooth transition of hormonal changes. Anxiety states and stress-related disorders, which could include heart trouble, angina and high blood pressure are all obvious candidates for the naturopath, if surgery or drugs are to be avoided.

An understanding of the naturopathic system can, most importantly, remove people's fears of bugs and disease: they are shown that they have control and power over their body. Once they view ailments as an expression of their body fighting back, rather than as an external invasion, then they cope better with the problem and this in itself aids recovery.

PSYCHOTHERAPY

Psychotherapy is essentially 'talking' treatment, although the more modern varieties incorporate an element of 'doing' as well. Most forms involve two people, a therapist and a client. The term client is preferred to patient for two reasons. First, it emphasizes the fact that psychotherapy is not just for sick people, but for healthy people with problems. Secondly, it encourages the person seeking help to regard the therapist as their social and intellectual equal. This aims to avoid the aloof manner and technical jargon often attributed to doctors. Some therapies — group therapy — can accommodate a number of clients simultaneously; the essential element of all of them, however, is the desire of one subject to talk to and listen to another with the expectation that they will derive emotional benefit from this.

WHAT IS PSYCHOTHERAPY?

Therapies differ so much in technique that it is difficult to identify common features. The most fundamental one is a belief on the part of the therapist that they will be able to modify their client's feelings and ideas about themselves or others by what takes place in the course of the therapy.

The simplest division of psychotherapy is into three types in ascending order of complexity: supportive psychotherapy, exploratory psychotherapy and specialized psychotherapy. Virtually all the named therapies — psychoanalysis, Gestalt therapy, for example, fall into the most complex category, but understanding the simpler forms will help you set these in a wider context.

SUPPORTIVE PSYCHOTHERAPY

This is the simplest and least intrusive. You may be surprised to hear that you have been both practising and receiving supportive psychotherapy for years. It consists of allowing a person to talk and air their problems in an atmosphere of trust and warmth, and in the knowledge that what they say will neither be judged or later used against them. It has been said that psychotherapy of this kind is no different from a neighbourly chat over the garden wall or a winding-down drink with a colleague after a hectic day at work. The reason for seeking professional help for this might be that a person has no such friendly neighbour or cannot be sure that their colleague will treat their revelations with absolute confidence. At this level of psychotherapy the job of the therapist is merely to provide an attentive and sympathetic ear. Their skill lies more in the timing of what they say rather than in the content of what is said. One of the most sought-after therapists in a hospital department of psychotherapy where I worked was a South American doctor who knew hardly a word of English, but had an uncanny knack of interspersing 'ums' and 'ahs' at exactly the right moment, presumably based on observation of gesture and facial expression.

Supportive therapy is open-ended. It can be as frequent as the client wishes and can last a life-time. It can be practised by anyone who is a natural listener. In my experience it should be a vital ingredient in all medical and natural health consultations, whether the illness is acute or chronic, curable or incurable. Unfortunately, many modern doctors are so preoccupied with investigations and drugs that they neglect it, and one of the advantages of a holistic health approach should be to provide the right balance between correct diagnosis and treatment and supportive psychotherapy.

EXPLORATORY PSYCHOTHERAPY

Most people seeking professional help for emotional or physical complaints will have already tried such supportive outlets. They will expect a more active therapist. Exploratory psychotherapy is the next step. Here, the client is encouraged to explore the problem rather than merely air it. The therapist is not just a passive recipient of the client's woes, as in supportive psychotherapy, but actively intervenes to point out inconsistencies, evasions and neglected aspects of an issue. If this is done diplomatically and without losing any of the warmth and lack of bias which are the hallmarks of supportive psychotherapy, explorative psychotherapy can be a powerful instrument for change.

In my experience it is most effective in relatively normal people who have problems in one or two fairly circumscribed areas of their life. For example, a 30 year old woman consulted me because she had developed a fear of visiting her parents at weekends, which she had done regularly ever since leaving home 12 years before. We explored together all the aspects of her relationship with her mother and it transpired that she and her mother had never got on and her visits were duty visits which neither party enjoyed. When she realized this, she reduced her visits to once a month: she felt better, and the relationship with her mother actually improved.

This form of psychotherapy is more appropriate for psychological problems, but can be useful in some cases of physical ill-health, particularly if it is situational. A simple example is the case of a farmer who suffered from asthma. On detailed enquiry he was surprised to discover that his attacks mainly occurred when he entered his barn or whenever he had an argument with one of his farm-workers. It also emerged that if an argument took place within the barn he had a particularly severe attack. As well as neatly demonstrating that most physical illnesses have a physical component (in this case allergy to hay) and emotional component (in this case anger), it also shows that someone can be quite unaware of apparently obvious precipitants of their physical distress. Usually the link between situations and illness is not as glaring as this, but exploratory psychotherapy may uncover aggravating factors in many cases.

This sort of therapy should have a structure. The therapist should discuss with the client from the outset the number and length of the sessions that are planned (weekly one-hour sessions over six weeks is a good start) and the goals that are expected. It should be within the competence of any good social worker, marriage counsellor or general psychiatrist.

SPECIALIST PSYCHOTHERAPIES

The named psychotherapies, from classical Freudian psychoanalysis through to the modern Californian ones such as est are distinguished from supportive and exploratory types in two main respects. First, they are based on a theory of how the mind and body, emotions and personality, relate to one another. This the therapist directly or indirectly communicates to the client and expects them to accept.

Secondly, the procedure or rules of the therapeutic process are strictly laid down. In classical psychoanalysis the client has to lie on a couch five times a week for an hour for at least three years and is encouraged to discuss their dreams and their feelings for the therapist. In primal scream therapy, the emphasis is more on doing than talking, with an intensive three-week course leading up to a final scream. Sometimes the therapy is far from gentle. In est, for example, the therapist may insult the client, refuse permission for the relief of bodily functions despite marathon sessions, and fine the clients for not applauding the therapist's interventions!

There are a large number of these therapies now on offer. Some are expensive, some are cranky, and some are frankly dangerous, unless, paradoxically, one is psychologically tough!

- **Psychoanalysis** was developed by Sigmund Freud, the Austrian psychiatrist, at the turn of the century. It was immensely popular in the USA throughout most of this century, but is now on the wane. It is expensive, lengthy, and time-consuming. It is superficially gentle (talking about dreams on a couch) but the analyst continually interprets what you say in terms of your childhood relationships with your parents, and this can be upsetting and leave you very vulnerable. In my view, it is not to be recommended unless you enjoy a protracted, intellectual battle. (Jungian psychotherapy, following the principles of Carl Jung, one of Freud's ablest pupils, is similar in its practical details, except that what is said is interpreted in terms of symbols and myths rather than childhood relationships.)

- **Gestalt therapy** was introduced by Fritz Perls in the USA also during the 1950s. It derived its theoretical basis from the Gestalt school of psychology. The central tenet of this school was that the whole is greater than the sum of its constituent parts. The therapeutic implication was that if one could encourage the client to view their symptoms within the wider context of normal emotions then these symptoms would become less insistent. If they could cry, for example, tension in the head causing headache might dissipate. This is the most relevant of the specialist psychotherapies for natural health as it provides a theoretical basis for the concept of holistic medicine, the idea that the individual symptoms should be seen as part of a Gestalt, literally the 'whole'.

- **Psychodrama** is therapy through dramatic enactment of emotional problems. It was first suggested by Jacob Moreno, an Austrian who emigrated to the USA between the wars. The idea was suggested to him by a friend who was in charge of a travelling theatre group. This friend had noticed that his wife, one of the actresses, who was usually irritable and continually rowing with him, would become calmer and their marital life less stormy whenever she played the part of an evil woman. Moreno concluded that playing the part of an angry or miserable or jealous person might reduce the strength of that emotion in a person's everyday life.

- **Bioenergetics** and **Rolfing** are adaptations of the ideas of Wilhelm Reich, one of Freud's early disciples. He encouraged therapists to become interested in the posture and tone of their patient's bodies as well as the content of their minds, and can be considered the father of many of today's holistic therapies. In **bioenergetics** a person is encouraged to experience their body in some action, eg kicking or stamping, and is then asked to recall similar experiences in the past. These memories are then related to an emotional event, for example, anger with father, which the person never really got over. Thus, the body is used to recall, then to relive, finally it is hoped, to neutralize the traumatic event or dissipate its harmful effect on their present life. The founder of this form of treatment, Alexander Lowen, believed that people who were suffering in this way and for whom bioenergetics would be effective could be identified merely by observing their posture. For example, a man whose chief personality characteristic was the withholding of emotions would be identified by a stooping posture. An important part of treatment is to encourage the person to experience their body moving as freely as possible, and to this end they are told to lie on a mattress and kick their legs up and down, sometimes for hours on end.

    Rolfing, founded by Ida Rolf in New York, has similar objectives, but the treatment takes the form of massage. The therapist tries to detect areas of energy imbalance within the body and tailors the massage technique accordingly.

- **Behavioural psychotherapy** or behaviour therapy developed out of a school of thought popular amongst academic psychologists in America before the last war. The essential feature is the belief that most neuroses arise because a person learns or is conditioned to some behaviour as a child, which although useful at that time, becomes a hindrance or 'maladaptive' when they grow up. For instance, a child may have an unpleasant experience with a fierce dog at a young age, from which it learns that dogs should be avoided. As an adult this behaviour may persist and 'generalize' so that the person becomes afraid to go out at all in case they meet a dog. Behaviour therapy aims to reverse this trend so that the person relearns that not all dogs are fierce. The actual techniques used may seem rather brutal but are often the only way to treat certain well-established phobias. Basically, the person is made to encounter the feared object — whether it be dog, cat, spider or open space — experience their anxiety and not run away. The anxiety diminishes and they then learn that the feared situation is not as bad as they thought. Gradually, after several closer and closer encounters with the object of their phobias, they gain confidence in dealing with it.

- **Cognitive therapy** is one of the most recent therapies of all, introduced by an American psychologist, Aaron Beck. Cognition is the general term covering perception, memory and thinking, and the aim of cognitive therapy is to alter someone's perceptions, memories and thoughts about themself if these are considered the root of their problem. To illustrate the technique, imagine yourself as an attractive and pleasant girl who believes, however, that she is unattractive and boring. When you go to a dance you hide in the corner and no-one asks you on to the floor. This then reinforces your belief that no-one likes you and a vicious circle is set up. The aim of cognitive therapy is to reverse this process. You are told to think and behave positively (even if you don't feel like it initially) and you then find that people come up to you and ask you to dance. You thus receive positive reinforcement that you are worth something, and your original low self-esteem disappears.

CHOOSING A THERAPY

In the context of natural health, some of these therapies are contra-indicated and some of doubtful benefit. The guiding principle should be the confidence you feel with the therapist. This is more important, in my view, than understanding the precise theoretical basis for the actual therapy.

Supportive psychotherapy may be all that some people need. Others may seek or need a more active approach. Some may prefer to work with their bodies, some with their minds. Some may enjoy analysing emotional nuances, some may prefer thinking through problems.

One final point: you will probably select a therapist who suits your personality and inclinations, but remember that some of the problems we encounter in life are the result of taking too narrow an approach. Someone who intellectualizes all the time will probably find psychoanalysis appealing, but that may be part of their problem. What they *need* rather than *want* is a more bodily-oriented therapy such as bioenergetics. Someone who is preoccupied with the state of their body, its every twinge or lump, might be better advised to explore their mind instead. So don't be afraid to experiment a little.

RELAXATION THERAPIES

We all need to relax; not just by going on holiday once or twice a year, but by training ourselves consciously to relax for a short period each day. Relaxing does not mean just falling asleep: it is a conscious state in which all your muscles are relaxed one by one and your brain clears, to as close a state of emptiness as possible.

Some people relax actively, by going swimming, for example; others relax passively, by watching television. Watching television does not always secure the desired effect, however, since you achieve a state closer to sleep than relaxation, very often slumped in an uncomfortable posture or are overstimulated by the programmes.

WHAT IS RELAXATION?

When you are properly relaxed, a number of changes take place in your body. You will feel a sense of relaxed, sometimes heightened awareness, and a physical feeling of warmth and heaviness. Your heart rate will decrease (which is one of the reasons why true relaxation is good for you) and, because your heart is pumping blood more slowly, you will start to feel your entire body slowing down. Your blood sugar and blood fat levels, which increase in response to stress, will slowly return to a healthy level.

ACHIEVING RELAXATION

Apart from physical exercise, there are a number of ways in which you can relax: they include autogenics, biofeedback, meditation and yoga. In addition, **hypnotherapy** (p. 80) achieves a state similar to that of autogenics and yoga, while **acupuncture** (p. 66) and **massage** (p. 86) are also relaxing. **The Alexander technique** (p. 69) teaches the optimum postures for keeping muscular tension to the minimum.

AUTOGENICS

This is a system of mental exercises, introduced by Dr Johannes Schultz, German psychiatrist and neurologist, in the 1930s, which is performed in order to relax the mind and body (autogenous means self-generating or originating within the body). Autogenic training (AT) is designed to switch off the stress 'fight or flight' response and switch on the rest, relaxation and recreation system associated with psychophysical relaxation. The exercises are extraordinarily simple and, once trained, you have a system which you can follow for life.

It is often recommended that you learn AT with a qualified practitioner, partly because a few people experience what is known as autogenic discharge, such as temporary twitching, feelings of dizziness, lethargy, anger, sadness or hilarity, which may be unexpected although nothing to worry about.

THE EXERCISES

You will be taught to experience the sensations of heaviness and warmth, to regularize the heartbeat and the breathing, to induce a feeling of warmth in the abdomen and a feeling of coolness on the forehead. You will be instructed first to repeat, 'my right arm is heavy and warm, my heartbeat is calm and regular, my breathing even,' and so on, dealing first with the right arm and the other five directions, then with the left arm and the five directions and so on through the body.

Autogenic training, when properly learned, produces a remarkable relief from tension and fatigue, both in day to day terms and in terms of eliminating stress that may have built up over years: this is thought to be the explanation for autogenic discharge. As with biofeedback, autogenics has been shown to be effective for any stress-related disorder, notably indigestion and ulcers, heart problems, asthma, migraine and anxiety.

BIOFEEDBACK

Biological feedback is essentially a system in which the body provides feedback or information about its condition by means of monitoring devices. The information you receive, which can be related to stress levels and anxiety, can be used to control and reduce these levels. The biofeedback instrument can measure skin temperature, muscle tone and even the amount of hydrochloric acid produced in the stomach.

The most common way in which the body provides feedback is through the sweat rate. Anxiety makes you sweat and

---

Relaxing for beginners

This basic relaxation exercise slows the heartbeat and the breathing rate and consequently refreshes and renews you. You need only half an hour for this exercise to begin with, and as you become practised, you will need even less time.

- Turn off the radio or television, disconnect the telephone and try to empty your mind of thought or emotion.
- In a warm room, lie flat on a very firm bed or on a rug on the floor. Close your eyes and take three deep, slow breaths in and out.
- Stretch your left leg along the floor away from your body as hard as you can, pointing your foot and contracting the calf, thigh, buttock and lower back muscles. Hold yourself in that position until you feel a slight trembling in the muscles, then relax. Repeat with the right leg; then with both legs, and relax.
- Stretch your left arm down your side, spreading your fingers and pushing from the big muscles at the back of the neck and shoulder, contracting all the muscles of the upper arm, forearm and hand. Relax.
- Repeat with the right arm and relax. Repeat with both arms and relax.
- Stretch both arms and legs together and relax.
- Take five deep breaths and repeat the cycle again. Repeat the cycle four more times.
- Relax totally for 10 minutes, preferably with a blanket within reach, since body temperature may drop as a consequence of slower heart beat and lower breathing rates.

sweat decreases the electrical resistance of the skin. This resistance can be measured through metal contacts or pads attached to the body and connected to a visual or audible signal, so that it is possible to tell when you are feeling stressed and anxious and, consequently, to make conscious efforts to control your body's stress levels.

Many people are not aware when they are under stress: indeed, one of the most pernicious aspects of stress is that you can become bound up in a situation and not recognize the damage you are doing to your body. The adrenaline builds up, without the facility for discharging itself either in fight or flight, and the body's heart rate, respiratory rate and levels of blood sugar and blood fats all increase to meet the challenge. All these changes contribute to heart disease.

THE HARDWARE

The different sorts of biofeedback machines include those that measure skin resistance (ESR), muscle tensions (EMG or electromyograph) and brain waves (EEG). Each of them will indicate, by buzzing at an increasingly high note as your stress level rises, what you will gradually be able to recognize for yourself without the aid of machinery: when you are calm, your skin is cool and dry (your skin resistance goes up) and the audible indicator will soften to a muffled click and them stop; when you are more agitated, the buzzing assumes a higher note; when you are really anxious, and your adrenaline is causing a cold sweat and palpitations, or when you are hot and flushed in response to the body's noradrenaline, which is released when you are angry, the buzzing becomes higher and higher until it screeches.

The biofeedback ideal is to learn to monitor your stress levels without gadgetry—when driving, for example—and to learn how to relax through deep breathing, good posture and observing regular daily relaxation periods.

Biofeedback has become part of mainstream medicine and is used particularly in cardiac units and in migraine clinics. Its other applications includes hypertension and insomnia.

Chemofeedback

This is a fairly recent step in preventitive medicine, and is allied with biofeedback. The person being screened provides a small blood sample (a simple fingerprick). The sample is then analysed for blood sugar levels (which alter with stress), cholesterol levels, clotting factor, and the presence and concentration of stress hormones (adrenaline and noradrenaline). Chemical changes in the blood brought about by liver damage can also be detected.

Data from the blood analysis is collated with the answers given to a questionnaire about work, family life, finances, eating and drinking habits, degrees of tiredness etc to give an overall profile.

In all, the test only takes half an hour, and requires nothing of the person being screened but cooperation. You do not have to learn any exercises or monitor your reactions. Chemofeedback can only forewarn of a predisposition to certain illnesses and conditions (stress, tension, depression, alcoholism, heart disease, stroke, high blood pressure). It is a diagnostic tool rather than a therapy per se. Once you have the profile, it is up to you to initiate the relevant self-help therapy.

MEDITATION

Meditation has always been an integral part of Indian religions, as well as of Roman Catholicism (in saying the rosary), in Tibetan Buddhism (concentration upon the mandala) and in the Orthodox Church (concentration upon the icon).

All forms of meditation seek to harmonize the way things are (reality) and the way they ought to be (the ideal). There is a great variety of systems of meditation and each put the emphasis to a greater or lesser degree on the main components, which are:

- to appreciate clearly the ideal order of things through greater awareness
- to develop receptiveness to that established order
- to be active in putting that order into practice

In the West, the greatest emphasis has been placed on the vision of the ideal order, on visualizing it in silent contemplation, and by concentrating upon it. All meditation techniques are based on the need to develop a particular kind of awareness, which can be described as a state of restful alertness where the mind is emptied of everything. To help the individual accomplish this, the various forms of meditation focus concentration on to a single subject and this concentration is accompanied by the continual repetition of a word or phrase, known as a mantra in some systems of meditation.

This rhythmic chanting is said to enhance meditation by exerting a vibrating and hypnotic effect upon the mind, leading to trance; together with meditating itself, it is said to exert positive health effects, such as decreased heart rate and consequently lower blood pressure and a slower and more even respiratory rate, both of which will mitigate the possibility of heart disease, anxiety and stress-related disorders.

TYPES OF MEDITATION

Some forms of meditation are almost or totally devoid of content and the individual is encouraged to transcend thought entirely in order to cultivate a total receptiveness for the cosmic vision of the ideal order of things. These forms include the Japanese Zen Buddhism of 12th-century Chinese origin (which concentrates upon breathing, especially for beginners); the Taoist T'ai-Chi (which concentrates upon carefully designed and rhythmically precise movements to intensify and refine innate vital energy); and Transcendental Meditation (TM), a development of ancient Indian traditions, seeking to empty the mind entirely through entering the trance state, introduced to the West in 1959 by Maharishi Mahesh Yogi and enormously popular in the 1960s as a consequence of such luminaries as The Beatles taking it up.

YOGA

Yoga is used loosely in the West to describe many forms of relaxing exercise and meditation, accompanied by certain distinctive postures known as *asanas*. Yoga with a capital Y denotes the Hindu system of philosophy which aims at the mystical union of the self with the Supreme Being in a state of complete awareness and tranquillity through certain physical and mental exercises. Yoga can also mean, broadly, any method by which such awareness and tranquillity are attained, especially a course of related exercises and postures designed to promote a physical and spiritual wellbeing, but which is not necessarily formally religious.

The five main types of yoga, which are accepted by all schools of Indian philosophy are *karma yoga, jnana yoga, bhakti yoga, raja yoga* and *hatha yoga*. Hatha yoga is the basis of the modern practice of yoga in the West and is the system of yoga that concentrates upon longevity and health. There are other well-known types of yoga rest therapies that have become popular

---

Meditation for Beginners

The following exercise is a synthesis of meditative systems devised by Dr Herbert Benson of Harvard Medical School and has been found useful in treating stress.

- Sit, lie or recline in a comfortable position, making sure there are no external distractions such as radio or television.
- Shut your eyes.
- Relax all your muscles as in the basic relaxation exercise described earlier.
- Breathe deeply through your nose and try to clear your mind of all thought. Repeat the mantra word, 'one', either aloud or in your head. Breathe deeply and evenly and continue for 10–20 minutes, ignoring distracting thoughts and repeating the mantra.
- At the end, remain still, with your eyes shut for one or two minutes, then in the same position with your eyes open.

  Some forms of meditation can cause sudden outbursts of emotion, such as tears and laughter. This is said to be a sign that the meditation is working.

in the West, but these are merely the offshoots of hatha yoga that have been more energetically promoted and commercialized.

THE YOGA SYSTEM

Yoga is carried out in two levels: the first, known as *kriya yoga*, is the yoga of observances of physical accounts and this is carried out in five stages:

- adoption of restraints, or control, from evils (*yama*)
- adoption of religious observances (*niyama*)
- use of posture (*asana*) suitable for meditation
- restraint of breath or controlled breathing (*pranayama*)
- withdrawal of the senses from their objects (*pratyahara*)

The second chief level of yoga, known as superior or royal yoga, is carried out in three stages:

- concentration (*dharana*) of the intelligence on an object
- meditation (*dhyana*) as an uninterrupted mental state and awareness of that object
- trance (*samadhi*) in which the individual is fully identified with the object of meditation, so that they become as one

True Yoga, then, is a profoundly religious and spiritual system of philosophy which has existed in India for thousands of years and which has, only comparatively recently, been taken up in the West in abridged form.

HOW CAN IT HELP?

Many people take up yoga here simply because it teaches relaxation techniques, mobility and flexibility. The series of postures (*asanas*), which are an integral part of true Yoga, promote inner and outer harmony and grace and have the added benefit of reducing stress and tension, making you sleep better and leaving you calm and relaxed with a clear, uncluttered mind.

Yoga is suitable for people of all ages from young children to the elderly and arthritic. It is a particularly good form of exercise for the elderly because it is fairly gentle. It should be done regularly for maximum benefit and, when starting out, it is better to have personal supervision from a teacher before practising at home.

Set aside 15–20 minutes each day for deep breathing and some of the simple *asanas*. Many people have found that these basic exercises have helped them to cope better with daily pressures and the relief of tension, without even moving on to more advanced postures.

Whatever the origins of yoga and its various systems, and indeed of meditation as well, there can be no doubt that these therapies are not only benign—provided that they do not relieve the participants of too much in fees—but can be positively health-giving in their role of reducing stress.

For the many people who suffer from chronic stress symptoms, such as migraine, asthma and hypertension, hobbies, exercise and beneficial sleep are not enough. For them the answer lies in systematic relaxation. Some of the simple techniques of relaxation are useful for almost everyone, however, since temporary stress, at least, is sometimes unavoidable.

Whilst it is always best to learn yoga from a competent teacher, some of the simple postures can be a great help at times of stress crises. True yoga is a combination of the physical and the spiritual, but simply adopting these positions and maintaining them for as long as is comfortable will help to break the cycle of stress → physical tension → discomfort → more stress. As with nearly all relaxation techniques breathing is a vital component of yoga. Once you have achieved the required position, focus your concentration onto your breathing, trying to establish a relaxed, regular rhythm.

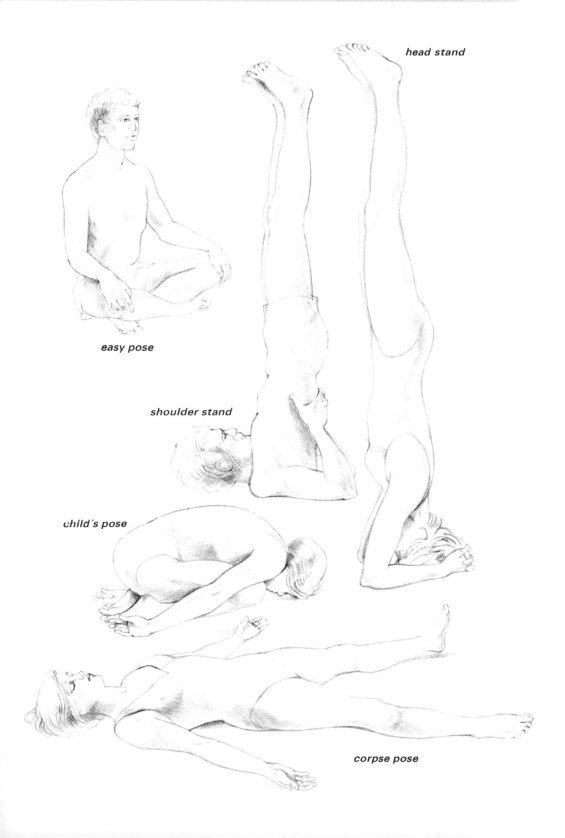

head stand

easy pose

shoulder stand

child's pose

corpse pose

PART III

THE A–Z
OF DISORDERS

INTRODUCTION

The purpose of this A–Z is to provide a quick and easy guide to diseases and their symptoms and to indicate the appropriate natural therapeutic response. Of course, consulting a complementary medical practitioner will be the long-term solution to a wide range of health problems, but knowing, how to take immediate, safe, sensible and effective steps which will help both you and your family without hindering the body's own healing powers is of paramount importance. The A–Z has no pretensions to being a medical textbook and you will not find every known disease or symptom listed here; neither is it a guide to self-diagnosis. It is intended to help the reader understand more about illness and to encourage a greater awareness of the holistic approach to restoring the body to health.

How the A–Z works
At first glance, it may seem that a section based on symptoms and their treatment contradicts the whole concept of complementary medicine, but this is not the case. The entries are arranged this way to guide the reader more efficiently towards a natural, less invasive drug-orientated approach to health problems. Under each heading you will find alphabetically listed the appropriate natural therapies and how they can help. Some entries are very specific, some more general: compare, for example, the acupuncture advice on angina to that given for allergies; angina is a specific disease with specific remedies; allergies present a much more diffuse problem and the treatment depends on a large number of variables.

There are also self-help directions for many common ailments. Often that is all that is needed. There are some situations, however, for which self-help is inappropriate and where professional advice should be sought from a qualified health practitioner WITHOUT DELAY. Such instances are signalled with a large exclamation mark in the margin.

It will probably help you to read the Major Therapies Chapter (pp. 65–101) before you consult the A–Z, but below are some practical notes on the recommended therapies to save duplication within the entries.

ACUPUNCTURE
Of course, you cannot apply your own acupuncture (even acupuncturists rarely

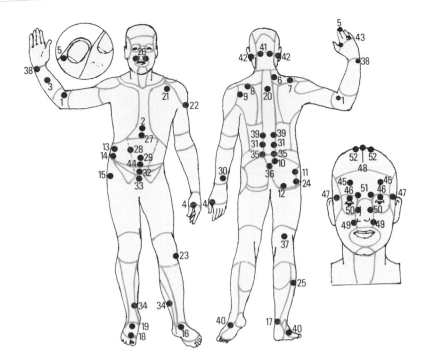

do it to themselves) but you will find reference throughout to acupressure. This refers to spots on the body which you can press either with your fingers or with the blunt end of a ball-point pen, to relieve pain. Above you will see an illustration showing 56 acupressure points mentioned throughout the A–Z.

When applying acupressure, bear the following points in mind:

● Never use severe pressure on any of the points.

● Make allowances for the age and strength of the person you are working on; don't treat anyone who is in a state of fatigue or emotionally upset.

● Use only light pressure on pregnant women and avoid the abdomen, especially in the first three months of pregnancy.

● Don't treat anyone who is under the influence of alcohol or drugs, or who has just eaten a large meal.

● Always treat people when they are lying down, in case there are reactions such as tiredness and giddiness.

HERBALISM

In the herbalism sections, instructions are given for the making of decoctions, infusions, teas, tisanes and poultices. Spe-

cific methods are given in the text where appropriate but here are some general rules. The basic proportion is 25 g/1 oz finely chopped herbs to 0.5 l/1 pt liquid. Where a combination of herbs is recommended, the total quantity (25 g/1 oz) is the same. Herbal teas and tisanes will keep for up to three days, covered tightly in the fridge.

Infusions

These are made from the leaves or flowers of the herb, occasionally the whole thing, excluding berries or seeds. Pour 0.5 l/1 pt boiling water onto 25 g/1 oz of fresh chopped herbs in a warm pot and cover to prevent steam escaping. Strain through a fine sieve or a coffee filter paper. Make a smaller quantity by adding a teacupful of boiling water to a teaspoonful of dried herbs (double the quantity for fresh herbs).

Decoctions

These are made from the root, bark or berries of the herb. Add 25 g/1 oz of the chopped or crushed remedy to 0.75 l/1½ pts cold water, bring to the boil and simmer gently until the liquid reduces to 0.5 l/1 pt. Leave to cool then strain. Use an enamel or stainless steel pan and distilled water if you live in an area supplied with fluoridated water.

Dosage

Unless otherwise stated the dose is 45–60 ml/3–4 tbsp (about a wineglassful) first thing in the morning, mid-afternoon and just before you go to bed.

Teas

Tea is made from the fermented leaves or stalks of one or more plants mixed with boiling water. The fermentation process produces the tannin, and the taste and effect of a tea and a tisane (see below) made from the same herb are entirely different. You can buy teas from the herbalist, ready fermented. Many are available in tea-bag form (chamomile, peppermint, fennel, rosehip, raspberry leaf, buckwheat etc).

Tisanes

Like infusions, these are made by adding boiling water to fresh or dried (but *not* fermented) plant matter, normally green leaves. To dry your own leaves, pack them on a wire rack in your airing cupboard or in a warm airy place for about 48 hours. Store them in airtight dark glass jars. They should last for a year. Don't use your usual teapot because tannin left in it from your tea will spoil the delicacy of the tisane.

Poultice

This is made by crushing or pounding the remedy and mixing it into a spreadable paste with a little hot liquid, usually water. Herbs can be mixed into carrier paste such as flour, cornmeal or bran in the proportion of 60 g/$2\frac{1}{2}$ oz to 500 ml/20 fl oz loose paste. Sandwich the mixture in thin cloth before applying it to the skin.

Aloe vera gel and pulp is mentioned in some herbalism sections. It comes from the aloe vera plant, which grows freely and easily as a house plant in Australasia and other warm climates, but does not thrive in northern Europe or the UK. Substitute with commercially available aloe vera gel and cream where appropriate.

HOMEOPATHY

In some cases, you are recommended to consult a homeopath. This usually means that you have a general or chronic rather than a local problem and need a constitutional remedy which is difficult and unpracticable for you to choose for yourself.

When remedies are mentioned, they are usually for use until you can get to your homeopathic physician. Lack of space means that only a limited number of remedies can be provided under each heading, and these should be seen as examples only. The remedies listed can be bought from homeopathic chemists, some orthodox chemists and many health food shops. The dosage is normally the 6 c potency; 30 c and above are difficult to obtain without prescription.

NATUROPATHY

Under the naturopathy section, mention is made of fasting and exclusion diet. Below is an example of a fast, provided by a qualified naturopath.

Exclusion Diets

An exclusion diet is used to try and pinpoint a food to which you have an intolerance or an allergy. These are quite difficult to carry out unsupervised, and you should consult a naturopath or clinical ecologist who will help you. The diet usually involves 2 or 3 (more if necessary) days on distilled water and then the gradual reintroduction of foods. Adverse reactions can be noted and the source of the allergy or intolerance isolated. Detailed information can be found in *Clinical Ecology* (*see* Bibliography).

PSYCHOTHERAPY

The psychotherapies section (pp. 92–6) gives a brief run down of the kind of psychotherapy available. However, you may experience some confusion about the practitioners. The 'Know Your Therapist' panel will help you sort out the different kinds.

VITAMINS AND MINERALS

Please note that dosages given under the vitamin and mineral treatment sections are therapeutic doses only and should not be regarded as normal for the healthy person.

Fasting

The following short fast may be undertaken to rest the body physiology and detoxify the tissues from time to time, or when you have minor ailments, such as a cold, skin rash, or digestive upset. If you are in doubt about your ability to undertake this programme consult your doctor or a naturopath.

Days One and Two
Juices only. Use freshly squeezed fruit or vegetable juices, or canned or bottled juices which are pure, unsweetened, and free from additives and preservatives.
Take one tumblerful of juice four or five times through the day. (You may prefer to dilute the juice with mineral or spring water—recommended for canned pineapple juice.) If thirsty at other times drink mineral or spring water with a slice of lemon.

Day Three
On rising: Pure fruit or vegetable juice.

Breakfast: Dish of plain goats-milk yoghurt. Fresh fruit, such as grapes, apples, pears, melon, peaches or paw-paw.

Mid morning: Pure juice

Lunch: Fresh fruit.

Mid afternoon: Pure juice.

Evening meal: Mixed raw salad consisting of a selection of vegetables in season. Lettuce, chopped cabbage, Chinese leaves, chopped cauliflower, grated carrots or beetroot, chicory, endive, parsley, tomatoes, and cucumber are just some of the possible ingredients. Garnish with spring onions and herbs and add a dressing made with vegetable oil, lemon juice or cider vinegar, and yoghurt or tahini.

On retiring: Fruit juice drink.

Day Four
Breakfast: As for day three.

Between meals: Fruit juice or herb tea.

Lunch: Mixed raw salad as above or vegetable stew, flavoured with yeast or vegetable extract or soya paste (miso). Fresh fruit as dessert.

Evening meal: As for lunch or vegeterian savoury with two or three conservatively cooked vegetables. Fresh fruit as dessert.

On retiring: Fruit juice, herb tea or savoury extract in hot water.

Note: For the first day or two there may be some hunger feelings and light-headedness. It may be best to start at the weekend when you can take more rest. Mild headaches, coated tongue, or looseness of the bowels, are signs that the body is beginning it's cleansing work and need give no cause for concern.

Know Your Therapist

A **psychiatrist** is always medically qualified and has passed a further exam in mental illness and psychological problems. They are allowed to prescribe drugs as well as practise psychotherapy.

A **psychologist** has always obtained a basic university degree in psychology but this is mainly theoretical, and they may or may not have had experience in dealing with actual people suffering psychological problems. They are not allowed to prescribe conventional drugs.

A **clinical psychologist,** in addition to their basic university degree, has passed a further exam in psychological problems and their treatment by psychological means. They mainly practise behaviour therapy and cognitive therapy and cannot prescribe conventional drugs.

A **psychotherapist** is anyone— doctor, psychologist, lay-person—who practises any variety of psychotherapy. Some are trained, some are not.

A **psychoanalyst** is anyone—doctor, psychologist, lay-person—who has trained in the practice of psychoanalysis. This requires them to be psychoanalysed themselves.

A

ACNE

Acne is a distressing skin disease which afflicts about 80% of all those between the ages of 12 and 24. Changing levels of the sex hormones (androgens) during adolescence increases the activity of the sebaceous glands in the skin, which may go into over-production of the fatty substance sebum (the skin's natural lubricant and moisturizer). Acne can be aggravated by emotional upset, stress and, it is thought, by certain foods and drink.

SYMPTOMS
Acne is most commonly found on the face, neck, top of the shoulders and back.

It first appears as blackheads and whiteheads (plugged sebaceous glands). If these become infected by bacteria, they form angry, painful pustules. Scratching or squeezing with dirty fingers will spread the infection, which may become serious.

ORTHODOX TREATMENT
Skin-drying lotions; UV light; antibiotics.

HERBAL TREATMENT
Help rid the bloodstream of waste and impurities with a decoction of 2 parts each burdock root, dandelion root and red clover flowers and 1 part each yellow dock root and poke root. Take 45–60 ml 3–4 tbsps three times daily.

An infusion of clivers herb will cleanse the skin.
- *For oily skin* a weak infusion of lavender or marigold flowers can be used twice a day as a lotion.
- *For dry or normal skin* use a limeblossom infusion.
- *For an astringent* use elderflower infusion or distilled witch hazel.

Scars can be gradually reduced with aloe vera gel (from the fleshy leaves of the plant) applied twice a day.

HOMEOPATHY
Consult a homeopath for severe conditions. Local remedies include:
- *Hepar sulphuris* Where there is a tendency to form pus.
- *Calcium sulphuris* Where there are tender blind boils that never erupt and subside after a while.
- *Silica* Where there is scarring.

MASSAGE
Lymphatic drainage massage can be helpful. Go to a qualified masseur.

NATUROPATHY
Diet: Introduce a diet of whole grains, fresh fruit and vegetables, limit dairy produce, particularly milk, exclude refined carbohydrates.

A cleansing programme of raw fruit and salads for 2 or 3 days, followed by the gradual introduction of whole grains and cooked vegetables, should be repeated every 2 or 3 weeks.
Hydrotherapy: Stimulate healthy skin function on arms and trunk by cold friction rubs — rubbing down the skin with a loofah and cold water.

PSYCHOTHERAPY
Extreme cases of acne can be an embarassing cause of disfigurement to adolescents. Psychotherapy may be useful in overcoming the difficulties of interpersonal relationships which are likely to arise.

Bioenergetics (see p. 95) in particular, appeals to young people.

VITAMIN AND MINERAL TREATMENT
Adolescent acne may respond to oral vitamin A (2,500 iu's 3 times daily) plus 5 mg zinc as amino acid chelate (3 times daily). Difficult cases may need additional Oil of Evening Primrose (500 mg with each meal).
Pre-menstrual flare-up may respond to 50 mg vitamin B$_6$ daily for one week before menstruation and during it.

ADDICTION

(SEE ALSO LIVER PROBLEMS)

Addiction is the unavoidable dependence on a substance or an activity. The common factor in all addictions is that they alter the body chemistry of the addict, producing inevitable mood changes.

While there are some personality types more likely to become addicts, addiction can affect any person of any age. Many common addictions are to seemingly innocuous substances like tea, coffee and chocolate, while at the other end of the scale addiction to the hard drugs such as heroin and cocaine are an ever-increasing menace. Between these two ends of the spectrum — the compulsive tea drinker and the mainline heroin addict — are found the anorexic addicted to laxatives, the exercise fanatic addicted to running, the adolescent hooked on all forms of solvent abuse from glue to marker pens, the tranquillizer-dependent patient and the alcoholic.

The dependence which addiction produces may be either physiological or psychological; the body chemistry becomes dependent on the drug and the addict believes that they cannot function without their preferred addiction. In either case, the end results are the same; any attempt at removing the addictive factor from the addict's lifestyle results in withdrawal symptoms of a greater or lesser nature.

EVERYDAY ADDICTIONS

While society increasingly condemns the addict who uses illegal substances, it condones mass addiction to many substances in common use. The caffeine which occurs in tea and coffee and all cola drinks is a powerful stimulant. Aspirin is available over the counter or out of machines in every High Street and many people cannot start the day without their dose of aspirin in case they get a headache. The stimulant effect of nicotine and the social use of alcohol are not only accepted but heavily advertised and generate a large source of revenue to governments.

PRESCRIBED DRUGS AND TRANQUILLIZER ABUSE

The problems of addiction to the morphine-based pain killers and barbiturate sleeping pills is well known and these drugs are largely under the control of hospital doctors rather than general practitioners, but an epidemic of addiction to the newer drugs is sweeping through the Western world. Those particularly involved are the tranquillizers and the anti-depressants. These are the commonest cause of physiological drug dependence through prescription, while the non-barbiturate sleeping pills commonly cause psychological dependence. The ease with which these drugs are prescribed and mindless regularity with which repeat prescriptions are issued are responsible for the fate of a growing number of our population whose lives are governed by the bottle of pills in their pocket, handbag or on the bedside table. Today, there are probably more tranquillizer addicts than alcoholics.

The difficulties that arise when the addict tries to reduce their use of behaviour modifying drugs can be enormous. The tranquillizer addict may suffer from PALPITATIONS, APPETITE LOSS, TENSION and even INSOMNIA. This dependence can arise in some people after three or four weeks of taking tranquillizers and most people are liable to become dependent after two or three months of regular use.

ALCOHOL ABUSE

Contrary to popular belief, alcohol is not a stimulant but a very powerful depressant. It acts by depressing the activity of the body's nervous system and the insidious way in which the occasional drinker who uses alcohol to relieve stresses and tensions progresses to the heavy social drinker who progresses in turn to the alcoholic. Peer pressure, especially among youngsters, and some sections of the business community, is a powerful factor in the creation of the alcoholic. At best, the alcoholic risks social degradation, destroying family relationships and losing employment; at worst, irreversible and frequently fatal liver disease, nutritional deficiency diseases and, all too commonly, fatal road traffic accidents.

(See *also* **Positive Health** p. 63)

> At least 26,500 people die every year in the UK as a result of alcohol abuse.
> One in 5 of all hospital admissions are alcohol related.
> One in three drivers involved in road accidents were over the legal limit.
> 52 per cent of deaths by fire were caused by someone who was drunk.
> 33 per cent of all domestic accidents are alcohol related.
> 30 per cent of all drownings are alcohol related.

SMOKING

The detrimental (and sometimes fatal) effects of smoking are well documented, and yet the message is still ignored in some quarters. Hardened tobacco addicts have turned their faces against sense and seem to adopt a seige mentality. Public attitudes are at last beginning to change — more 'no smoking' compartments in trains, areas in cinemas, tables in restaurants, influential public people are no longer seen smoking publicly and advertizing has retreated to billboards and, ironically, sports sponsorship.

Even though the once glamourous image of smoking is now tarnished, the smokers themselves are still addicts and still have to come to terms with it before they can kick the habit. (See **Positive Health** p. 63 for more information on 'giving up graciously'.)

ILLEGAL DRUGS

Heroin, cocaine and glue sniffing are all growing menaces in our society. They are all addictive and they can all lead to fatal end results. The abuse of illegal substances frequently starts at school, when children may be encouraged by others to experiment or maybe coerced into drug taking by their peers. The majority of children do not ever experiment with drugs and many of those who do seldom do it more than once or twice, but a few become addicted. It may be extremely difficult to tell when someone is using drugs occasionally unless you catch them in the act or they are showing obvious signs of intoxication. Sudden mood changes, irritability, aggression or appetite loss, are frequently just signs of normal growing up but combined with other strange behaviour may need investigation (see **Positive Health** pp. 60–1).

GETTING OFF IT

It does not matter whether the addict is legal or illegal, in either event their lives become dependent upon the particular substance or activity which dominates their lives and the first and vital step in overcoming the addiction is for the addicts themselves to recognize their problem. Without their willing co-operation there can be no solution.

Family support is vital in the successful treatment of addiction and counselling the family as a whole is a useful starting point.

The self treatment of all addictions must be approached with commitment and patience. Sleeping pills, tranquillizers and anti-depressants should be withdrawn slowly and gradually by reducing the doses over a period of weeks or sometimes months. Substitution with herbal or homeopathic remedies is very helpful. Care must be taken however, not to replace one dependency with another.

ACUPUNCTURE

Acupuncture can be extremely valuable in the relief of withdrawal symptoms, particularly for the treatment of smokers and both prescribed and illegal drug abusers.

HERBAL TREATMENT

A serious addiction to any toxin requires skilled treatment and a desire on the part of the addict to be free of the addiction. Strong will power is essential. Blood cleansing herbs such as burdock root, fumitory, echinacea together with agents to ensure optimum function of liver and kidneys are needed. You should consult a herbal practitioner.

Homeopathy
Consult a homeopath. Both the underlying cause(s) of the addiction and the addict's constitutional type must be assessed and discussed before any remedy can be prescribed. *Nux vomica* has proved effective where feelings of tension, pressure and irritability have led to the use of tranquillizers or alcohol in the search for relief.

Naturotherapy
Whatever addiction you are trying to escape from, maintaining a good nutritious diet can be very helpful for building up the body's stamina.

Psychotherapies
As each addiction has its own special problems, generalizing about the role of psychotherapy in managing addictions is not easy.

In alcohol and heroin addiction, group therapy has been the most widely recommended psychotherapy. It is the basis of self-help groups such as Alcoholics Anonymous and its aim is both to support the addict and to point out the evasions and covering up which many addicts indulge in. It may not suit everyone because it takes a strong evangelical approach to the problems.

In the 1970s, **behavioural psychotherapy** (see p. 95) was tried with alcoholics. They were trained to control their drinking, by recognizing when they were drunk, being shamed by being shown videotapes of themselves when drunk and occasionally being given nausea-inducing drugs which, it was hoped, would be an aversive stimulus. Aversion therapy has occasionally been used for smoking.

Neither group therapy nor behaviour therapy are very effective in combating addictions, and the factors which have been shown to be most effective are sheer personal will-power, a total change in lifestyle and education about the dangerous effects on health. It is essentially an attitude of mind which needs to be fostered.

Relaxation Techniques
Meditation (p. 98) and **yoga** (p. 99).

Vitamin and Mineral Treatment
Addictions respond to high dose vitamin C, 10 g daily for short periods reducing to 3 g daily long-term in cases of drug addiction.

Addiction to mild tranquillizers may be overcome with a high potency vitamin B complex (10 mg of each vitamin with relevant potencies of B_{12} and folic acid) 3 times daily plus 500 mg vitamin C daily.

Alcoholism should be treated with high potency vitamin B complex (10 mg of each vitamin) 3 times daily plus 15 mg zinc and 300 mg magnesium daily as amino acid chelates or as gluconates. Vitamin C (500 mg three times daily) is taken to detoxify the alcohol.

Tobacco smokers need to take extra vitamin B_{12} (10 μg), vitamin C (500 mg), vitamin B_1 (10 mg) and vitamin B_6 (10 mg) daily to overcome deficiencies induced by the components of tobacco smoke. Beta-carotene (13.5 mg daily) should be taken as a preventative against lung cancer.

Adenoids *see* TONSILS AND ADENOIDS

Alcoholism *see* ADDICTIONS

Alopecia *see* HAIR AND SCALP PROBLEMS

ALLERGY

An allergy is the inappropriate response by the body's immune system to a substance that is not normally harmful. The immune system is the highly complex defence mechanism which helps us to combat infection. It does this by identifying 'foreign bodies' and mobilizing the body's white cells to deal with them. In some people, the immune system wrongly identifies a non-toxic substance as an invader, and the body's white cells overreact and do more damage than the invader: the allergic response becomes a disease in itself. Common responses are ASTHMA, ECZEMA and HAYFEVER.

The substances which cause allergies are called *allergens*. Almost any substance can cause an allergy to someone somewhere in the world, but the most common allergens are **grass pollen, the faeces of the house dust mite, certain metals** (especially nickel), **some cosmetics, lanolin, some animal hair, insect bites and stings, some common drugs** (penicillin, aspirin), **some foodstuffs** (strawberries, eggs, shellfish), **some additives** (tartrazine, benzoic acid, sulphur dioxide), **chemicals in soap and washing powder.**

No-one knows why some people are allergic to substances to which the rest of us are immune. Allergies run in families, so there may be a hereditary element; it is also claimed that babies fed on cow's milk rather than breastmilk tend to develop allergies. There may be an emotional cause to the problem as well; anger, especially when suppressed, is a frequent contributing factor.

A growing number of practitioners now believe that many other conditions — including MIGRAINE, hyperactivity, DEPRESSION and CYSTITIS — may be the results of an allergy.

SYMPTOMS

- *In the chest* Dry cough, wheezing (the primary symptom of ASTHMA).
- *In the nose* Itchy, stuffy runny nose with sneezing. Different from a COLD as the symptoms last longer and the mucus is more watery and thinner.
- *In the eyes* Tears, itchiness and redness (both eyes affected).
- *In the skin* Possible rash as well as scaling and swelling (*see* DERMATITIS and NETTLE RASH).
- *In the ear* Possible partial or intermittent deafness, and sometimes a watery discharge.
- *In the digestive tract* CRAMPS, NAUSEA, vomiting, DIARRHOEA and/or a great deal of intestinal gas or 'wind'.

NB Very severe allergic reactions may produce a dramatic fall in blood pressure, irregularities of the heart beat and SHOCK.

ORTHODOX TREATMENT
Antihistamine drugs; steroids; patch tests; desensitizing injections.

ACUPUNCTURE
Constitutional acupuncture treatment may be needed to balance the organ energies so that they can handle allergenic substances effectively.

HEALING
Allergies tend to respond well to healing, although improvement can occasionally be slow.

HERBAL TREATMENT
All means of building up the general health and vitality of the body must be carried out, including remedies to improve liver and kidney function, to clear catarrh if that is present and to maintain good bowel action. A herbal practitioner will provide the individual remedies necessary, and will advise on diet.

HOMEOPATHY
Always consult a homeopath, as an allergy is usually only a symptom of a more general imbalance.

HYPNOTHERAPY
Hypnosis can reduce sensitivity by helping to control the symptoms by suppression of the body's auto-immune responses.

VITAMIN AND MINERAL TREATMENT
The effects of allergy may be reduced by vitamin C (500 mg 3 times daily on a short term basis, reducing to 500 mg once daily as a prophylactic.) Respiratory allergy (ASTHMA, HAYFEVER) needs vitamin B_6 (25 mg twice daily, reducing to 25 mg once daily).

See *also*: ASTHMA; DERMATITIS; ECZEMA; FOOD INTOLERANCE; NETTLE RASH.

Allergic rhinitis *see* HAYFEVER

Amenorrhoea *see* MENSTRUAL PROBLEMS

ANAEMIA

Anaemia is a reduction in the oxygen-carrying capacity of the blood. This can occur for a number of reasons:
- loss or a lack of iron because of heavy and/or prolonged periods, PILES, bleeding ULCERS or increased need due to pregnancy and periods of growth, resulting in iron-deficiency anaemia; responsible for 90 per cent of all cases of anaemia.
- loss/lack of other essential nutrients, such as vitamin B_{12} (resulting in what is called 'pernicious anaemia'); folic acid (common in pregnant women), which may prevent bone marrow from producing sufficient amount of blood, and vitamin C, which is necessary for the body to absorb iron.
- destruction of red blood cells, either because they are abnormally shaped (sickle cell anaemia and thalassaemia) or because the body wrongly 'recognizes' them as 'foreign' and attacks them.
- loss of a relatively large amount of blood through an accident or during surgery.

SYMPTOMS
Tiredness, BREATHLESSNESS and pallor, particularly inside the eyelids, the inside of the mouth and lips and the finger-nails. Severe cases will cause DIZZINESS, FAINTING, buzzing in the ears and, in the case of pernicious anaemia, 'pins and needles' in the hands and feet. Slowly developing anaemia may first show itself by a loss of appetite, HEADACHES, CONSTIPATION, irritability and difficulty in concentrating.

ORTHODOX TREATMENT
Iron or folic acid supplements; vitamin B_{12} injections (*pernicious anaemia*); blood transfusions; removal of spleen (rare).

SELF-HELP
When the body demands extra iron and folic acid — during periods of growth in children, in pregnancy and in old age — take supplements to avoid iron-deficiency anaemia (see VITAMIN AND MINERAL DEFICIENCY)

HERBAL TREATMENT
Drink nettle tea or an infusion of equal quantities of nettles, dandelion leaves and finely chopped roots, comfrey leaves and vervain. Nettles can also be cooked as a vegetable, rather like spinach.

A daily salad should include young dandelion leaves, parsley, watercress, fresh chickweed and any other fresh culinary herbs—chives, lovage or fennel. Fruits should include elder-berries in season, either as a syrup or stewed with apples and blackberries.

HOMEOPATHY
To help the body use the various supplements, homeopathic remedies may be given, especially in the form of tissue salts (see p. 79).

NATUROPATHY
To ensure that the body gets enough iron, folic acid and vitamin B_{12}—eat enough of the following rich sources:
- *Iron*: liver, black pudding, kidney, bread and other cereals, pulses, leafy greens, dried apricots, molasses, beef, other dried fruits.
- *Folic acid*: leafy greens, liver, wheatgerm, unpasteurized milk, peanuts, almonds, tomato purée, beef and yeast extract, brewer's yeast.
- *Vitamin B_{12}*: all foods of animal origin (especially offal). Of special importance to organs are fortified non-animal foods, eg many brands of yeast extracts, some breakfast cereals.

Much folic acid is lost in cooking water; the latter should be added to soups and stock, and salads of leafy greens should be eaten. Iron absorption is helped by eating foods rich in vitamin C at the same meal—eg a salad with an omelette, an orange with an egg sandwich. Iron absorption is also hindered by coffee, strong tea, cola.

VITAMIN AND MINERAL TREATMENT
The following are in addition to any supplements

Iron-deficiency anaemia is treated with 25 mg elemental iron 3 times daily, 2 mg of copper daily and 100 mg vitamin C with each dose of iron.

Anaemias due to the destruction of red blood cells: in babies, 10–30 iu vitamin E in water-soluble form daily; in adults, up to 600 iu vitamin E daily as oil, or 200 iu in water-soluble form, daily.

ANGINA PECTORIS

'Angina' is a pain behind the breastbone, which may radiate into the left shoulder and arm, or up the neck into the jaws. It is frequently excruciating, but may also be experienced as 'indigestion'. It is due to the narrowing or obstruction of one or more of the coronary arteries (*see* ATHEROSCLEROSIS) and the subsequent reduction in blood supply to the heart muscle. The pain lasts for only a few minutes and then, after a short rest, the person can carry on normally. However, always remember that it is an acute symptom of HEART DISEASE.

ORTHODOX TREATMENT
Glyceryl trinitrate; beta blockers; coronary bypass surgery.

SELF-HELP
See HEART DISEASE.

ACUPUNCTURE
Spasm is reduced by treating the vessels of Conception (midline of the abdomen), Spleen/Pancreas and Pericardium (the membrane covering the heart). In some, a point on the Heart meridian is also used.

As a first aid measure, massage the front of the wrist of either hand, especially on any point that is painful (on the pathways of the Heart, Pericardium or Lung), usually where the pulse is taken. Gentle pressure may also be applied to points 1 and 2 (see pp. 104–5).

HERBAL TREATMENT
Consult a herbal practitioner. Substitute herbal tisanes such as chamomile, lime-blossom or rosemary in place of coffee or tea. Hawthorn may also be beneficial (*see* HEART DISEASE). Ginseng may have a tonic effect on the heart.

HOMEOPATHY
Consult a homeopath. First aid remedies include:
- *Aconite* When the pain is accompanied by great fear.
- *Cactus grandiflora* For the classical symptoms of a tight band round the chest, with a cold, sweaty forehead.
- *Glanoine* When the main feature is a violent throbbing as if the heart would burst open, with cold, sweaty limbs.
- *Spigelia* When there are marked palpitations, with shooting, stabbing or darting pains down to the left elbow; especially if the attack comes on after smoking or drinking.

HYPNOTHERAPY
Hypnosis can relieve the pain and, in some people, may have even deeper effects.

MANIPULATIVE THERAPIES
Treatment to the mid-dorsal area of the spine and to the joints and muscles of the rib cage can be of considerable help. By improving the flexibility of the rib cage and the vertebral joints attached to it, it is possible to improve breathing and thereby increase the amount of oxygen in the blood. Improvements in posture can also be beneficial.

NATUROPATHY
Overexertion and trying to drive yourself through the pain barrier should be avoided. Give up smoking, if you haven't already. Gentle, vigorous (but not violent) exercise that is stopped

short of the point where the anginal chest pain comes on can benefit the heart.

RELAXATION TECHNIQUES
Autogenics (p. 97) and **meditation** (p. 98).

VITAMIN AND MINERAL TREATMENT
This is treated with high doses of vitamin E (800 iu or more, depending on response). In addition, lecithin granules—5 ml/1 tsp with each meal—plus 3 daily capsules of concentrated fish oils and magnesium will complement the action of the vitamin E.

Ankylosing spondylitis *see* ARTHRITIS

ANOREXIA NERVOSA

Anorexia simply means loss of appetite. This can be caused by a variety of problems (*see* APPETITE LOSS), but anorexia nervosa, is a common symptom of anxiety neurosis. It is a serious disease whose main symptom is an abhorrence of food and an absolute rejection of eating sufficient quantities to maintain normal bodily functions.

This often results in long-term damage to the digestive system. Girls, particularly, run the risk of becoming infertile. Anorexia can sometimes be fatal.

CAUSES OF ANOREXIA
Although emaciated, sufferers are normally obsessed with the idea that they are fat. This can result from excessive teasing by their peers or parents. The children often display great fear at the prospect of growing up and with young girls there is frequently a very difficult mother/daughter relationship. The girls almost always suffer from AMENORRHEA and as a forerunner to the disease there is often a history of emotional trauma.

Divorce or death of a parent or loss of a sibling can often be the precipitating factors.

All forms of treatment are normally rejected by the anorexic and no amount of common sense or persuasion will force them to change their mental image of how they look. The malign influence of the media, especially upon young girls, cannot be over-emphasized here. The body image created by glamorous advertisements and fashion features reinforce the belief that being excessively thin is a passport to a better world.

ORTHODOX TREATMENT
Psychotherapy.

HEALING
Anorexia nervosa and bulimia tend to respond more to self-healing than the traditional laying-on of hands.

HYPNOTHERAPY
Hypnosis should be able to modify the anorexic's attitude to eating, especially things like an irrational revulsion when presented with food.

NATUROPATHY
After psychotherapy, nutritional rehabilitation will be necessary. Gradually introduce a wholefood diet with a range of supplements recommended by an experienced naturopath.

PSYCHOTHERAPY
Anorexics must be treated by an experienced and sympathetic child psychiatrist. Psychotherapy usually centres on deep issues of identity, freedom and sexuality. The work can be done individually or with the anorexic and their family. It is important to perceive anorexia not as an illness that can be taken away, but as a symptom of a misdirected effort to solve conflict.

RELAXATION TECHNIQUES
Meditation (p. 98) and **yoga** (p. 99).

VITAMIN AND MINERAL TREATMENT
For both anorexia and bulimia: high doses of zinc (50 mg 3 times daily) until sense of taste and smell return. Then reduce zinc intake to 15 mg 3 times daily until appetite returns to normal.

Bulimia nervosa

Bulimia is also an eating disorder. Sufferers alternatively diet and binge, sometimes eating more than enough for six people, then purging themselves with laxatives or emetics and going back to their diet.

It is not always easy to spot them: they are usually older than anorexics (mid 20s is the usual age); they are independent of home; they are not emaciated like anorexics; and their 'diet' is usually socially acceptable.

Bulimia is prompted by much the same things as anorexia: poor self image, demands from over ambitious parents, lack of attention. There is often considerable underlying depression and anxiety.

Treatment, once the bulimic has admitted the problem, is usually by psychotherapy. **Behavioural therapy** (p. 95) is often used initially, and **cognitive therapy** (pp. 95–6) shows good results.

ANXIETY

(See *also* DEPRESSION and TENSION.)

A person with an anxiety neurosis experiences fears and anxieties out of all proportion to reality.

That there is some inherited tendency towards anxiety neurosis, but emotionally traumatic experiences during childhood are the most common causes.

General anxiety neurosis may turn into some form of PHOBIA when this anxiety is psychologically linked directly to one event—for example, an acute fear of flying.

SYMPTOMS

Constant anticipation that something unpleasant is going to happen; this is usually accompanied by feelings of tension (both emotional and physical), sweating and a speeding-up of the heart rate.

Anxiety makes decision-making difficult, and hyperactivity, irritability, restlessness and obsessional fears about serious illness are often observed. APPETITE LOSS, disturbed sleep patterns and weight loss are frequent. Hyperventilation (overbreathing) commonly occurs and sufferers show a marked increase in perspiration.

ORTHODOX TREATMENT

Counselling; tranquillizers; sleeping pills; antidepressants.

ACUPUNCTURE

General acupuncture treatment aims to balance the energies, mostly involving those of the large intestine, liver and water organs, which are traditionally associated with the emotion of fear.

Acupressure on certain points on the pathway of pericardium — eg point 3 (see pp. 104–5) about halfway between the wrist and the elbow on the inside of the arm, or on the nail point 5 may help. Relaxation can be induced by gentle massage of point 4, in the web between the thumb and the index finger.

ALEXANDER TECHNIQUE

This can help reduce anxiety by improving posture.

HERBAL TREATMENT

Teas that combine a number of herbs which help to soothe irritated, jangled feelings, can be taken occasionally during the day as well as at bedtime.

An infusion of balm will be relaxing and will ease colic and palpitations of nervous origins, while vervain taken 2 or 3 times daily will relieve gloom and depression.

Valerian has long been used for its sedative effect on nerves, as has skullcap. These are more easily taken in the form of anti-spasmodic tincture than as infusion; 2.5–5 ml/$\frac{1}{2}$–1 tsp in a little warm water sweetened with honey will quickly give comfort.

See also the decoction described under APPETITE LOSS; reinforce this with 1 cup of peppermint tea daily.

HOMEOPATHY

Those suffering chronic anxiety should

consult a homeopath. For acute, short-lived anxiety:

- *Aconite* Intense feeling of fear, sudden onset after a fright.
- *Gelsemium* Stage fright with weak, trembly feeling in legs.
- *Argentum nitricum* feeling of butterflies in stomach with diarrhoea and craving for sweet things.
- *Arsenicum album* very restless, exhausted, fussy, complains of the cold excessively.
- *Pulsatilla* hot-blooded, very emotional, bursts into tears over nothing.

HYPNOTHERAPY
Hypnosis can reduce anxiety levels and modify reactions to a stress-creating situation.

MANIPULATIVE THERAPIES
Deep neuromuscular massage, correction of posture and manipulative techniques can help relieve some of the physical aspects of stress.

MASSAGE
Massage, especially with essential oils, can be greatly beneficial. Visit a masseur or ask a friend to massage gently the muscles of the neck, shoulders and back to help reduce tension and encourage feelings of well-being.

PSYCHOTHERAPIES
Anxiety neurosis is well treated by psychotherapy. Learning to understand the roots of the problem and explaining interpersonal and family relationships, together with improvement of self-image, self-confidence and self-esteem, are all factors that will be dealt with by a psychotherapist. Coming to terms with repressed anger and aggression and learning to use these powerful emotions positively will form part of the treatment.

RELAXATION TECHNIQUES
Meditation (p. 98), **yoga** (p. 99) and **autogenics** (p. 97).

VITAMIN AND MINERAL TREATMENT
High-potency vitamin B complex (up to 50 mg), 2 or 3 times daily, reducing gradually to one daily plus vitamin C (200 mg) with each meal.

Arteriosclerosis *see* ATHEROSCLEROSIS

APPETITE LOSS

Most appetite loss (except for ANOREXIA NERVOSA) is the result of illness: MOUTH ULCERS, tooth problems, DIGESTIVE DISORDERS, acute infection, exhaustion for example. It is a common result of high FEVER and any condition which causes NAUSEA and vomiting; it can also be the side-effect of drug therapy.

During acute illness, appetite loss is the body's natural response and should be respected as such.

HERBAL TREATMENT
When symptoms have subsided, a decoction of equal parts gentian root, poplar bark, meadowsweet herb and centaury herb can be taken in doses of 45–60 ml/3–4 tbsps 2 or 3 times daily. An infusion of sweet cecily herb in 45–60 ml/3–4 tbsp doses before breakfast and at bedtime will restore appetite and act as a tonic.

For emotional problems, reinforce the above with a cupful of peppermint tea each day and nerve remedies as for ANXIETY.

HOMEOPATHY
In an acute situation, consider:

- *Lycopodium* When hunger is present, but the patient is full up after a mouthful or two.
- *Pulsatilla* With lack of thirst and an aversion to fatty, rich food.
- *Lignatia* For complete loss of appetite from grief or hysteria.
- *Rhus tox* For complete loss of appetite.

NATUROPATHY
Although the loss of appetite is not caused by food, it may lead to a vicious

circle of poor nutrition. While the underlying cause is tackled, foods with concentrated nutritional value can be stressed: foods with lots of calories, vitamins and minerals in little bulk. Fatty foods and large portions will be rejected. Go for freshly made fruit and vegetable juices; puréed soups (good if chewing is a problem) made from briefly cooked ingredients; and wheatgerm, yoghurt and peanut butter (although this is oily). Small frequent meals are better than the normal three times a day.

Take a multivitiamin/mineral supplement as an insurance against deficiency.

Vitamin and Mineral Treatment

Vitamin B_{12}, one 10 mg tablet half an hour before meals with a glass of water, together with 15 mg zinc chelate.

For more extreme cases see ANOREXIA NERVOSA.

Arteriosclerosis *see* ATHEROSCLEROSIS

Arthritis

There are many types of arthritis — over 200, in fact — but all of them involve some sort of malfunction of a joint or joints and, usually, pain and swelling.

Osteoarthritis

This is the degenerative 'wear and tear' variety of arthritis, in which the cartilage covering the bones in a joint becomes eroded and the once-smooth surface becomes rough, resulting in friction. The tendons, ligaments and muscles holding the joint together become weaker, and the joint itself becomes deformed, painful and stiff.

Osteoarthritis is a natural result of ageing — although it does run in families and is much more common in women than men. It can occur earlier in those who joints have been deformed at birth or have been injured since, or because of excessive stress on joints.

Rheumatoid Arthritis

In this type of inflammatory arthritis, the synovial membrane lining the joint cavity becomes inflamed and thickened, and develops folds. It spreads over the cartilage and, together with enzymes in the synovial fluid, virtually eats away the bone underneath. The joints become unstable, painful and swollen, and then greatly deformed. The body as whole also suffers, the person feeling weak, tired, feverish and generally ill, with a loss of appetite.

Gout

Gout results when the body produces too much of the waste product *uric acid* or the kidneys are unable to excrete it properly. It crystallizes into needle-like formations that settle in joints (producing arthritis), the kidneys (producing stones) and/or the outer ear (producing nodules).

The person will be shivery and feverish and then a joint (usually the one in the big toe) will become red, swollen and extremely painful.

Ankylosing Spondylitis (AS)

This affects certain joints of the spine (*see* BACK PAIN) which become inflamed and then stiff, rigid and fused together. It begins in the lower back, with pain and aching felt in the thighs, buttocks and small of the back. Sometimes this is the only sign of the disease and it then disappears, but the symptoms may worsen, and the person becomes generally unwell. As the inflammation dies down, healing around the vertebrae takes place and bone develops on either side of the affected joints. This results in stiffness and fusing of the spine, which is usually quite painless and, if confined to the lower back, will cause virtually no limitation of movement. Unfortunately, sometimes the whole of the spine may become rigid and bent, and the effects on the hips may also be quite disabling. If the joints between the ribs and spine are affected, there will be severe breathing problems as the expansion of the chest wall is limited. Postural deformities are common.

Systemic Lupus Erythematosus (SLE)

SLE is a malfunction of the body's immune system. For some reason, the body produces antibodies that act against itself. They can find their way to the skin, causing rashes; can clog blood vessels, or can be deposited in the joints, lungs, heart, kidney and brain, where inflammation can then develop.

SLE has many features but one of the most common is painful and inflamed joints and tendons. However, unlike rheumatoid arthritis, which it can mimic, the joint disease of SLE is not a crippling one—it rarely results in permanent damage.

Orthodox Treatment

Anti-inflammatory drugs; steroids; immuno-suppressive drugs; surgery.

Self-help

- *Exercise* is important. Joints must be used or else they will become immobile. In general, it is better to perform any sort of activity (eg gardening, walking) with short rests in between, and to ensure that all your joints go through their full range of movement at least twice a day. Swimming is particularly good.
- *Learn simple techniques for protecting your joints and avoiding pain.* These can include such things as how to sit down and get up correctly, how to lift and carry things.
- *Lose weight (see* OBESITY), if you need to; your weight-bearing joints will be under less stress.

Acupuncture

Arthritis can be seen as the blockage of energy brought about by excesses of wind, cold or dampness and by poor nutrition. Local symptoms are a reflection of the obstructed Chi or of sluggish blood. Acupuncture treatment is based on the correct analysis of the cause of the arthritis, and aims to open up the pathways so as to permit the flow of Chi and blood.

Acupressure on points 6, 7, 8, 9 can relieve pain in arms, shoulders and fingers, and on points 13, 14, 15, 16 can help pelvis, hips and lower limbs. General pressure points for arthritis that are worth trying are 17, 18 and 19 (see pp. 104–5).

Herbal Treatment

Celery-seed tablets are useful for their anti-rheumatic alkaline properties, as well as for being antiseptic, and can be beneficial when rheumatoid arthritis leads to depression. Parsley tea can be taken for its diuretic effect, helping to eliminate acids and toxins from the body. To make it, add 5 ml/1 tsp chopped parsley to a teacupful of boiling water; cover and leave to cool. Strain and drink the liquid at intervals during the day, until a cupful has been drunk.

Extract of willow and primula combined with yeast extracts is a powerful anti-inflammatory formula for the treatment of arthritis and rheumatism, and has none of the serious side-effects of modern non-steroidal drugs even when used over a very long period.

Aloe vera barbadensis juice taken internally has given some people relief.

Eating two or three fresh leaves of the feverfew shrub not only relieves many headaches but, in a large percentage, also alleviates joint pain.

Many herbs are used in liniments, which are massaged throughly into joints and muscles to stimulate circulation, relax and tone stiff muscles and help bring about greater mobility of joints. Aloe vera barbadensis is particularly useful; rub on fresh gel, or make a pulp from ground leaves to be heated and packed in a muslin bag and applied to painful joints.

Homeopathy

Consult a homeopath for chronic cases. In acute cases, the following can be considered:

- *Arnica* after injury.
- *Bryonia alba* When pains are worse in warmth and during the slightest movement, and better during pressure and cold applications.
- *Pulsatilla* where pains flit from joint to joint, and the patient is thirstless and feels worse in a stuffy room.
- *Rhus toxicodendron* When pains are

worse after rest, during first motion and in cold, damp weather, and better during continued motion.

MANIPULATIVE THERAPIES
Osteopathy and chiropractic have a great deal to offer. The maintenance of good posture and the restoration of maximum possible movement to affect joints are all of benefit, both in the relief of pain and discomfort and in the long-term course of the illness.

However, manipulative therapies should *not* be used when inflammation is present, as in rheumatoid arthritis, SLE and AS.

MASSAGE
A soothing massage, using 15 drops of oil containing rosemary, lavender and marigold combined with 50 ml of almond oil, will alleviate pain. Pressure point massage can be carried out on relevant key points.

A poultice of pounded fresh ginger and be applied to painful areas.

NATUROPATHY
Diet: A vegetarian diet excluding refined carbohydrates may prove beneficial. Some people (especially those with rheumatoid arthritis) may need to exclude milk products, citrus fruits and other possible allergenic foods.
Hydrotherapy: General stiffness and muscular pain may be eased by Epsom salts baths: dissolve 3–4 tbsp of commercial Epsom salts in a bath of hot water; soak for 20 minutes. Swelling and inflammation of individual joints may be relieved by cold compresses.

VITAMIN AND MINERAL TREATMENT
Rheumatoid arthritis may respond to calcium pantothenate with regime of 500 mg daily for 2 days; 1,000 mg for 3 days; 1500 mg for 4 days; and 200 mg a day after that for 2 months or until pain is relieved. Then daily intake should be reduced to the minimum needed to maintain relief.

Rheumatoid and *osteoarthritis* may also respond to vitamin C (4000 mg daily) in divided doses; high doses (3–6 g daily) if nicotinamide or nicotinic acid.

As a preventative supplementary intake try 100 mg calcium pantothenate, 500 mg vitamin C and 100 mg nicotinamide daily.

ASTHMA

See *also* ALLERGY; FOOD INTOLERANCE

Asthma attacks are paroxysms of breathlessness and wheezing. The main difficulty is breathing out. This is because spasms in the muscles surrounding the bronchi (small airways in the lungs) constrict the outward passage of stale air. The effort of pushing it out produces the characteristic wheeze. The muscular spasms (together with increased mucus) are brought on by histamine produced by the body's immune system during an allergic response (see ALLERGY). Therefore any kind of allergen can precipitate an asthma attack. One of the most virulent is the faeces of the house dust mite.

Childhood asthma occurs in allergic individuals. There is frequently a family history of allergy and the child may also suffer from other allergic responses such as ECZEMA and HAYFEVER.

In some childhood asthmatics, food and food additives are an important factor. Fish, eggs, dairy produce, yeasts and wheat are common foods which can trigger an asthma attack; artificial colourings, flavourings and preservatives have all been reported to have similar effects.

Late-onset asthma is not normally an allergic response to the environment, but is triggered by something within the body.

As well as exposure to an allergen, there are a number of other things that can bring on an attack:
- emotional stress and anxiety.
- sudden vigorous exercise.
- chest infections.
- sudden changes in breathing patterns—eg laughing.

- irritants such as paint fumes and tobacco smoke and chemicals.
- sudden changes in temperature.
- chemical sensitivity to metabisulphites or sulphur dioxide gas.

SYMPTOMS

The main symptom is the wheeze as the sufferer tries to breathe out; there will also be a cough, tightness in the chest, shortage of breath, rapid breathing, FATIGUE, and severe distress in some cases.

ORTHODOX TREATMENT

Bronchodilator drugs; *disodium cromoglycate* (Intal); steroids.

SELF-HELP

- **Turn off central heating** in asthmatics bedroom. (It creates currents of air that circulate allergen particles which are inhaled by the sleeping occupant.)
- **Don't smoke** if you are asthmatic; don't allow smoking in the home if any member of the family suffers from asthma.
- **Avoid furry** pets and cage birds.
- **Always take medication** as prescribed, as much of this is preventitive and will be useless if an attack occurs.
- **Take up a sport** which will exercise and strengthen the lungs. Swimming is excellent for the development of the ribcage and the secondary muscles of respiration.
- **Encourage children** to take up a wind instrument, to establish good breathing habits.

See also self help under ALLERGY.

ACUPUNCTURE

Bronchial asthma is associated with the energies of the Lungs, Spleen and Kidneys. When wind and cold invade the lungs, Chi energy is prevented from making its natural journey downwards because of the formation of phlegm and dampness in the lungs. Acupuncture treatment is aimed at relieving wheezing by encouraging the 'stuck' energy to descend. Eventually phlegm has to be eliminated, and correct nutrition is one of the essentials in ensuring an unobstructed flow of lung Chi.

Acupressure during acute attacks, on points 4, 18, 20–23 (see pp. 104–5) will help.

ALEXANDER TECHNIQUE

This is an effective therapy for improving breathing.

HERBAL TREATMENT

Comprehensive treatment is necessary as so many factors can affect asthma. Consult a herbal practitioner.

HOMEOPATHY

Always consult a homeopath. The following acute remedies should be used only until trained medical help arrives:
- *Arsenicum album* Great restlessness and exhaustion, usually worse between midnight and 2 A.M., thirsty for small sips of warm fluids.
- *Ipecachuana* Nausea and loud rattly cough.
- *Kali carbonicum* Attacks occur between 3 and 5 A.M.
- *Aconite* After exposure to cold, dry wind, accompanied by great fear.

MANIPULATIVE THERAPIES

This can be of exceptional value to asthma sufferers. The early-onset asthmatic is liable to develop curvatures of the spine and a pigeon-tipped chest as a result of years of breathing difficulties. Manipulative treatment can improve the mobility of the rib cage and spine, and can prevent or correct postural changes. A therapist can also help enormously by teaching a patient correct breathing exercises.

MASSAGE

Massage to the back and neck will help to release muscular tensions and improve difficult breathing.

NATUROPATHY

Diet: Introduce wholefood diet that excludes cows' milk products and sugar. For **catarrhal asthma**, increase fresh fruit and vegetable intake. Garlic (fresh or as tablets) and onions will help reduce mucus. **Nervous asthma** without expectoration may require more wholegrain produce and non-dairy protein.

Heat/Cold Treatment: Hot and cold fomentations to the chest and back will promote lung function.

PSYCHOTHERAPIES

There is often a psychosomatic component to asthma, and psychotherapy will help to expose the deep-seated problems that may beset the asthma sufferer. These can be strongly associated with difficult child/parent relationships, deep feelings of insecurity and attention-seeking mechanisms.

VITAMIN AND MINERAL TREATMENT
See ALLERGY

ATHEROSCLEROSIS

Atherosclerosis occurs when atheroma, a waxy, cheese-like substance, and fibrous tissue are deposited in the walls of arteries. This can happen in all the large and medium-sized arteries, and particularly in the coronary arteries that supply the heart muscle and in the cerebral arteries that supply the brain. The gradual increase of these fatty deposits obstructs the blood flow, causing a rise in BLOOD PRESSURE and an increase in the possibility of blood clots forming.

THE CAUSES OF ATHEROSCLEROSIS
Cigarette smoking is one of the greatest potential factors in the development of this condition.
Alcohol in excessive quantities will raise the level of fats in the blood, although a very small intake—a small glass daily—does seem to have some protective effect.
Diet is the fundamental key to both prevention and treatment of atherosclerosis. A diet high in saturated (mainly animal) fats and low in dietary fibre has been strongly implicated in its development.

Lack of exercise is another common factor causing this condition.
High blood pressure can damage the walls of blood vessels, encouraging the development of atherosclerosis.

In the USA alone, it is estimated that the cost of treating atherosclerosis is in the region of $56 million per year. Atherosclerosis of the coronary arteries may account for over 20% of all deaths in the Western world.

THE EFFECTS OF ATHEROSCLEROSIS
● *When the arteries of the limbs* are involved, there will be a reduction in the peripheral circulation, causing pain and swelling in the limbs.
● *In the arteries of the legs* atherosclerosis can lead to a condition known as *intermittent claudication*: in this, extreme pain in the calf muscles is apparent during even the slightest physical effort.
● *In the coronary arteries*, atherosclerosis will gradually lead to ischaemic heart disease, which in turn will develop into heart failure.
● *If the blockage* of a coronary artery occurs suddenly a heart attack will occur.
● *In the small arteries of the brain* arterial narrowing or a clot will produce a stroke.

ORTHODOX TREATMENT
Anti-coagulant drugs; surgery.

SELF-HELP
See HEART DISEASE.

HERBAL TREATMENT
This condition requires professional treatment. However, raw and cooked garlic and onions can reduce blood levels of cholesterol, yarrow herb lessens the risk of blood clots forming, and hawthorn berries may reduce the amount of atheroma in the arteries.

NATUROPATHY
All dietary fibre is of benefit to the body, but the water-soluble type found

in oats and pulses has the distinct advantage of reducing excess cholesterol. Ginger also has a specific effect on reducing cholesterol levels, and it also inhibits blood platelets from sticking together to form clots. Ginger can be used as a condiment and added to many dishes.

See HEART DISEASE for general advice on diet.

VITAMINS AND MINERALS
Sufferers of atherosclerosis should take 5 ml/1 tsp of lecithin granules with each meal. In addition, they should take 400 iu vitamin E twice daily, up to 3 g vitamin C daily and 7500 iu vitamin A daily.

ARTERIOSCLEROSIS
The term *arteriosclerosis* is frequently but wrongly used to describe atherosclerosis. In fact, arteriosclerosis—commonly called 'hardening of the arteries'—is a normal process of ageing, in which degenerative changes in the walls of the arteries leads to them becoming hardened and thickened due to deposits of calcium and the effects of long-standing high blood pressure. There is no proven treatment for this condition.

Athlete's foot *see* RINGWORM

B

BACK PAIN

Each year, thousands of patients parade their bad backs through osteopath's rooms throughout the country. They nearly all have two things in common: fear and ignorance.

Fear for their future, since their minds are filled with old folk-tales, half-truths and misunderstood information from other practitioners, *to say nothing of the mental picture of the wheelchair in which they confidently expect to end their days.*

Ignorance of even the most basic knowledge of their own bodies and, in particular, the spine. For some reason, the spine has become imbued with almost as much mystique as the soul and the osteopath with the legendary powers of Merlin.

There is nothing magical or mystical about your back or the right treatment for your problem. The spine is a mechanical structure and the osteopath a good mechanic.

Half the population have had back pain.
More than 10% of the population has back ache all the time.

THE CAUSES OF BACK PAIN
- *A damaged or worn disc* can bulge at the edges when under extreme pressure. This can squeeze against the posterior ligaments of the spine, which are pain-sensitive.
- *Pressure on a nerve root* causes acute pain which is also the fault of a degenerative disc. The wall of the disc becomes damaged and allows the soft jelly in the centre to bulge out and cause direct pressure on the nerve. This results in the severe pain, often travelling down the legs, that is called *sciatica*, as well as pins and needles, and loss of sensation, reflexes and muscle strength.
- *Vertebral dislocation* resulting in spondylolisthesis (see below).
- *Inflamed joints* The rear portions of the vertebrae form the 110 joints, or articulating surfaces, of the spine. As with any joint, the membrane that links these surfaces is highly sensitive and can become swollen and inflamed to cause pain.
- *Muscle spasm*, produced by bad posture, injury or strain, can in itself cause pain. If there is also disc damage, the vice-like pressure of contracted muscle will cause even more compression of the disc and subsequent ligament pain as well.

Back pain can also be a symptom of other disorders: gynaecological problems, DIGESTIVE DISORDERS, GALLSTONES, kidney disease, tumours, even certain kinds of CANCER. Therefore, it is *vital* that a detailed medical history is taken before any treatment is begun. Lumbago is a loose term used to describe any low back pain.

ORTHODOX TREATMENT
Bedrest, traction, corsets, drugs, injections, physiotherapy; surgery.

SELF-HELP
● Train yourself, and be ever vigilant, to lift and carry things properly as well as sit and stand in such a way that you do not put undue strain on your back.
● Choose a firm, supportive bed, and not one that sags and pulls your spine out of position.
● Keep your weight down; this will reduce the strain on your back.
● Keep active, even if you do not follow a full exercise programme, to ensure that those joints remain in good working order (see **Positive health/Back Pack** pp. 53–9).
● Consult a properly qualified osteopath or chiropractor immediately. If you do not receive help speedily, then your acute back pain could become chronic back pain.

ACUPUNCTURE
The acupuncturist must make an analysis of the reasons for the back pain before initiating treatment accordingly. This may involve the major meridian of the back (known as the 'Governor') as well as the Bladder meridians alongside. Treatment may be carried out with needles, moxibustion or cupping (see **Acupuncture** pp. 66–8).

Acupressure can be carried out by sufferers themselves on Bladder point 17 on the outside of the foot below the ankle. For lumbago, try pressure on the side of the leg at 24, the side of the lower leg at 25, and any point on the low back that is painful but feels good on pressure (see p. 102–3).

ALEXANDER TECHNIQUE
This is a suitable treatment, particularly for prevention.

HEALING
Back pain is probably the most common ailment to be treated by healers, who can often relieve the pain or cure the condition.

MANIPULATIVE THERAPIES
It is in the treatment of back pain that the osteopath and chiropractor come into their own. The manipulator's highly developed sense of touch and intimate knowledge of the structure and function of the spine enable them to take a broader view of back problems.

X-rays are frequently a vital aid to correct diagnosis, and unlike orthodox doctors, the osteopath and chiropractor will always X-ray the spine when the person is *standing*. This enables small measurements to be made of abnormalities in posture that would not appear on X-rays taken with the person lying down.

Manipulation to correct small disturbances in the position of the vertebrae and to relieve pressure on nerve roots and surrounding tissue is only part of the osteopath's treatment. Soft-tissue massage, remedial exercises and advice on posture, working positions, lifestyle and nutrition all form part of the holistic approach to the treatment of back pain.

It is essential for the osteopath or chiropractor to take a detailed medical history of the patient in order to establish exactly how the problem began, which factors aggravate it and which alleviate the discomfort. An examination of the entire body is vital since a simple problem—such as an untreated corn that affects the way the patient walks, and in turn changes the posture and weight distribution—can be a cause of chronic backache. In this situation, no amount of manipulative treatment will relieve the condition unless the underlying cause is identified and dealt with.

To achieve the best results, combine manipulation with one or more of the other therapies, particularly relaxation and psychotherapy, where appropriate.

MASSAGE

For back pain that does not arise from an abnormality of the spine or other parts, massage and acupressure on pressure points can be used to soothe away tension. Areas to concentrate on are the back, legs, feet and stomach. Exercises will be recommended to strengthen the back and stomach.

NATUROPATHY

Pain and stiffness may be relieved by the application of hot and cold fomentations to the affected areas: apply a hot fomentation for 3 minutes, followed by a cold one for 1 minute, and repeat this routine for 20–30 minutes, at least once daily.

Sleep and rest on a reasonably firm, flat surface to prevent undue stress and pressure on affected joints. (Put a board under your mattress or put the mattress on the floor.) Stiffness may be relieved by gentle exercise, but pain is a warning that you should stop.

PSYCHOTHERAPIES

Psychosomatic factors can play a major part in back pain, but it is sometimes difficult to establish whether chronic pain causes the psychological disturbances or vice versa.

However, it is true that back pain can be a psychosomatic way of avoiding unpleasant stress and unwanted obligations and responsibilities. Some people have a vested interest in maintaining their back pain.

In addition, back pain is sometimes an overt expression of deeply repressed anger and frustration, which causes postural changes and alters the 'body image' — eg clenched jaws, hunched shoulders, stiff neck, belligerent posture.

In all these situations, psychotherapy — particularly **bioenergetics**, **Gestalt** and group therapy (see **Psychotherapy** p. 92) — can be very useful in helping the sufferer understand and deal with the roots of the problem.

SPONDYLOLISTHESIS

This is a condition in which one vertebra slides forward on the vertebra beneath it, frequently causing chronic back pain. The most common is when the last vertebra slips forward on the top of the tail bone (sacrum). There are various causes of this which range from congenital defect to traumatic injury, degenerative disease and other bone diseases such as tuberculosis or cancer.

SYMPTOMS

Pain which radiates into the hips, thighs and sometimes into the feet; pain in the sacroiliac joints is common and most of the pain is the area of the low back. There is often muscle spasm and considerable stiffness of the lower part of the back. The lumbar lordosis (*see* POSTURE PROBLEMS) is usually accentuated and there is sometimes an actual depression above the sacrum which can be felt.

TREATMENT

As long as there is no bone disease, manipulative therapy can be useful in all but the most severe cases. Mobilization to improve the flexion of the lumbar spine, corrective exercises to improve posture, particularly the back flattening exercises (see **Positive Health/Back Pack** pp. 53–9) together with the appropriate massage to the muscles in spasm will all help.

Baldness *see* HAIR AND SCALP PROBLEMS

BEDSORES

Bedsores are deep ULCERS caused by pressure over bony areas of the body restricting circulation and leading to the death of the cells in the overlying tissue. They are most commonly found on the heels, buttocks, hips, sacrum and shoulder blade. They always occur during periods of prolonged bed rest and so particularly afflict the comatose, paraplegic or bedridden elderly.

ORTHODOX TREATMENT
Antibiotic dressing and irritant drugs; surgery.

SELF-HELP
Bedsores are totally preventable.
- Keep the pressure points off the surface of the mattress by using pillows to plug the gaps between bed and ankles etc so that the body is supported but pressure on sensitive areas relieved.
- Lamb's wool fleeces (for the patient to lie on) minimize bedsores.
- Turn the patient regularly. (If you are doing this to a bedbound person at home, ask your doctor or visiting nurse to show you how to do it properly.)
- Give frequent alcohol rubs to stimulate the circulation and prevent the blood vessels from closing up. (Use rubbing alcohol, available from chemist, and cotton wool.)

HERBAL TREATMENT
Calendula cream and comfrey ointment can be used externally. Buckwheat tea and limeflower tea are also helpful.

HOMEOPATHY
Apply *hypericum* oil locally. Internally, try
- *Arnica* After injury and bruising.
- *Crotalus horridus* Where there is a marked sloughing of skin
- *Lachesis* Where surrounded by dark purple skin and accompanied by marked pain.
- *Sulphur* In chronic cases.

MASSAGE
Effleurage (see p. 87) will encourage better healing.

NATUROPATHY
Diet: Increase the quality of nutrition, especially protein from wholegrains and pulses.

Treatment: Make a honey dressing (honey on lint or gauze) for the sores.

VITAMIN AND MINERAL TREATMENT
Take Vitamin C (500 mg 2 times daily) and vitamin E (100 iu daily) to promote cell growth and improve circulation. A supplement of vitamin A and the B complex will also help.

BEDWETTING

(NOCTURNAL ENURESIS)

This is more common in boys than girls. Most children have grown out of bedwetting by the time they are four, but for some this distressing problem can continue or recur through to adolescence at which time it nearly always resolves itself. Bedwetting is rarely caused by disease or deficiency in the urinary system but in persistent cases medical help should be sought to rule out the possibilities. The problem is nearly always the result of stress or some form of behavioural disturbance.

Occasionally postural or muscular problems in the lower back can cause irritation to the nerves which supply the bladder.

ORTHODOX TREATMENT
Counselling; psychotherapy.

SELF-HELP
- Make sure the child passes urine before going to bed.
- Wake the child and take him to the lavatory just before you go to bed yourself.

There are some warning devices on the market, designed around pads connected to an electric buzzer which is triggered when moisture hits the pad. There are not very satisfactory and best avoided: they do not wake the child until urine has already been passed.

HOMEOPATHY
Usually, you should consult a homeopath but also consider:

- *Silica* Especially if the child is of a reserved nature and has cold, smelly, sweaty feet.
- *Lycopodium* Where the child is very apprehensive of being left alone or going to school.
- *Arsenicum album* For the fussy, chilly, restless, overanxious child.

HYPNOTHERAPY
Hypnotherapy is able to investigate the underlying anxieties and set up systems to wake the child in time and/or reduce the incidence of bedwetting.

MANIPULATIVE THERAPIES
These can help if the bedwetting is caused by problems in the lower back.

PSYCHOTHERAPIES
Continence is a learned skill, like riding a bicycle, and some children learn it faster than others. ANXIETY or other emotional upset can easily disturb the pattern that has just been learned and then bedwetting starts.

Behavioural therapy concentrates on relearning the skill, and it is often a good start providing the initial upset is self-limiting. If it is not, then the problem will be more persistent, and an individual therapy for the child of family therapy or counselling for the parents could be useful.

RELAXATION TECHNIQUES
Any of these, adapted for children's use, can dispel TENSION and so help to solve anxiety-induced bedwetting.

BLEEDING

The acute, sudden loss of large quantities of blood—*haemorrhage*—can be serious and life-threatening. The sudden fall in BLOOD PRESSURE that this causes can lead to SHOCK, and the loss of body fluids can prove irreversible and fatal. Haemorrhage may be caused by injury, or may be due to a medical condition such as a perforated gastric ULCER.

Gradual chronic blood loss, however, may pass unnoticed. This can be caused by excessively heavy periods (*see* MENSTRUAL DISORDERS), severe PILES, ulcerative COLITIS, CROHN'S DISEASE, GINGIVITIS and vitamin K deficiency (*see* BRUISES). In addition, small amounts of blood can be lost from the stomach as a result of excessive intake of alcohol or long-term treatment with aspirin or other non-steroid anti-inflammatory drugs.

All these forms of chronic gradual blood loss may lead to ANAEMIA, and possibly to the RESTLESS LEGS syndrome.

Professional advice must be sought at the first signs of blood in urine or sputum, or if large amounts of bright red blood or even small amounts of very dark black blood appear in stools.

Vaginal bleeding not associated with the normal menstrual cycle—and especially during or after the menopause—is also a cause for concern and should be investigated immediately.

HOMEOPATHY
- *Aconite* Associated with panic.
- *Arnica* After injury.
- *Belladonna* Bright red, hot blood; hot head and cold extremities.
- *Carbo vegetabilis* Associated with collapse, cold sweats and gasping for breath.
- *Phosphorus* Bright red blood, with craving for iced drinks and ice cream.

NATUROPATHY
For bleeding from cuts or bruises, apply a dressing soaked in a few drops of *calendula* tincture.

VITAMIN AND MINERAL TREATMENT
May respond to vitamin K, but medical control essential. Vitamin C may help bleeding gums, but consult a naturopath.

BLOOD PRESSURE

Blood pressure is the direct measurement of the amount of work being done

Measuring Blood Pressure

Your blood pressure measurement actually tells you how much pressure it takes to *stop* the flow of blood through your arteries. This is assumed to be equivalent to the pressure at the pump end, the heart.

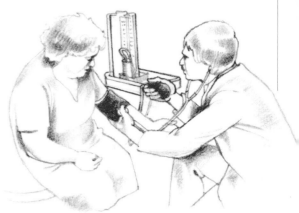

Blood pressure is measured at two points in the heart's pumping rhythm: *systolic pressure* is taken when the heart is actually beating; *diastolic pressure* is taken when the heart is at rest between beats. The combined pressure is usually expressed as a fraction—120 (systolic) /80 (diastolic) for example. The normal systolic pressure for a healthy adult is 120 (100 for a child).

The figures refer to the height a column of mercury reaches under a certain pressure. The measurement is taken with a *sphygmomanometer*. This is a soft inflatable cuff attached to a column of mercury (calibrated in millimetres). When the cuff is wrapped around your upper arm and inflated, the pressure in it pushes the mercury up the column. Systolic pressure is measured when there is no longer a pulse in the arm beyond the cuff; then the cuff is deflated and the diastolic pressure taken when the blood flows freely once more.

by the heart as it pumps blood through the arteries. Throughout daily life, the blood pressure varies considerably depending on what is needed. The brain needs a constant 750cc a minute, regardless of what the body is doing. If the arteries harden or get silted up with cholesterol, the flow is blocked, the heart pumps harder to push the blood through, and your blood pressure rises.

HYPERTENSION (high blood pressure)
In the Western world, hypertension is the chief cause of premature death. High blood pressure exceeds 140/90.

The level of diastolic pressure (the smaller number) is considerably more important in the diagnosis of hypertension because this shows the minimum pressure that the artery walls have to sustain continuously. If this is too high, the walls will suffer progressive damage in the form of ATHEROSCLEROSIS,

which in turn can lead to ANGINA and HEART DISEASE. Arteries are placed under severe strain, and the smaller arteries of the brain may rupture, causing a stroke.

Hypertension can be caused by disease of the kidney and the thyroid gland. Gout (*see* ARTHRITIS), OBESITY, the oestrogen hormone in many oral contraceptives and a diet high in salt and saturated fat are often contributory factors. Smoking is another aggravating cause, as is caffeine.

ORTHODOX TREATMENT
Beta-blockers; diuretics.

SELF-HELP
● Adjust your diet to eliminate salt and animal fats.
● Take regular exercise—any form of aerobic exercise (cycling, swimming, walking) will increase

the efficiency of the circulation system (see **Fit for Life** p. 29).
- Stop smoking; nicotine makes the blood vessels contract, impeding the flow of blood.

ACUPUNCTURE
Deviations of blood pressure from the normal require investigation and can usually be treated.

Acupressure in the crease of the folded elbow and below the knee on the outside of the leg (point 25) could help (see pp. 102–3).

ALEXANDER TECHNIQUE
This may prove to be beneficial.

HERBAL TREATMENT
Take 45–60 ml/3–4 tbsp of lime blossom, rosemary or nettle tea 2 or 3 times daily, to help lower blood pressure. Reinforce it with 2 garlic oil capsules at bedtime (this will also reduce blood cholesterol).

Dandelion, parsley and celery are natural diuretics.

Passiflora or hawthorn tablets can be taken to relieve high blood pressure due to stress or TENSION. Substitute China, Luaka or Earl Grey teas and dandelion coffee for everyday tea and coffee; avoid alcohol.

HOMEOPATHY
Consult a homeopath.

HYPNOTHERAPY
Therapy to induce relaxation will help.

MANIPULATIVE THERAPIES
A manipulative therapist can help those with high blood pressure considerably by improving posture, thereby creating more space in the chest cavity, improving breathing and inducing muscle relaxation, which can be a first step in breaking the vicious circle of emotional stress and physical tension.

MASSAGE
Massage with repetitive, rhythmic strokes to soothe and relax.

NATUROPATHY
Seek professional advice and guidance. Eat a wholefood diet, reduce salt, exclude sugar, coffee and other stimulants. Avoid all meat for three months.

PSYCHOTHERAPIES
Over-commitment, repressed anger, sexual frustration and job dis-satisfaction, together with difficulties in personal relationships, are common either as causes or contributory factors in high blood pressure. They can all be helped by psychotherapy (*see also* HEART DISEASE).

RELAXATION TECHNIQUES
Mildly raised blood pressure is best dealt with by attention to lifestyle and the regular use of relaxation techniques. **Biofeedback** (p. 97), **autogenics** (p. 97), **yoga** (p. 98) and **meditation** (p. 99) are all helpful.

VITAMINS AND MINERALS
High blood pressure may respond to choline (up to 100 mg per day) or lecithin (up to 15 g per day). Claims have also been made for rutin (up to 600 mg daily) and tyrosine (400 mg) 3 times daily for both hypo- and hypertension.

HYPOTENSION (low blood pressure)
Despite the popular belief that low blood pressure is common and the cause of many vague symptoms such as DIZZINESS, lethargy and lack of stamina, this condition rarely causes any physical symptoms whatsoever.

The commonest problem is *postural hypotension*. In this, a sudden change from lying down to sitting or standing can cause a temporary but dramatic fall in blood pressure that lasts only seconds. This can result in FAINTING or even a blackout, but the blood pressure quickly returns to normal and the person recovers.

SELF-HELP
See FAINTING for advice on dealing with postural hypotension.

ACUPUNCTURE
Acupressure used to vigorously stimu-

late the tip of the nose can influence low blood pressure.

Herbal Treatment

Low blood pressure, a frequent sequel to prolonged illness and debility, can often be resolved by a course of ginseng capsules.

Naturopathy

45–60 ml/3–4 tbsp of beetroot juice, 3 times daily, is helpful.

Boils and Carbuncles

A boil — medically called a *furuncle* — is an area of acute bacterial infection, usually in a hair follicle or sweat gland. Sometimes the infection spreads to neighbouring follicles, other boils are formed and this collection is called a *carbuncle*. A boil that occurs in the follicle of an eyelash is called a STYE.

Diabetics are prone to boils when the concentration of sugar in their blood is high; this provides the bacteria with the perfect environment for breeding.

It is important to see your practitioner if:
● you develop a carbuncle.
● you develop a high temperature and/or feel generally unwell.
● you are very young or old.
● you suddenly start having recurrent boils.

First Aid

Bring a boil to a head by bathing it in hot water or applying a kaolin poultice to it. Heat the kaolin paste in a pan of boiling water until it is moderately hot, then spread it on a dressing and apply it to the boil.

When the boil bursts, magnesium sulphate on a dry dressing will help to draw out the pus.

Herbal Treatment

A blood-purifying decoction similar to the one recommended for ACNE should be taken in doses of 45–60 ml/3–4 tbsp 3 times daily, or 2 echinacea tablets daily, for a period of several weeks until the boils have cleared completely.

Powdered marshmallow root or powdered slippery elm, mixed to a stiff paste with boiling water, should be spread on lint and then applied as a hot poultice; this should be changed every 24 hours, until the boil has burst and discharged its contents completely. The slippery elm will help it to heal, and should be used as a cold poultice for several days.

Proprietary herbal drawing ointments are available from either health food shops or herbal suppliers.

Homeopathy

● *Belladonna* For early stages, when the boil is bright red, throbbing, very tender and worse when cold.
● *Hepar sulphuricum* As the boil starts to 'point', this will 'ripen' it more quickly.
● *Silica* Once the boil bursts, this promotes the discharge of pus.
● *Tarentula cubensis* For severe stinging pain with throbbing, especially under the arm. For recurrent cases, consult a homeopath.

Naturopathy

Diet: The underlying condition should be treated with attention to the diet: eat a wholefood diet excluding sugar and other refined carbohydrates and limiting milk and other dairy products. A cleansing programme of fruit, raw vegetables and wholegrains for 2–7 days can quicken healing.

Heat/Cold Treatment: Local treatment may include the application of small poultices of finely chopped cabbage.

Vitamin and Mineral Treatment

Treat with extra zinc at levels of 25–50 mg daily to accelerate healing, then prevent recurrence with 15 mg daily on a continuous basis.

Breast feeding *see* PREGNANCY AND CHILDBIRTH

BREATHLESSNESS

Breathlessness while you are at rest or doing very little may be a symptom of lung disease or HEART DISEASE, but it is not the first one to appear. It is also a symptom of ANAEMIA, ASTHMA, BRONCHITIS, CATARRHAL INFECTION and EMPHYSEMA.

It is often a psychological problem, induced by ANXIETY. The person is anxious, breathing becomes faster, they hyperventilate (overbreathe) and this makes them highly anxious and panicky.

ACUPUNCTURE
The ideal treatment for problems involving fullness in the chest and shortness of breath is dependent on a full analysis of the causative factors. (See *also* ASTHMA.)

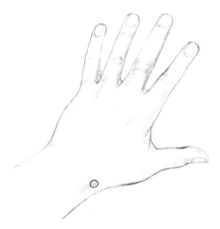

The 'anatomical snuff box'
The natural hollow at the point where your thumb joins onto the side of your wrist is known as the anatomical snuff box since when you spread your hand as wide as possible a small hollow is formed between the tendons of the thumb from which it is possible to sniff your snuff.

Acupressure on the anatomical snuff box may benefit some sufferers.

ALEXANDER TECHNIQUE
This can be beneficial.

HYPNOTHERAPY
This may help by identifying the cause of the underlying anxiety.

NATUROPATHY
Diet: Cut down on dairy produce and maintain a diet based on fruit, vegetables and wholegrains.
Exercises: Breathing exercises may increase lung capacity; so will regular cycling, walking or swimming.
Heat/Cold Treatment: In cases of catarrhal congestion, hot and cold fomentations should be applied for 20–30 minutes at least once daily.

PSYCHOTHERAPIES
Sufferers should be treated as for ANXIETY.

RELAXATION TECHNIQUES
Yoga (p. 99).

BRONCHITIS

This is an infection or obstruction of the tiny airways in the lungs, the bronchi.

Acute bronchitis usually follows upper respiratory tract infections such as INFLUENZA or a heavy COLD. The body's resistance to bacteria is lowered, the bronchi become prone to infection and its corollary, inflammation. The sensitive membranes step up mucus production to deal with the inflammation and this in turn becomes infected.

Chronic bronchitis is 'the English Disease'. It is commoner in England than anywhere else in the world. It results from frequent irritation of the lungs: smoke, fog, dampness and fumes can all irritate, stimulating overproduction of mucus in the lung tissue. This is not infected but so abundant that it clogs the airways. Gradually, the area of lung available for the exchange of oxygen and carbon dioxide diminishes, and the heart has to work harder to keep the volume of blood high. This can result in HEART DISEASE. Chronic bronchitis is made worse by an attack of acute bronchitis on top of it.

SYMPTOMS

Common to both is BREATHLESSNESS, the cough as the lungs try to get rid of the excess mucus, and the thick greenish yellow sputum. Acute bronchitis also produces wheeziness, FEVER and general malaise.

ORTHODOX TREATMENT

Antibiotics, anti-flu vaccine, cough medicine (acute); broncho-dilators (chronic).

SELF-HELP

- Give up smoking; if you are the parent of bronchitic children, ban cigarettes from the house.
- Avoid cold air, smoke, fog and exertion.
- Use steam inhalations (with olbas oil if you like) to make the air you breathe warm and moist.
- Keep away from people with colds to reduce the risk of reinfection.
- Deal promptly with colds, coughs and catarrh if you are prone to bronchitis.

Chronic bronchitics must learn to help themselves, as there is little that can be done unless the irritant substances that cause the mucus to clog the air passages are eliminated. As this is normally cigarette smoke, the message should be clear.

ALEXANDER TECHNIQUE

This can be very beneficial.

HERBAL TREATMENT

Consult a herbal practitioner.

For acute bronchitis, rub warm liniment into the chest (back and front) and throat. A hot infusion of equal quantities elderflower, hyssop and white horehound taken in 45–60ml/3–4 tbsp doses every 2 hours will promote perspiration, soothe the inflamed bron-

chi and encourage expectoration. When the temperature is normal, take the infusion cool 4 to 5 times daily. A combination of white horehound and elecampane in 15 ml/1 tbsp doses night and morning will clear mucus and ease the bronchial cough.

Garlic capsules every night during winter and the herbal teas above taken cold twice daily will help prevent a recurrence of acute bronchitis.

For chronic bronchitis, consult a herbal practitioner, but herb tea (as above) taken regularly will help.

HOMEOPATHY

Chronic bronchitics should consult a homeopath.

For acute bronchitis:

- *Aconite* At first sign of fever, especially after dry cold winds.
- *Bryonia* For painful cough, great thirst, feel worse when moving.
- *Kali bichromicum* When the mucus is stringy.
- *Mercurius solubilis* For increased sweating which offers no relief, tendency to dribble on the pillow at night and sensitivity to temperature change.
- *Pulsatilla* For dry cough at night when lying down, loose green sputum in the morning and lack of thirst.

MANIPULATIVE THERAPIES

Any treatment which will improve the available air space within the chest cavity will help to a certain degree. Manipulations to the dorsal spine and the rib attachments together with breathing exercises, postural exercises and massage to relieve muscular spasms all have a part to play.

NATUROPATHY

Diet: A good wholefood diet excluding dairy products will minimise the mucus production.

Heat/cold treatment: Use cold packs to stimulate breathing; avoid overheated very dry atmospheres.

RELAXATION TECHNIQUES

Any of these will be beneficial.

VITAMIN AND MINERAL TREATMENT
Take vitamin C (500mg 3 times daily) particularly during the winter months.

The Smoker's Cough
The smoker's hacking morning cough accompanied by sputum is the tell-tale symptom of chronic bronchitis. It is caused in the main by smoking, although industrial effluent, fog and smog can play a part.

The cough is the lung's effort to get rid of the excess mucus. Normally small hairlike projections (*cilia*) in the bronchi sweep mucus up the windpipe and into the throat, where it can be swallowed. In chronic bronchitics, there is so much mucus that the cilia are swamped and immobilized. The only way to move the mucus is coughing. If the smoker continued to irritate the lungs with cigarette smoke, the mucus production increases and the vicious circle goes on. The chronic bronchitic who does *not* give up smoking will deteriorate little by little over the years, declining into a miserable old age of chronic and permanent disablement.

See ADDICTIONS

BRUISES

If no specific disorder can be found, the tendency to bruise easily may indicate vitamin K deficiency. Vitamin K is essential to the formation of the blood clotting protein which prevents haem-orrhage (see BLEEDING).

FIRST AID
- If bruising is severe, raise the affected part to reduce the blood flow through it.
- Apply a cold compress or ice pack—frozen peas are ideal.
- Apply arnica ointment if the skin is not broken.

HERBAL TREATMENT
Make a solution of distilled witch hazel, 10ml/2tsp tincture of arnica to a cup of cold water and an infusion of calendula.

Soak a lint or gauze pad in the mixture and keep it in place over the bruise with a bandage. Apply more solution until the swelling subsides.

Aloe vera gel smoothed on to the bruise twice a day will heal the bruise quickly.

HOMEOPATHY
- *Hypericum* When associated with crush injuries, especially to fingers and toes.
- *Ledum* When the bruise is associated with a puncture wound.
- *Rhus tox* When associated with sprains and strains of muscle.

NATUROPATHY
To combat vitamin K deficiency, eat yoghurt every day to encourage the micro-organisms that manufacture the vitamin. Eat plenty of green vegetables — cabbage, cauliflower, spinach, broccoli and kale. Drink pineapple juice and eat fresh pineapple: the enzymes in it (also available in tablets called Bromelain) encourage dispersal of the bruise.

VITAMIN AND MINERAL TREATMENT
Adequate intakes of vitamin C (500mg daily) and bioflavonoids (50mg 3 times daily.)

Bruxism *see* TEETH GRINDING

Bulimia nervosa *see* ANOREXIA NERVOSA

BUNIONS

Bunions are caused by wearing badly-fitting or badly-shaped high fashion shoes, and/or socks which are too small. Some people's big toes bend naturally towards the other toes, and ill-chosen footwear will exacerbate this.

SYMPTOMS
The joint becomes inflamed, swollen, painful and very distorted.

ORTHODOX TREATMENT
Anti-inflammatory drugs; surgery.

131

- Wear only the most sensible shoes and go barefoot wherever possible.
- Small foam rubber pads placed between the big toe and the second toe help to push the affected toe into a better alignment, but this treatment must be instituted before the joint becomes too fixed and rigid.
- Mobilize the joint for yourself, especially during or just after a warm bath.
- Foot exercises involving rolling the feet backwards and forwards on a bottle, exercising with a wide elastic band looped over both big toes, picking up pencils with the toes and heel to toe walking in bare feet can also help (see **Positive Health** p. 52).

ACUPUNCTURE

Relief of pain can be achieved by inserting acupuncture needles in selected points of the foot, but only if further causative pressures such as tight shoes are avoided.

ALEXANDER TECHNIQUE

This can be beneficial.

HERBAL TREATMENT

See ARTHRITIS.

MANIPULATIVE THERAPIES

Manipulation of the big toe joints can be of the greatest benefit to relieve stiffness, rigidity and inflammation.

MASSAGE

Massage the foot gently to improve mobility and relax muscle tension.

NATUROPATHY

Stiff, sore toe joints may be relieved by hot Epsom Salts footbaths (1 tbsp commercial Epsom Salts dissolved in hot water). Soak for 20 minutes daily.

See also ARTHRITIS

BURNS AND SCALDS

Large or severe burns and scalds are very serious, especially in babies and small children who could go into SHOCK. Seek professional help *at once*.

For temporary first aid and for minor burns and scalds:

- **Immediately apply cold water** to the burn for at least 10 minutes. Place under a running tap, immerse in a bath or pour cold water over the affected area.
- **After scalding, remove hot wet clothing** very carefully.
- **Chemicals will continue to burn** if they are still soaked into clothing that is touching the skin. Remove clothes at once, protecting your own hands.
- **Give the person small, frequent sips of cool water** to drink to replace lost fluid.

DO NOT:

- **Remove burned clothing**. This may be stuck to the skin, and its removal will cause more damage.
- **Use grease or ointments** on any new burn.
- **Cover burns with sticky plasters** or adhesive dressings.
- **Apply cotton wool or other** fluffy material to burns.
- **Break blisters.**
- **Give hot drinks** or alcohol.

HERBAL TREATMENT

Apply any of the following on soft cotton fabric or the smooth side of lint:

- infusion of elderflowers or marigold flowers
- distilled witch hazel
- diluted lemon juice (1 part juice to 3 parts water). Honey also has healing properties and has been used effectively on burns. Calendula cream is soothing for minor burns if they still smart after some hours.

Aloe vera can give relief and will heal burns and scalds quickly without pain.

HOMEOPATHY

- *Cantharis* Blistering, painful burning sensation.
- *Urtica urens* Milder burns without blistering; more of a stinging nettle sensation.

If the skin is unbroken, cover with *Urtica urens* or *Hamamelis* ointment.

NATUROPATHY
Use an ionizer for half an hour at a time as frequently as needed; this will relieve pain and hasten healing. Apply essential oil of lavender (2 drops to 5 ml almond oil) to assist healing.

VITAMINS AND MINERALS
Vitamin E cream should be applied directly but not until skin begins to heal. Keep the burned area lightly covered, adding more cream every 8 hours.

C

Callus *see* CORNS AND CALLUSES

CANCER

Cancer is a process by which cells, for whatever reason, become changed, lose their normal identity and structure, multiply out of control, invade the surrounding area and may spread to parts or organs of the body relatively far away from the original cancer. Usually, the body's defence, or immune, system mops up these abnormal cells — which, according to some authorities, may number in the thousands at any given time in each of us — but if the immune system is inefficient, then a cancer develops.

Certain agents can stimulate this cancer process. These are called carcinogens, *and there are a number of widely accepted ones, including radiation, a range of industrial compounds (such as asbestos), overexposure to sunlight in susceptible individuals (eg the pale-skinned) and smoking. Smoking is particularly guilty (see* ADDICTIONS*): smokers are up to 25 times more likely to develop lung cancer, and in recent authoritative hearings at the United States Congress, it was stated that no less than 30 per cent of all cancers can be linked to smoking.*

At the same hearings, it was stated that an even higher percentage of cancers (35 per cent) were linked to diet. However, it is notoriously difficult to pinpoint any particular foodstuff as being responsible, and indeed, it may well be that how we eat is as important as what we eat.

It is hardly surprising that diet is so important when one considers that, every six months, 95 per cent of the body has been completely replaced. It is like rebuilding a house over and over again, and obviously the quality of the bricks is vital.

THE CANCER PERSONALITY
As well as the physical condition of a person, the psychological make-up may have something to do with whether or not they develop cancer. Much has been written about the 'cancer personality', notably by Lawrence LeShan, an American psychotherapist who has worked with over 200 cancer patients.

According to LeShan, the typical personality had an emotionally deprived youth, followed in later life by a period of fulfilment in an intense relationship or through all-involving work, followed by the loss of that relationship or work and consequent despair. It is during this latter period, when the person has lost their *raison d'être*, that the cancer occurs. The other main characteristic is the person's inability to express anger, particularly in their own defence; such a person is often described by others as being 'like a saint'. (There is evidence that those people who angrily fight the disease do much better than those who accept or become fatalistic about the situation. Those who simply deny their illness fare somewhere between these extremes.) LeShan believes that this pattern fits 76 per cent of his patients.

PREVENTION
Cancer prevention takes in diet, a healthy lifestyle, avoidance of stress, a strongly positive mental attitude and (although not strictly *preventive*) methods of catching any cancer that may develop at a very early stage.

The guidelines for a cancer preventive diet are really no different from those for healthy eating in general (*see* **Nutrition** pp. 18–19).

As for supplements, beta-carotene — the precursor of vitamin A, found mainly in plants — is probably beneficial, since it may make cancer cells more vulnerable to the body's immune system. A protective effect against lung cancer is the most strongly reported relationship. Carrots and dark green leafy vegetables are particularly rich in carotene, as are some fruits such as apricots. Vitamin A supplements can cause liver damage and so should only be taken under medical supervision.

Adequate levels of vitamin E may also be important in cancer prevention — for example, low levels of vitamins E and A have been linked with a higher risk of developing breast cancer. However, if a cancer is diagnosed, medical advice *must* be sought about the use of vitamin E because it may encourage the growth of any tumour.

So if you avoid the known carcinogens and pay attention to your diet, what else may be beneficial for cancer prevention? Basically, there are a number of general self-care principles that can act to improve your immune system. This aspect cannot be overemphasized. Louis Pasteur, one of the greatest medical scientists of all time, said on his deathbed: 'The microbe is nothing — the terrain is everything' — in other words, your own healing processes are much more decisive in whether you fall ill than the infectious agent itself. This goes a long way towards explaining why some people seem to remain healthy while all around them fall ill.

These general self-care principles include regular exercise (and it matters little what it is; often the best is the type one enjoys most), diet (as discussed above) and periods of relaxation, with or without using specific relaxation techniques (*see* pp. 96–101). Another important factor, and often the most difficult to achieve, is developing a positive approach to life.

DETECTING CANCER EARLY

A cancer that is discovered early is, naturally, much easier to treat. Cancer of the cervix in women (or pre-cancerous but abnormal cells) can be revealed by a simple cervical 'Pap' smear. Ideally, every woman should have a smear test every year, but certainly at intervals of not longer than every five years. Cancer of the breasts is even easier to detect, since all women should perform a breast self-examination once a month, just after a period if they are still menstruating.

There is, therefore, much for which you can take responsibility to minimize the risk of developing cancer, and the role of doctors should be more that of guides and sources of encouragement than someone to 'treat' you.

SYMPTOMS

Just as there are so many different types of cancer, so there are a multitude of ways in which it can produce symptoms. However, the American Cancer Society has come up with the **'Seven Warning Signals of Cancer'**—that is, those symptoms that are found to be significant in the more common types of cancer.

1 A change in bowel or bladder habits.
2 A sore that does not heal.
3 Unusual bleeding or discharge, especially from the rectum or vagina.
4 A thickening or lump in a breast or elsewhere.
5 Indigestion or difficulty in swallowing.
6 An obvious change in a wart or mole.
7 A nagging cough or hoarseness.

To these can be added an eighth 'warning signal': any unexpected and unexplained loss of weight.

If you have any one or more of these symptoms, you must see your doctor at once. Although the presence of such a symptom is not positive proof that you have cancer, only your doctor and hospital specialists can find out for sure. If you wait in the hope that the trouble will go away, you may find that you have missed an opportunity that could have saved your life.

DIAGNOSIS

What will happen when you go to your doctor with a suspected cancer? First, the diagnosis has to be confirmed, and usually will involve investigations such as X-rays and/or minor surgery at your local hospital. Once the diagnosis is confirmed, you will need to explore its implications and plan a course of treatment. Your doctor will be able to discuss with you the many different approaches available, both conventional and otherwise, and help you to decide which ones are the most appropriate for you.

ORTHODOX TREATMENT

Surgery; radiotherapy; chemotherapy; hormone therapy; stimulating the immune system.

NATURAL THERAPIES

Whereas most conventional techniques have focused on healing the body, largely ignoring the mind and spirit, the focus of these approaches is the opposite. This is not to say that one approach is better than the other, but merely that they are different routes to the same goal — namely, *health*.

Many people feel guilty about having cancer, especially when they are aware that so much of it is preventable. While that may be true, the positive side is that there is much one can do to help oneself, and now is the time to start. The outlook is better than it has ever been, and a positive approach is essential, and is encouraged by the use of these natural approaches.

HEALING

From a scientific standpoint, no trials have been done, but many people are convinced of the benefits of healing, and it is increasingly being used. It is important that it should be carried out in conjunction with, and not separately from, other forms of treatment.

HOMEOPATHY

There are many homeopathic remedies for cancer but the treatment should only be dealt with by a skilled homeopath.

NATUROPATHY

One of the main principles of a cleansing diet is to detoxify the body and thereby mobilize its own healing powers. Such diets focus on raw food — unprocessed food, with no additives or colourings, that is uncooked (or little cooked) and eaten as fresh as possible. This provides a high-nutrient, low-calorie diet, since it contains fresh vegetables, fruit, nuts and seeds. Its high fibre content helps the detoxification process. Processed foods, white flour, white rice and stimulants are avoided.

PSYCHOTHERAPIES

As well as the DEPRESSION and anger that can follow the news that a person has cancer, the elements that make up the 'cancer personality' can also be helped by counselling and other forms of psychotherapy.

In addition, this characteristic personality pattern of behaviour can be reflected in the family of the cancer patient. Many families are concerned that they may in some way be guilty that one of their own has developed cancer. There is no evidence that how a family behaves can cause cancer, although each family will obviously react differently to such a crisis. Psychotherapy can also be aimed at mobilizing the family's resources, helping them to look at issues raised and offering them support and counselling.

RELAXATION TECHNIQUES

General relaxation is important, and training is becoming more widely available in such techniques as diaphragmatic breathing, auto-hypnosis, **biofeedback**, **autogenics** (p. 97) and exercise (which, where possible, should be broadly encouraged rather than restricted for cancer patients).

Techniques are often taught in groups, which also provide a meeting point for mutual support. **Meditation** (p. 98), visualization and psychotherapy are often practised together by groups.

VISUALIZATION

Visualization is seeing with the 'mind's eye'. It is a process in which one purposely uses one's imagination to create visual images. The basis for its effect is that energy follows thought—like positive thinking. In cancer therapy, it is used to 'see' cancer cells either dissolving away or being attacked by the body's own defence cells. Pioneered in Texas by the radiotherapist Dr Carl Simonton and his wife Stephanie Simonton, it is claimed to have had some remarkable successes.

VITAMIN AND MINERAL TREATMENT

It is well recognized that many cancer sufferers are deficient in certain vitamins. Vitamin C supplements (a minimum of 2 g per day) are generally accepted as being worthwhile, but there is controversy over the dosage. High doses (10 g per day) have been used and claims made about their success. In controlled trials, no overall survival advantage was noted, but the appetite and sense of well-being of cancer sufferers improved over 4–6 weeks. Nobel Prize winner Linus Pauling recommends doses up to 25 g per day on the basis that vitamin C is cancer-destructive, but the evidence so far is inconclusive.

The use of laetrile (also known as amygdalin and vitamin B_{17} although it is not a vitamin) has long been controversial. The claims made for it have focused on it being a 'natural' or 'herbal' alternative to cancer chemotherapy, since it destroys more cancer cells than healthy ones: the cancer cells lack an enzyme that changes the cyanide produced from the laetrile into a less toxic substance. Taken by mouth, however, the cyanide in the blood can rise to toxic and even lethal levels. There has so far been no drug trial that clearly shows a benefit in outcome, although it has been reported that people feel better subjectively when using laetrile with other therapies.

Carbuncles *see* BOILS AND CARBUNCLES

Candidiasis *see* THRUSH

CATARRH

When the mucus membranes of the nose and throat are irritated by, say, smoke, fumes, the viruses that cause the common COLD or the allergens that produce HAY FEVER among other allergic reactions (see ALLERGY), the membranes produce excess mucus to fight off the irritation or infection. This is catarrh.

Excess mucus can lead to a feeling of a 'full' head, and can also block the Eustachian tubes leading to the middle ear, making an infection likely (see EARACHE). Infection of the sinuses which may result can cause severe HEADACHE and pain above and below the eyes.

ORTHODOX TREATMENT

Nasal decongestants (not suitable for children); antihistamines.

SELF-HELP

● Avoid all fumes, pollution, etc that can irritate the airways.
● STOP SMOKING.
● Avoid potential allergens (see ALLERGY).
● Blow the nose regularly to clear it and reduce the possibility of infection (blow only one nostril at a time).
● A walk at night just before bed will help clear the air passages for an hour or two and will help you to sleep.
● Thick, tenacious catarrh may be loosened by steam inhalations (see COUGHS). Add a few drops of herbal aromatic oils to the water.

ACUPUNCTURE

Nasal catarrh requires treatment of the Large Intestine and Lung meridians.

Acupressure on the back of the skull and points 26 on each side of the nose and point 4 on the web of the hand will clear the head (see pp. 104–5).

HERBAL TREATMENT

To clear the temporary catarrh that

results from a cold or influenza, try following measures:

- Two garlic oil capsules (which act as a natural antiseptic and clear mucus) should be taken each night.
- An infusion of hyssop herb should be taken in 45–60 ml/3–4 tbsp doses three times daily, occasionally alternated with an infusion of agrimony herbs to tone and strengthen the lax, spongy lining of the nasal passages.
- An infusion made up of equal quantities of eyebright, yarrow and hyssop can also be taken in the same dosage. These teas should be cool in the daytime, and hot at bedtime.

HOMEOPATHY

- *Natrum muriaticum* When the catarrh is associated with a great amount of sneezing, and the mucus is like the uncooked white of an egg.
- *Kali bichromicum* When the mucus is yellow or white and very stringy.
- *Hydrastis* When there is a constant drip from the back of the nose, and deafness due to blockage of the Eustachian tube.
- *Arsenicum iodum* When the sufferer is generally under the weather with a dripping nose that burns the upper lip.
- *Graphites* When the person is chilly, constipated and suffers from DERMATITIS, particularly around the nose and the back of the ears.

MANIPULATIVE THERAPIES

Manual drainage of the sinuses by massage and cervical manipulation are used to treat catarrh.

MASSAGE

Massage can encourage the drainage of the sinuses, and will relax the muscles of the neck and shoulders.

NATUROPATHY

Diet: Eat a wholefood diet with abundant fresh fruit, salads and vegetables. Exclude all dairy products and limit starchy and sweet foods.
Treatment: Beetroot juice is a very mild

astringent. Mix together 1 part juice to 2 parts tepid water in a shallow container. Sniff this through each nostril alternately, sucking the solution into the mouth and spitting it out. Two or three sniffs through each nostril can provide relief for several hours.

VITAMIN AND MINERAL TREATMENT

When catarrh is induced by allergy or after infection, it may be relieved by vitamin C (500 mg, 3 times daily) and vitamin B_6 (25 mg, 3 times daily), reducing the dosages to 500 mg vitamin C and 25 mg vitamin B_6 once a day.

CHICKENPOX

This highly infectious childhood illness is caused by the same virus (*Herpes zoster*) that causes shingles (*see* HERPES). It is usually transmitted from one child to another via droplet infection—but it can be passed from a person with shingles. In addition, a child with chickenpox can cause an adult (especially an elderly person) to develop shingles if that person has had chickenpox in the past. For this reason, infectious children should be kept away from elderly relatives. However, one bout of chickenpox confers a lifetime immunity against the illness.

SYMPTOMS

Symptoms develop between 10 and 21 days after exposure to the virus (the incubation period). There may be FEVER, HEADACHE and, possibly, vomiting and aches in the legs although these symptoms are usually mild. Sudden high temperatures must be referred to a professional practitioner. Within 24 hours, a rash of tiny pimples will spread from the mouth and throat to the trunk, arms and legs. These pimples quickly turn into blisters, filled with virus-laden clear fluid. By about the fourth day, these will burst, forming crusts which eventually drop off by themselves.

The blisters and crusts are infectious and can be very itchy, and care must be taken for the child not to scratch them as this could lead to infection.

Complications are few and rare, usually only occurring in those who are on long-term steroid treatment or have certain seriously debilitating diseases. Chickenpox cannot damage an unborn child.

ORTHODOX TREATMENT
Calamine lotion, antihistamines to soothe itching; antibiotics for secondary infections.

SELF-HELP
For general care, *see* CHILDREN'S ILLNESSES.

Scratching must be avoided, to prevent the spread of infection. Keep your child's nails short; small children may need to wear cotton gloves (tied at the wrist), particularly at night-time.

HERBAL TREATMENT
Herbal teas of yarrow, limeblossom, chamomile flowers or meadowsweet, sweetened with a little honey, can be given 3 or 4 times daily to reduce fever: dessertspoon doses for children aged 6–10; 10 ml/2 tsp for younger children.

Garlic and eucalyptus are herbal antibiotics. Take garlic raw or as perles. Make an infusion of eucalyptus by boiling 25 g/1 oz of leaves in 1 l/1¼ pts water for 1 minute. Stand covered for 10 mins, strain and cool; give 5 ml/1 tsp 3 times a day.

Sponging an infusion of elderflowers on the rash as often as needed will help soothe the irritation. Aloe vera gel will relieve itching and lessen the chance of scarring.

HOMEOPATHY
- *Antimonium tartarricum* If the child is very irritable, whining and demands company, and there are very large blisters.
- *Rhus tox* If the child is very restless.
- *Pulsatilla* If the child is very clingy, weepy and thirstless.
In addition, see remedies under FEVER.

NATUROPATHY
Fasting (under supervision), which increases the blood's white cell count, high fluid intake (especially fresh fruit juice) and the use of tepid sponging to control temperature (*see* CHILDREN'S ILLNESSES) are the initial treatments in the first 48 hours of acute infectious illness.

The body's way of fighting infection is to increase the number of white cells and raise body temperature. The naturopath will encourage these mechanisms and avoid supressing them with drugs such as aspirin and antibiotics insofar as this is consistent with the needs of the sufferer.

VITAMIN AND MINERAL TREATMENT
To enhance a child's natural anti-viral resistance, take vitamin C (100 mg), 3 times daily. During convalescence, take a low-potency multivitamin/multimineral preparation.

CHILBLAINS

These are sore, itchy, inflamed and often swollen patches of skin on the backs of the fingers or tops of the toes, although they can occur on ears and other parts. They are caused by poor peripheral circulation which restricts the blood supply to the extremities resulting in damage to the cells.

ORTHODOX TREATMENT
Soothing creams.

SELF-HELP
- Improve your circulation by regular exercise, naturopathic treatment (*see below*) and cutting down on coffee and smoking, as caffeine and nicotine constrict the blood vessels.
- Keep feet and hands warm when the weather is cold.

HERBAL TREATMENT
If the skin is unbroken, apply distilled witch hazel with a few drops of tincture of myrrh added, rub with the surface of a cut lemon which has been dipped in sea salt or apply a compress of elderflower infusion.

If the skin is broken, use comfrey ointment or oil or calendula cream to ease the pain and promote healing.

To improve circulation, take 5 ml/1 tsp of composition essence in hot water night and morning or a cayenne tablet each morning. Yarrow tea and prickly ash bark will both improve circulation. 45–60 ml/3–4 tbsp of either taken 2 times daily will be adequate.

Aloe vera gel will soothe and heal.

HOMEOPATHY

Tamus ointment can be used directly on the chilblains.

- *Agaricus muscaria* When aggravated by cold and with burning itching sensation.
- *Calcarea carbonica* When feet are damp and cold.
- *Petroleum* When associated with cracks in the skin at the finger tips.
- *Pulsatilla* When aggravated by heat or letting the legs hang down.

MANIPULATIVE THERAPIES

Manipulation to the neck and lower part of the spine can help to promote good circulation in the extremities.

MASSAGE

Massage your feet after soaking them in a footbath containing calendula oil.

NATUROPATHY

Hydrotherapy: Bathe feet in warm water for 2–3 minutes followed by cold for 1 minute. Repeat each evening for 15–20 minutes. Friction rubs will help general circulation.

VITAMIN AND MINERAL TREATMENT

Take vitamin E (100 iu capsules 4–6 a day) and vitamin C as bioflavanoids (1–3 g a day).

Treat with nicotinic acid or vitamin B_3 (25 mg) and acetomenaphthone or vitamin K (10 mg) 3 times daily. Creams containing methyl nicotinate (vitamin B_3) may be applied directly.

Childbirth *see* PREGNANCY AND CHILD-BIRTH

CHILDREN'S ILLNESSES

Almost all children develop, from time to time, COLDS *and* INFLUENZA *as well as, during the first 10 or so years of life, what are called 'childhood illnesses' — measles, mumps and the like. These are mainly passed on via 'droplet infection' — that is, a fine spray of saliva bearing the virus or bacteria is emitted by one child during a cough, sneeze or even just breathing and this is breathed in by another. Such infections can also be transmitted by contact with infected stools or urine or through contaminated food or drink.*

An illness lasts from the time when the child picks up the particular bug until he or she is well again. The incubation period *— is the time it takes for the child to develop symptoms once they have been exposed to the virus or bacteria. The* period of contagion*—is the number of days (or even weeks) during which a child could transmit the illness to another.*

For a full description of each childhood illness see CHICKENPOX, COLDS, CROUP, DIARRHOEA, GERMAN MEASLES, GASTROENTERITIS, INFLUENZA, MEASLES, MUMPS, SCARLET FEVER, SORE THROAT, TONSILS AND ADENOIDS, WHOOPING COUGH.

GENERAL CARE

In addition to any specific treatment bear these general rules in mind.

Fluids A child with a fever loses fluid much faster than an adult so encourage them to drink as much as possible, even if this is painful or just not wanted. Even more important, a child who is vomiting or has DIARRHOEA or both is in great danger of dehydration and of impaired kidney function and upsetting the balance of their body chemistry. A simple remedy is to dissolve 5 ml/1 tsp salt and 15 ml/1 tbsp sugar in 0.5 l/1 pt just boiled water. Allow to cool and store in a screw top bottle in the refrigerator. Give the child the mixture in teaspoonful.

Common childhood illness			
Disease	*Source*	*Incubation*	*Period of contagion*
Chickenpox	Virus	10–21 days	From 1 day before rash appears until all the scabs have dried
German measles (Rubella)	Virus	14–25 days	From start of symptoms until up to a week after the rash has appeared
Influenza	Virus	1–3 days	From just before the onset of symptoms up to 10 days maximum
Measles	Virus	7–14 days	From 4 days before rash appears until 5 days afterwards
Mumps	Virus	14–21 days	From several days before feeling unwell until all swelling has gone (usually 10 days)
Scarlet fever	Bacteria	1–7 days	From several days before symptoms until 24 hours after the beginning of antibiotic treatment
Whooping cough (Pertussis)	Bacteria	5–21 days (usually 10 days)	From first symptoms until 6 weeks after onset of cough under

Food A sick child will usually not want to eat very much, if at all. Most Western children can go for a relatively long time without food without showing any ill effects — provided they have enough fluid. Fasting increases the white cell count.

Rest If a child has a mild case of childhood illness, there is no reason to make them stay in bed, as long as the room in which they stay in is warm and draught-free.

Fevers Many children can develop very high fevers for no physical reason — say, during exuberant play — while others, particularly babies, can be quite ill with no sign of a raised temperature. Therefore, if you take your child's temperature, be careful that you treat the result as simply one of many symptoms — not the whole illness.

However, sudden high temperatures in children are not suitable for self-help treatment. Seek professional guidance immediately.

TIPS FOR REDUCING FEVER
● Tepid sponging; remove all clothes and sponge child liberally with tepid (not cold) water. Do not dry off, but allow the water to evaporate: that is the main cooling effect.
● Don't wrap the child in blankets, or keep the room too warm. Normal pyjamas, comfortable warm room and a light blanket are all that is necessary, even if child is shivering.

TREATMENT
Bacterial infections can be treated with antibiotics but these drugs are of no use at all in the treatment of virus infections. Occasionally a virus infection may result in secondary bacterial infection for which antibiotics may be prescribed. Virus infections create an immunity from subsequent attacks by the same virus.

Cirrhosis *see* LIVER PROBLEMS

Cold sores *see* HERPES

COLDS

The common cold is caused by virus infection. This is usually followed by subsequent bacterial infection. Colds spread rapidly from person to person, and are most likely to be contracted in crowded public places. Any general debility that produces a lowered natural resistance will increase the probability of catching a cold.

ORTHODOX TREATMENT
Decongestants; aspirin or paracetamol to relieve pains and HEADACHE.

HERBAL TREATMENT
Take herbal infusions: hot to promote perspiration, cool when the cold is streaming and the temperature is back to normal.

Elderflower, peppermint and composition essence is available as a bottled remedy, or an infusion can be made of equal quantities of the two herbs with the addition of 5 ml/1 tsp of composition essence to each teacupful.

Yarrow herb is generally useful. Boneset herb helps aching limbs. Lime-blossom quenches thirst and is effective when there is much sneezing in the early stages.

Hyssop will give relief in a cold on the chest — more so if combined with white horehound. Hyssop can also be taken later as a cool infusion if catarrh is present.

HOMEOPATHY
For recurrent colds, consult a homeopath. For the occasional one:
- *Aconite* Early stages, especially after to cold, dry wind.
- *Gelsemium* For influenza-like cold with trembling, weakness and chilliness.
- *Nux vomica* When nose pours like a tap; irritability very noticeable.
- *Natrum muriaticum* For early stages with much sneezing, and nasal discharge like raw white of egg.
- *Allium cepa* For burning discharge from nose with sneezing.
- *Arsenicum album* For burning discharges from eyes and nose; chilly and weak.

NATUROPATHY
As a cold is a manifestation of the body's attempt to eliminate accumulated poisons, it should not be suppressed. Withhold all milk products and starchy foods; exclude sugar and refined carbohydrates. Two or three days on fruit and raw vegetables will encourage speedy resolution of the cold with less residual catarrh. Eat plenty of raw garlic.

VITAMIN AND MINERAL TREATMENT
Increase vitamin A intake to 7500 iu daily during period of illness. Treat with vitamin C at an intake of 1 g every 4 hours until relief is obtained; then gradually reduce this over one week to 1 g per day, and then to a 500 mg maintenance dose.

Symptoms have been relieved by *sucking* lozenges each containing 23 mg zinc gluconate every 2 hours while awake. Zinc tablets that are swallowed have no beneficial effect in relieving cold symptoms.

COLIC

Colic is an acutely painful spasm of the hollow organs of the digestive system. The cause can be as simple as CONSTIPATION or the colic can arise as a result of numerous DIGESTIVE DISORDERS. FLATULENCE, IRRITABLE BOWEL SYNDROME, COLITIS, DIVERTICULITIS, DIARRHOEA, GASTROENTERITIS and food poisoning are all possible causes of colic. Obstruction can also cause colic. GALLSTONES blocking a bile duct will cause colicky pains.

Colic in babies is frequently associated with wind but it has been shown that bottle-fed babies are more likely to suffer from colic, and breast fed babies whose mothers consume large quantities of cows' milk have a far higher incidence of colic than babies whose mother's drink little or no milk. A connection with ALLERGY and FOOD INTOLERANCE should not be overlooked.

Recurring spasms should be examined by a medical practitioner to make sure there is no serious underlying cause.

ORTHODOX TREATMENT
Diagnosis and treatment of underlying cause.

HERBAL TREATMENT
Adult colic: For the occasional attacks, try the following teas: chamomile, peppermint or catmint served hot and sipped slowly; seed tea. Mix equal quantities of fennel, aniseed and caraway seeds; crush 5 ml/1 tsp of the mixture and add to a cupful of boiling water. Cover and infuse for 10 minutes, then strain. Drink it hot.

Antispasmodic tincture or tincture of ginger in hot sweetened water will relieve pain and disperse flatulence. An infusion of powdered ginger taken warm in 15 ml/tbsp doses will also relieve intestinal spasm. Peppermint oil and licorice are also known for their antispasmodic properties.
Infant colic can be relieved by any of the above, given warm in 5 ml/1 tsp doses.

HOMEOPATHY
● *Chamomilla* Especially for babies.
● *Colocynth* For pains brought on by anger, better for pressure, restless, cutting pains.
● *Ipecachuana* When there is great nausea.
● *Magnesia phosphorica* When there are sharp pains better for pressure and heat.
● *Nux vomica* After overindulgence in alcohol and fatty spicy food; associated with constipation.

COLITIS

This is the inflammation of the lining of the large intestine, or colon. The condition may be acute or chronic — when it is called *ulcerative colitis* — and is frequently associated with stress and ANXIETY. Colitis can sometimes be associated with bacterial infections of the colon, or may be caused by the changed sensitivity of the intestinal lining due to adverse reactions to some foods (see FOOD INTOLERANCE).

SYMPTOMS
Pain in the abdomen, DIARRHOEA and sometimes the passing of blood or mucus with the stool are the common symptoms.

ORTHODOX TREATMENT
Antibiotics; steroids; surgery.

ACUPUNCTURE
Treatment aims to remove excesses of activity in various pathways, possibly the Liver, Stomach and/or Bladder pathways. The umbilicus (navel) may also be treated by warming salt and pouring this into the umbilical hollow.

To remove such excesses, go on a brief fast and drink only water until relief is obtained, usually after 1–3 days.

Acupressure on a point on the outside of the leg below the knee (point 23), will control muscular movement of the intestine; acupressure on a point halfway between the umbilicus and the sternum (breastbone) (point 27) will help some acute cases. (See p. 103)

ALEXANDER TECHNIQUE
This may prove beneficial.

HERBAL TREATMENT
Slippery elm, taken twice daily, will soothe irritated intestinal walls. Alternate it with astringent teas such as agrimony — either alone or combined with an equal quantity of avens herb — 45–60 ml/3–4 tbsp of the tea taken cold, 3 or more times daily.

Include fresh chickweed in the daily salad, or take it as a warm infusion, for its soothing healing properties.

HOMEOPATHY
● *Colocynthis* When there is much colic.

- *Sulphur* When colitis is worse in the morning.
- *Arsenicum album* When symptoms are worse between midnight and 2 a.m. and are associated with restlessness, exhaustion and chilliness.

MANIPULATIVE THERAPIES

Treatment of the lower regions of the spine can be helpful in stimulating the nerve supply to the digestive system.

NATUROPATHY

Eat a diet of conservatively cooked vegetables or vegetable stews and broths. Gradually introduce raw vegetables such as finely grated carrots, to increase fibre. Limit the intake of wheat but use other grains such as brown rice and millet.

RELAXATION TECHNIQUE

Colitis caused or aggravated by stress and tension may respond well to **autogenics** (p. 97).

VITAMIN AND MINERAL TREATMENT

Take a high-potency multivitamin preparation, plus extra vitamin C (500 mg daily) and vitamin B$_6$ (25 mg daily), particularly when on steroid treatment.

CONJUNCTIVITIS

(Pink Eye)

An acute inflammation of the *conjunctiva* (the mucous membrane covering the outer surface of the eyeball and lining the eyelids.) Conjunctivitis can be caused by bacterial or viral infection or by some irritating foreign body in the eye. Frequently it is an allergic reaction especially to grass pollens or animal dander. Viral conjunctivitis can become a serious problem and requires urgent medical attention. This is a highly infectious condition and can sweep through closed communities in an epidemic.

ORTHODOX TREATMENT

Regular bathing (separate solution for each eye); antihistamines; antibiotics.

HERBAL TREATMENT

An infusion of elderflowers can be used to bathe the eyes or on compresses over the eyes. Simmer the flowers for 5 minutes in water and leave to stand (covered) for 10 minutes then strain through muslin or a coffee filter.

Chamomile flowers can be used the same way, but add the flowers to cold water, bring to the boil then leave to stand for 20 minutes before straining.

Chickweed also makes a good bath or compress. Take a handful of the fresh herb, wash the soil off, discard discoloured leaves, cover with boiling water, leave to cool (covered) then strain.

Use a fresh eye-bathful for each eye to avoid reinfection.

HOMEOPATHY

- *Aconite* For the early stages before discharge, especially if brought on by exposure to a cold, dry wind.
- *Apis* For blistering on white of eye and severe stinging pains.
- *Argentum nitricum* When there is a pus discharge.
- *Arsenicum album* Water from the eye which is so hot it burns the cheek.
- *Euphrasia* For the catarrhal stage with hot thick discharge from eye and constant watering.

VITAMIN AND MINERAL TREATMENT

Vitamin A (7,500 iu daily) may help prevent a chronic condition, but only take large amounts of vitamin A under professional supervision.

CONSTIPATION

Constipation is one of the commonest and yet most misunderstood conditions in Western society: the faecal mass moves too slowly through the large bowel, resulting in the infrequent passing of small, very hard stools not dissimilar to rabbit droppings. This problem is related absolutely to the lack of fibre in the Western diet. The muscular pushing effort required to evacuate the hard stool from the bowel is the forerunner of a number of much more serious complaints: DIVERTICULITIS, appendicitis, PILES, *hiatus* HERNIA and VARICOSE VEINS. There is also evidence to suggest that chronic constipation may be a forerunner of bowel CANCER.

Frequency of bowel movement is not necessarily an indication of constipation. It is the consistency of the stool which is passed which is of the utmost importance: a soft stool effortlessly passed on alternate days is acceptable, whereas a hard stool evacuated with much strain and effort is a sure sign of constipation, even if passed three or four times a day.

Constipation which occurs suddenly in someone with previously regular normal bowel movements is always a cause for concern since this can be an indicator of some obstruction in the bowel. Where this type of constipation is interspersed with episodes of diarrhoea there is always the possibility of cancer of the bowel and this should be investigated immediately.

CAUSES OF CONSTIPATION

Most constipation is caused by insufficient fibre in the diet and too little fluid intake.

Constipation may also be a common side effect of some drugs particularly anti-depressants, pain killers and iron tablets. It is also frequent during PREGNANCY. Psychological factors play an important role: ANXIETY, stress, TENSION and not infrequently obsessional attitudes towards bowel behaviour and defecation are frequently found in chronic sufferers.

ORTHODOX TREATMENT

Purges; laxatives; suppositories; diagnosis of underlying cause.

SELF-HELP

Stepping up your fibre intake to at least 40, preferably 60 g a day and your fluid intake to 1.5–2 l/$2\frac{1}{2}$–3 pts.

- Change to wholemeal bread, whole grain breakfast cereal and add extra bran to your daily intake (*see* NATUROPATHY below).
- For an isolated attack, eat prunes, dried apricot, figs or syrup of figs.
- Do not repeatedly ignore your body's signal to defecate.

ACUPUNCTURE

The proper functioning of the bowel is partly dependent upon the health of the small intestine from which it receives waste material for the separation of fluids from solids. These will end up as disposable urine and faeces. It also relies on an efficient stomach and spleen, the organs first called upon to extract the essence of the Chi energy from the food eaten. Acupuncture treatment of constipation is not, therefore, concerned with the use of laxatives to force a bowel movement but with the correction of causative energy imbalances.

In yin-yang terms, foods need to be selected according to the nature of the constipation, which can be either flaccid or spastic. **Acupressure** can be applied to points 4, 23, 28 and 29 (see p. 104–5).

HERBAL TREATMENT

If constipation occurs, following a change of routine or diet, the remedies below will be useful as a temporary measure.

Soak 15 ml/1 tbsp of linseed overnight in water (or use the proprietary remedy Linusit Gold) and add to breakfast cereal.

Crush 5–10 senna pods and add to a cupful of boiling water with a small piece of licorice root. Leave to soak, strain and take before breakfast.

An infusion of dandelion leaves and chopped dandelion root will be gentle laxative effect influencing the liver and kidneys. The dose is 45–60 ml/3–4 tbsp daily, but it can be adjusted as required.

MANIPULATIVE THERAPIES

These are frequently beneficial if the treatment is concentrated at the lower part of the spine.

MASSAGE

Rhythmic massage movements starting at the bottom right hand corner of the abdomen, going up to the ribs, across the diaphragm and down the left side of the abdomen will help stimulate contractions of the colon.

NATUROPATHY

Diet: Increase dietary fibre by introducing wholegrains, fresh fruit and raw vegetables and legumes. It is better to eat more food in its natural state than just sprinkle bran on top of a refined carbohydrate diet, but bran can be helpful as an interim measure. Take it in conjunction with a higher fibre diet and foods with natural laxative properties (dried fruit, linseed).

Bran can cause uncomfortable bloating, so take very small amounts at first; start with 10–15 ml/2–3 tsp a day and slow build up to a maximum of 12 g/½ oz. One reason for not relying heavily on bran long term is that when raw it contains an ingredient (phylates) which can combine with useful minerals and lock them into compounds that the body cannot absorb. As bran contains generous amounts of mineral itself, this is not important in the short term, but could be for vulnerable people, such as pregnant women who have a tendency to constipation while needing extra iron, zinc and calcium, the three minerals involved.

Exercise: Make sure you are getting enough exercise, especially of the abdominal muscles.

> In the UK some £50 million are spent on laxatives each year and more than $400 million in the USA: these figures exclude laxatives prescribed by doctors.

PSYCHOTHERAPIES

A small proportion of constipation cases may certainly arise a consequence of withholding strong feelings (particularly hostile and aggressive ones). This is marked in children. Any therapy that helps the feelings to be released and resolved can be helpful.

RELAXATION TECHNIQUES

Yoga (p. 99) will help to strengthen the abdominal muscles.

VITAMIN AND MINERAL TREATMENT

Stubborn cases may respond to vitamin B_1 (10 mg daily) and potassium, magnesium aspartate (1,500 mg daily. The complete B complex is sometimes used to stimulate intestinal bacterial growth to relieve constipation, particularly when it occurs after antibiotic therapy.

CORNS AND CALLUSES

Corns are painful wedges of hard skin (keratin, the kind of skin that builds nails and hair) which result from excess and undue pressure on the skin's surface. Calluses are thickened patches of skin spread over a wider area.

Corns most usually occur on the feet and can be caused either by ill-fitting shoes or by deformities of the foot, for example hammer toes where corns are seen on the tips of the toes which are in contact with the sole of the foot.

Corns can also be a secondary cause of BACK PAIN since a painful corn will alter posture, walking and weight distribution to protect the painful part. This imposes unnatural strains on the structure of the spine.

The importance of treating corns cannot be over-emphasised. In the elderly especially, painful corns can reduce mobility thereby preventing the activity and exercise essential for a sound circulation and healthy respiratory system.

SELF-HELP

● Prevent calluses by washing the feet regularly and removing rough skin with a pumice stone.
● Prevent the development of corns by choosing sensible, well fitting shoes.

ORTHODOX TREATMENT

Corns are best treated by a qualified chiropodist, since self-treatment usually involves the removal of the top surface of the corn which will soon regrow.

ALEXANDER TECHNIQUE
This can be beneficial.

HERBAL TREATMENT
For small corns, either paint the area with fresh lemon juice or crush a garlic clove onto the gauze patch on a sticking plaster and apply directly.

VITAMIN AND MINERAL TREATMENT
Vitamin E cream will soften the hard skin of calluses.

COUGHS

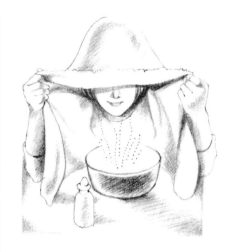

To relieve nasal congestion, sinus problems and chesty complaints, add boiling water to a bowl containing a little olbas oil. Cover head and bowl with a large towel, inhaling the vapour through the nose.

A cough is not necessarily the herald of disease. It is the first line of defence of the respiratory system. Particles of dust or mucus which settle on the surface of the larger airways can trigger off the cough reflex which eliminates obstructions from the upper airways.

However, the cough is the commonest of all respiratory symptoms: it may be short and painful or it may be loose and producing phlegm and mucus. It can occur in paroxysms of non-productive coughing especially in ASTHMA and chronic BRONCHITIS. Coughs are usually worse during the night or first thing in the morning and they are often irritated by changes in temperature or weather.
Any evidence of blood in the sputum, or a persistent cough in children should be investigated straightaway.

ORTHODOX TREATMENT
Expectorant or anti-tussive cough medicine.

ACUPUNCTURE
Coughs are usually associated with an excess or deficiency of Lung energy and acupuncture treatment will deal with this in the appropriate manner.

HERBAL TREATMENT
For a simple home remedy, simmer 25 g/1 oz elecampane root in 1 l/1¾ pts water for 15 minutes. Strain and add 15 ml/1 tbsp honey and 10 ml/2 tsp lemon juice. Drink a warm cupful 3 times daily.

Chopped raw onion eaten with a spoonful of honey will loosen a tight chest.

A herbal chemist will make you up a mixture of lungwort, white horehound, licorice, senega, elecampane root, marshmallow and a pinch of cayenne. This will soothe the cough and break up the mucus.

HOMEOPATHY
For chronic coughs, consult a homeopath. Specifically:
- *Aconite* For the first stage, after exposure to cold, dry winds.
- *Belladonna* When cough dry with a flushed hot face and high FEVER.
- *Bryonia* Hard, dry painful cough, head hurts when coughing; thirsty.
- *Drosera* For violent barking cough; often used in WHOOPING COUGH.
- *Ipecachuana* For moist, rattly cough with choking and nausea.
- *Kali bichromicum* When worse first thing in the morning and producing stringy sputum.
- *Phosphorus* For dry irritating cough.

MANIPULATIVE THERAPIES
Manipulation is always beneficial. Treatment to improve the mobility of

the dorsal spine, to improve the movement of the ribs and to increase the flexibility of the structure of the rib cage are all used together with the teaching of correct breathing exercises and posture.

NATUROPATHY
Diet: Increase fresh raw fruit and vegetables and exclude dairy products, starchy foods and sugar.
Heat/Cold treatment: Hot and cold fomentations to the chest and throat stimulate lung function and encourage expectoration.

Steam inhalations may help.

'Crabs' *see* LICE

Cradle cap *see* HAIR AND SCALP PROBLEMS

CRAMP

(*See also* RESTLESS LEGS)

A sudden and acutely painful contraction of muscles commonly occurring in the calves but possibly happening in any of the body's large muscles — neck, back, abdomen and even in the muscles in the face.

CAUSES OF CRAMP
Cramp can be caused by salt deficiency because of excessive sweating (athlete's cramp, stoker's cramp). It may be caused by poor circulation: narrowed arteries do not deliver enough blood for the activity or exercise on hand. Occupational cramp (writer's, typists etc) may be brought on by using the same set of muscles repeatedly over a long period. No-one knows what causes the agonizing cramp in the leg that happens in the middle of the night.

ORTHODOX TREATMENT
Small doses of quinine.

For the occasional acute cramp, stretching the muscle against the contraction is often a useful way of breaking the spasm.

HERBAL TEATMENT
Try cramp bark, the European cranberry (*viburnum opulus*) which grow in woods and hedgerows. Use up to 5 ml/1 tsp daily.

Mustard foot baths 3 times weekly can help. Take 15 ml/1 tbsp mustard powder and enough water to cover the feet. Bathe for 3 minutes, splashing calves.

To stimulate circulation to the calf muscles, make a drink of 5 ml/1 tsp each cloves, lemon juice, and honey, 15 ml/1 tbsp ginger wine and 125 ml/$\frac{1}{4}$ pt boiling water. Allow to stand for 24 hours. Drink 45 ml/3 tbsp at night time.

HOMEOPATHY
Chronic sufferers should consult a homeopath. For acute cases:
- *Arnica* When cramp is part of general tiredness.
- *Calcarea carbonica* Cramp associated with damp, cold feet and a tendency to be overweight.
- *Colchicum* For cramps in soles of feet.
- *Cuprum metallicum* For severe cramp.
- *Nux vomica* For night time cramps with no cause.

MANIPULATIVE THERAPY
Deep massage and **effleurage** (see p. 87) in order to encourage the circulation of blood to the affected area together with manipulative treatment and strengthening exercises are also useful.

NATUROPATHY
Hot and cold fomentations to the affected muscle will promote better circulation.

PSYCHOTHERAPIES
Many of the occupational cramps take the form of intention cramps and frequently have a deep psychological overlay. It is necessary to establish the root of the psychological problems and to teach a more relaxed use of the muscles involved in the specific occupation.

RELAXATION TECHNIQUES
Any of these can be useful.

147

Cramp induced by exercise should be treated with vitamin E (200 iu 3 times daily).

Night time cramps should be treated with vitamin E (200 iu in the daytime, 200 iu before sleep) plus vitamin C (500 g daily). Potassium (500 mg) calcium and magnesium (taken as dolomite, 1000 mg) before sleep may help.

CROHN'S DISEASE

This is a chronic inflammatory disease of the gastro-intestinal tract; its cause is unknown. Crohn's Disease can occur in all age groups, but commonly attacks young adults. It appears to run in families, but why and how is unknown. It's on the increase in Europe and Scandinavia.

ORTHODOX TREATMENT
Corticosteroid drugs; vitamin and mineral supplements; surgery.

ACUPUNCTURE
Treatment is given to maintain energy balance in the Colon meridian and to improve digestion by treating the Stomach meridian.

NATUROPATHY
Children will need an extremely healthy balanced diet, providing high level of unrefined carbohydrate intakes and good protein from sources other than red meat.

While some orthodox doctors accept the role of diet in the cause of Crohn's Disease, particularly diets which have a high intake of refined sugar and a low intake of fibre, most are not yet prepared to accept that FOOD INTOLERANCES may play a major role.

Naturopaths have for many years treated this condition by making radical alterations to the sufferer's diet. Recent research indicates that Crohn's Disease may be treated successfully by the use of an exclusion diet (see pp. 104–5). The work is still in the experimental stages but the foods which are most likely to adversely affect the Crohn's sufferer are wheat, corn, oats, dairy products, red meats, citrus fruits, onions, coffee, tea, nuts, chocolate, food preservatives and yeast. Crohn's sufferers who have excluded certain foods from their diet report great success.

VITAMIN AND MINERAL TREATMENT
All-round multivitamin/multimineral supplement preferably with fat soluble vitamins in water soluble form because of malabsorption problems.

CROUP

Croup is the abnormal noise which is made when air is breathed in through a constricted windpipe over inflamed vocal cords. This alarming noise occurs in young children, since their airways are much narrower than adults and frequently become plugged with mucus when there is an accompanying inflammation. Most commonly croup is caused by a cold or BRONCHITIS or ALLERGY, although it can happen as the result of a foreign body being inhaled.

Attacks frequently occur at night and produce laboured breathing with an accompanying croaking cough. The child will be distressed.

If the attack persists or if there is any suspicion of a foreign body having been inhaled, contact your doctor as soon as possible.

ORTHODOX TREATMENT
Antibiotics; removal of any foreign body.

SELF-HELP
Croup is aggravated by hot dry air, so turn off the central heating and open the windows. If the weather is hot and dry, take the child into the bathroom and turn on the hot tap or the shower to create a warm, moist atmosphere. Use humidifiers if your house is centrally heated, and make sure that bed-

rooms are adequately ventilated to prevent the hot dry atmosphere which causes so many respiratory and nasal problems.

Herbal Treatment
To make a soothing infusion, add 5 ml/1 tsp each of vervain and coltsfoot to 1 teacup boiling water. Cover and stand for 10 minutes then strain through a coffee filter paper. Reheat, adding 10 ml/2 tsp honey. Give it hot, 5 ml/1 tsp for infants under 5 and 15ml/1 tbsp for children over 5 years.

Rub a few drops of olbas oil into the chest. Inhalations with olbas oil in hot water are also useful, but cannot obviously be used by babies.

Homeopathy
Consult a homeopath.

Naturopathy
As with all respiratory problems, reduce dairy foods to inhibit mucus. Repeated attacks may be a sign of diminished natural resistance, so ensure that nutrition is adequate (see **Nutrition** pp. 14–15).

Vitamin and Mineral Treatment
Supplements of vitamin C will help to strengthen the body's own defences.

Cuts and Grazes

Even minor cuts and grazes can be possible sites of infection. If the injury has been caused by a dirty object, particularly in the garden, check on anti-tetanus protection (Call your doctor or visit the hospital casualty department, if in doubt). This is particularly important with puncture wounds, which can allow germs to enter deep into the body.

First Aid
● Make sure that your own hands are clean then clean the injury under running water to remove dirt, gravel, glass, etc. If you can't get all the foreign particles out, go to the doctor.

● Apply appropriate remedy.
● Cover with sterile or very clean gauze or lint, and bandage firmly into position.
● Watch out for any subsequent pus, swelling or inflammation. *See also* BLEEDING.

Herbal Treatment
The following can be applied to a clean dressing and then placed on the injury:
● distilled witch hazel.
● tincture of myrrh (1 part to 6 parts water): this stings but it is a good antiseptic.
● a few drops of calendula tincture.
● comfrey oil or an infusion of the herb.
● the gel from inside a leaf of aloe vera; twice a day.

Homeopathy
● *Arnica* Every 4 hours.
● *Calendula* If not healing; every 4 hours.
Bathe the injury in *Calendula and Hypericum Mother Tincture*: 3 drops in $\frac{1}{2}$ cup warm, boiled water.

Vitamin and Mineral Treatment
Vitamin E cream should be applied to minor cuts and grazes, to keep the affected area clean.

Cystitis

This is an acute or chronic bacterial infection of the bladder or the urethra. Cystitis is far more common in women and young girls than men.

It is hardly ever possible to isolate the specific organism which is causing the disease. In women, the cause may be ALLERGY or irritation caused by sexual activity. In men, cystitis may be initiated by inflammation of the prostate gland. (See PROSTATE PROBLEMS)

Generalized sensitivity to yeast organism (see THRUSH) is a frequent cause of and accompaniment to chronic or recurrent cystitis.

SYMPTOMS

There is frequent passing of urine accompanied by a scalding pain in the urethra in the female or penis in the male. Frequently there is pain just above the pubis just before, during and just after passing urine. There is also sometimes a feeling of wanting to pass urine again immediately after the bladder is emptied. The urine may have a strong unpleasant smell and look cloudy.

ORTHODOX TREATMENT

Antibiotics.

SELF-HELP

- Drink large quantities of fluid, especially water, but avoid alcohol, coffee and strong tea in excess.
- Eat live natural yoghurt regularly.
- Apply live yoghurt to the vaginal and urethral openings.
- Make sure you always wipe the anus front front to back, using clean white paper for each wipe to avoid transferring faecal bacteria to the urethra. Parents should teach their daughters to do this.
- Women with chronic cystitis should try to pass urine as soon as possible after sexual intercourse.

ACUPUNCTURE

Pressures, chills or infections can all lead to an inflammation of the bladder It is the causative factor that will be treated rather than the cystitis as such.

Acupressure on abdominal, low back and leg points (22, 33, 34, 37) may relieve cystitis.

HERBAL TREATMENT

Make a decoction of equal parts marshmallow leaves, bearberry (*uva ursi*), sage and horsetail mixed well together. Add 5 ml/1 tsp mixture to one large cupful of boiling water. Simmer gently for 5 minutes. Cover, cool. Drink it cool, 1 cup 3 times daily.

Barleywater is also soothing and gently diuretic. Boil 100 g/4 oz barley in a little water. Strain. Pour 0.5 l/1 pt water and the peel from half a lemon over the barley and simmer until barley is soft. Allow to stand until blood heat. Remove barley, add 50 g/2 oz honey. Drink as much as you like.

HOMEOPATHY

- *Aconite* For early symptoms, especially if brought on by dry cold.
- *Cantharis* Classical symptoms of burning pains on passing urine frequently.
- *Sarsparilla* When pain occurs only at the end of micturation.
- *Staphysagria* For so called 'honeymoon cystitis' after injury to the vulval area.

For chronic sufferers, long-term treatment especially with complex homeopathic remedies can be used under the direction of a homeopath.

NATUROPATHY

Reduce animal protein and citrus fruits in the diet. Avoid acidic foods (tomatoes, rhubarb, gooseberries, vinegar, pickles).

Chronic or recurrent cystitis should be approached ecologically. Treatment will involve an elimination diet (see pp. 104–5) to exclude all yeast-containing foods.

VITAMIN AND MINERAL TREATMENT

Maintain acid urine by taking 500 mg vitamin C 3 times a day until pain subsides, then 200 mg 3 times a day to prevent recurrence.

D

Deafness *see* HEARING PROBLEMS; *also*

DEPRESSION

Broadly speaking, depressive illness can be divided into two categories: *endogenous depressive illness* and *reactive depression*.

ENDOGENOUS DEPRESSIVE ILLNESS

Those who fall into this category exhibit mood variations from mild depression to black despair. INSOMNIA is a common factor. There is also an inability to make decisions, feelings of guilt, self-doubt, blame and or unworthiness that are totally unshakable, despite attempts by others to persuade or demonstrate that they have no basis in truth. Physical symptoms are also common, such as loss of weight, BACKACHE, CONSTIPATION, constant HEADACHES, APPETITE LOSS, a general slowing down of all physical activity and, in women, a loss of periods (see MENSTRUAL DISORDERS).

There is frequently a history of swinging mood changes and a rigid upbringing resulting in depression occurring in later life. Endogenous depression can be triggered by some physical disease such as INFLUENZA, but most frequently it occurs with no obvious external cause.

REACTIVE DEPRESSION

This more often occurs in young or middle-aged people, and is frequently accompanied by the symptoms of ANXIETY neurosis. There is an inability to get to sleep, and a preference for company rather isolation. Reactive depression is normally associated with some emotionally traumatic experience. In general, reactive depression is less serious than endogenous depressive illness, but in both groups, the illness can prevent very depressed people from expressing the true depth of misery to which they have sunk. There is often a fear of going mad, which is frequently intensified by the shame and guilt engendered by the suicidal feelings they are experiencing, and this must be seen as a very real problem and dealt with accordingly.

The real risk of suicide is high in those with severe depressive illness.

ORTHODOX TREATMENT

Anti-depressant drugs; tranquillizers; sleeping pills; ECT therapy in psychiatric hospital.

ACUPUNCTURE

The balance of yin and yang and the general energy levels are seriously disturbed in someone suffering from depression. Acupuncture treatment will aim to restore this balance, and maintain the equilibrium of Chi energy.

HEALING

Depression is perhaps one of the most frequently treated problems encountered by healers and certainly responds very favourably in many instances, although endogenous depressive illness tends to be more difficult to help than reactive depression.

HERBAL TREATMENT

Both borage and (particularly) vervain tea, taken once or twice daily, will lift the spirits. An infusion of 4 or 5 flowering lavender tops, with some honey added to taste, is a pleasant nerve tonic.

Many of the herbs used for ANXIETY will be beneficial for depression, together with tonics to improve general health and vitality. The following is one of the best of the latter: steep 12 g/$\frac{1}{2}$ oz each of finely chopped poplar bark and gentian root in 1 l/1$\frac{3}{4}$ pt water for 15 minutes; bring to the boil and add 12 g/$\frac{1}{2}$ oz each agrimony and centaury herbs; simmer for 10 minutes; leave to cool then strain; add honey to taste. Drink before meals in 45–60ml/3–4 tbsp doses.

HOMEOPATHY

If the depression is severe or recurrent, consult a homeopath. For short episodes:
- *Arsenicum album* When chilly, restless, anxious, exhausted; worse between midnight and 2 a.m.
- *Ignatia* For depression following disappointment in love, etc.; lump in the throat.
- *Natrum muriaticum* After bereavement, emotional upset; cannot cry easily unless alone.
- *Pulsatilla* When you weep easily, feel easily dominated; fear of insanity.
- *Aurum metallicum* When suicidal, especially after failure in business.

HYPNOTHERAPY

Hypnosis can be useful in treating depression.

D

MASSAGE

By inducing a feeling of well-being, massage can help to bring a sufferer out of depression.

NATUROPATHY

A physical basis for depression may lie in inadequate energy production for the brain and nervous system. Review your diet and introduce more wholefood ingredients and adequate protein. Exclude sugar, coffee and alcohol. Tyrosine or tryptophan tablets (1–2 g daily between meals) may prove helpful.

PSYCHOTHERAPIES

Psychotherapy aimed at improving self-awareness, group therapy, counselling, reviews of lifestyle can all be of great value. Above all, however, allowing sufferers to discuss their problems and feelings openly with a sympathetic person is the favoured option in the treatment of all depressive illnesses.

RELAXATION TECHNIQUES

Any one of these can help.

VITAMIN AND MINERAL TREATMENT

Mild depression may respond to vitamin B_6 (up to 100 mg daily) plus magnesium (300 mg daily). Once a response is obtained, maintain B_6 intake at 25 g daily and magnesium at 300 mg daily.

DERMATITIS (ECZEMA)

An allergic reaction in the skin, producing inflammation.

CONTACT DERMATITIS

The skin reacts to a substance with which it is in contact and becomes red and itchy. At worst, blisters may develop which then rupture and weep. The skin may become dry and scaly and may even swell, sufficiently to close the eyes when the face is the affected area. Typically, contact dermatitis develops where the skin is thinnest on the backs of the hands or the eyelids for example. Although it may arise from some irritant used for the first time, it more usually is the result of months or even years of continual exposure. The reaction may take two to seven days to appear.

Many substances may produce contact dermatitis but the commonest are nickel and other metals, some antibiotics, perfumes, rubber, chemicals, hair dye and even preservatives.

Metal Allergy Ten percent of women suffer from a skin reaction caused by nickel. Nickel is used in most metals and particularly foreign silver, gold plate and rolled gold. Cheap jewellery is the commonest cause of dermatitis on the wrists, neck and ear lobes and fingers. People suffering from contact dermatitis should make sure that the zips, clips, press studs, hooks and eyes on their clothes are made from plastic.

Perfumes These are a rich source of allergens. Most toiletries and cosmetics are perfumed and so are many deodorants. Adverse reactions to perfumes and toiletries can be aggravated by exposure to sunlight.

Cosmetics There are potential allergens in all cosmetics, even supposedly hypoallergenic ones. Preservatives and lanolin are present in nearly all and perfumes in many. Even nail varnish can cause contact dermatitis where the skin is touched frequently by the finger nails.

Hair dyes are a frequent source of problems. This arises mostly in people who have been dying their hair for a long period of time when dermatitis can appear behind the ears, forehead and neck.

Rubber can cause allergic rash over the back of the hands from wearing rubber gloves; rubber shoes can cause the same reaction to the feet. Frequently, people who already have skin problems wear rubber gloves for protection only to suffer an adverse reaction to the rubber.

Medicated creams and ointments used for the treatment of other problems are common causes of contact dermatitis. The worst amongst these are local anaesthetics, antibiotic creams and eye drops which frequently make the original condition worse.

Plants The American poison ivy (genus *Rhus*) and the British primula and chrysanthemum are common allergens. Even the lightest contact with these plants can cause severe reactions producing swellings and blisters on the area of contact and on the face and eyelids. Don't neglect the possibility of NETTLE RASH. Although, rare, there are some people whose skin reacts instantly to contact with certain foods particularly fish and eggs. The typical rash and weals are seen after contact with a stinging nettle.

With repeated exposure even on a limited area of skin, dermatitis can eventually spread to many parts of the body. The only treatment is to avoid the allergen. Sometimes it is not easy to isolate the specific substances involved and this should be done by allergy testing.

ATOPIC DERMATITIS

This is a chronic inflammation of the skin, the chief symptom of which is an exasperating itch. The inflammation itself may be quite mild but scratching to stop the itch makes it worse.

Sufferers are usually afflicted with ASTHMA and HAY FEVER as well. People with atopic dermatitis always will be susceptible (flare-ups may be triggered by emotional upset, stress TENSION, ALLERGY, FOOD INTOLERANCE or sudden change in the weather) but may also go for long periods with no problems. Unfortunately, bad patches of inflammation may leave scars or at least unpigmented skin patches.

ORTHODOX TREATMENT

Allergy tests; coal-tar ointments and moisturizing bath oil (atopic).

ACUPUNCTURE

Exposure of the skin to the aggressive aspects of wind, damp and heat can result in acute dermatitis. Chronic dermatitis represents an imbalance between Energy and Blood, when the person is in a deficient state. Treatment consists in the first case of dispersal of the untoward unfluences. For chronic dermatitis, the primary aim is to improve the general health. (It is useful to know that the state of the skin is one of the most important guides to analysis of the person as it so accurately reflects the internal imbalances.)

Acupressure on point 38 (see p. 104) can help allay itching but it is essential that general health measures are carried out, not least those of correct nutrition based on the organ energies that are aberrant. For example, energy deficiencies in the Liver meridian will impede elimination and aggravate the dermatitis, therefore a diet suitable for improving the liver function (no fats, alcohol or coffee) should be followed.

HEALING

This has sometimes been found to be useful.

HERBAL TREATMENT

You should consult a herbal practitioner, although the following lotions will give relief:

- A decoction of purple loosestrife (50 g/2 oz simmered gently for 5 minutes in 0.5 l/1 pt water and left to infuse for 10 minutes then strained) will relieve itching and heal cracks in broken skin.
- Fresh chickweed used as an infusion or an ointment will soothe and heal.
- An infusion of blackberry leaves will be astringent and dry the skin.
- An infusion of elder leaves will ease the condition; (25 g/1 oz crushed fresh leaves to 0.5 l/1 pt of cold water brought to the boil then left to stand for half an hour).
- Aloe vera gel will reduce itchiness and promote healing.

HOMEOPATHY

Chronic cases should consult a homeopath. For acute cases, care must be taken during treatment. Try one dose a week to begin with.

- *Graphites* When there is oozing of sticky fluid.
- *Petroleum* Associated with painful cracks on toes and fingers.
- *Rhus tox* For great itching and blister formation.

D

- *Sulphur* For dry dermatitis worse for hot baths and heat of the bed.

HYPNOTHERAPY
Hypnosis can help in reduction of sensitivity, and — over time — the reduction and even removal of the dermatitis itself.

MASSAGE
Some people are helped by a daily local massage with essential oils. Use either rose, geranium, juniper, lavender or hyssop. Mix 5 drops of essential oil with 30 ml/2 tbsp almond oil and massage well into the skin.

NATUROPATHY
This is often associated with lung dysfunction, so consult a naturopath for guidance.

Adopt a wholefood diet. Exclude possible allergenic foods such as dairy products (particularly cow's milk), sugar and food additives.

People suffering from atopic dermatitis may consider an exclusion diet (see p. 104–5) to find out if any food acts as an allergen for them.

PSYCHOTHERAPIES
If the dermatitis causes disfigurement (which may be the case with the chronic kind) psychotherapy may be useful in overcoming the difficulties of interpersonal relationships which are likely to arise. **Bioenergetics** (see p. 95) appeals to younger people.

RELAXATION TECHNIQUES
These can be beneficial.

VITAMIN AND MINERAL TREATMENT
Dermatitis may be related to lack of vitamin B complex or of vitamin A or of polyunsaturated fatty acids (vitamin F). Treat with high potency vitamin B complex (preferably prolonged release preparation) or 7,500 iu vitamin A or 3 capsules (500 mg strength) of evening primrose oil daily. The condition may need a combination of all three. Direct application of evening primrose oil cream to affected areas may also help.

DIABETES

Diabetes occurs in two forms: *diabetes insipidus* and *diabetes mellitus.*

DIABETES INSIPIDUS
A fairly rare metabolic disorder caused by a deficiency of pituitary hormone (usually the result of damage to the pituitary gland). Enormous amounts of urine are produced, regardless of the amount of fluid drunk. Pituitary hormone replacement is the usual treatment.

DIABETES MELLITUS
The most common form of diabetes; it is the result of insufficient insulin being produced by the pancreas. Without insulin, the body cannot use glucose; this means there is a high level of glucose in the blood and a low level of glucose absorption by the tissues.

Maturity-onset diabetes, or non-insulin-dependent diabetes, normally occurs in adults. Sufferers are mostly overweight (*see* OBESITY) with a family history of this disease. Excessive thirst, excessive urination, weakness, leg cramps, tingling in the hands and feet and reduced resistance to infection are common indicators.

Juvenile diabetes, or insulin-dependent diabetes, occurs mostly in young people, and it is thought that it may be linked with virus infections or chemical toxicity which damage the cells of the pancreas responsible for producing insulin.

In both forms of diabetes, there is always the risk to diabetic coma: too much sugar in the bloodstream due to a lack of insulin produces hyperglycaemic coma; a fall in blood sugar (due to excessive use of insulin) or lack of adequate food produces a hypoglycaemic coma.

Complications Severe problems affecting the eyes and the circulation to the extremeties can develop, as well as kidney disease, infections of the urinary system (particularly THRUSH) and skin problems (*see* BOILS AND CARBUNCLES).

ORTHODOX TREATMENT
Insulin; diet (mature onset); oral drugs.

SELF-HELP
- Eat regular meals and take regular exercise, both to help control the level of glucose in the blood and to maintain good general health.
- Keep warm (especially the extremities).
- Feet should be kept in good condition.
- Give up smoking (nicotine contracts the blood vessels).
- Carry a card—or wear a medallion or bracelet—that states that you are diabetic and what your treatment is.

HOMEOPATHY
Consult a medical homeopath.

NATUROPATHY
The treatment of diabetes by diet control has changed dramatically over the last five years. After many years of sufferers being given low-carbohydrate diets, they are now encouraged to obtain about half their calories from unrefined, high-fibre carbohydrates such as wholemeal bread, porridge, legumes and potatoes. This has been shown to improve diabetic control and may reduce long-term side-effects of diabetes, some of which may have been encouraged by the reliance of the previously recommended diet of high-protein foods, which also tend to be high in fats.

However, no diabetics, especially those taking insulin, should change their diet without the approval of their doctors/dieticians.

VITAMIN AND MINERAL TREATMENT
Supplementation with vitamin E (250 iu daily), chromium (200 mcg daily) incorporated into yeast, zinc (15 mg) and vitamin C (1 g daily) and manganese (4 g daily) may help prevent later complications.

DIARRHOEA

This is the frequent loose or even liquid evacuation of the bowel (sometimes involuntarily). It may also be accompanied by severe VOMITING.

CAUSES OF DIARRHOEA
- *Isolated bouts* can be caused by overindulgence in laxative foods (prunes, figs, apricots) or beer. They may also accompany fear, stress or ANXIETY.
- *Bacterial or viral infection* are the most common cause. This is why most people have diarrhoea when on holiday abroad. It's not the 'change of water' or unaccustomed food that is to blame, but exposure to bacteria against which the body has not developed an immunity. GASTROENTERITIS results.
- *Food intolerance* can cause diarrhoea in babies. If it occurs with vomiting and COLIC, it may indicate an allergy to milk and milk products. Gluten sensitivity should also be ruled out.
- *Infection* from inadequately sterilized feeding bottles.
- *Medication with antibiotics* is a frequent cause.

No change of otherwise normal bowel function should be ignored unless there is a very obvious cause and the normal bowel pattern returns in a short time (not longer than 36 hours). Recurrent bouts of diarrhoea for no reason, especially when alternating with bouts of CONSTIPATION are matters of concern and may indicate an underlying disease such as COLITIS, CROHN'S DISEASE, DIVERTICULITIS or IRRITABLE BOWEL SYNDROME. If diarrhoea persists beyond 48 hours, seek professional advice without delay.

All cases of diarrhoea in children should be referred to a practitioner immediately.

ORTHODOX TREATMENT
Anti-spasmodic drugs; specific therapy for the infecting organism.

SELF-HELP
For 'holiday tummy' diarrhoea, protect yourself from alien bacteria:
- Don't eat raw food that cannot be peeled (especially salad).
- Avoid tapwater and ice cubes.

- Avoid ice cream unless in the most hygienic of circumstances.
- Avoid the cold buffet: undercooked meat, poultry and raw fish often harbour bacteria.

For diarrhoea brought on by antibiotics, eat natural live yoghurt and take a short course of vitamin B complex for one week after the antibiotic treatment.

In all cases, remember that a side effect of diarrhoea is dehydration or fluid loss, which is particularly serious in babies and small children. It is vital to encourage fluid intake: give fluid in teaspoonsful every 10 to 15 minutes (it should be tepid, not ice cold.) To be certain, give the sugar and salt solution as in CHILDREN'S ILLNESSES (p. 139).

ACUPUNCTURE

When the energy of the Spleen, which should flow upwards to the lungs is 'rebellious', it flows downwards instead as diarrhoea.

Acupressure on 23, 29 and 39 will help to stimulate the Spleen, in addition to a brief fast if the diarrhoea is acute.

HERBAL TREATMENT

The following may help:
- Garlic oil capsules taken at night.
- Infusion of agrimony or plantain or geranium with a pinch of powdered ginger, cinnamon or crushed caraway seeds. Use 0.5 l/1 pt of water to 25g/1oz chopped herbs. Cover, stand for 15 minutes and strain. Take 3–4 tablespoonsful 3 times a day.

NATUROPATHY

Diarrhoea is the body's way of ridding itself of an unwanted substance and should not therefore be suppressed for at least 36 hours. Take care to keep fluid intake up.

Withhold food for 24 hours, giving only mineral water, apple juice or the salt/sugar solution. When diarrhoea subsides, introduce liquid food with a high food value (blended boiled rice and water, vegetable juice or soups). Live yoghurt will help the intestine return to its normal state of anti-infec-

tive flora. Start solid food with boiled rice, steamed carrots followed by bananas, hard boiled eggs and dry toast and then slowly back to normal.

For infants, use the above diet, but purée all food. Breastfeeding mothers should review their own diet for possible irritants.

VITAMIN AND MINERAL TREATMENT

Take mineral supplements (including potassium, magnesium and sodium) to replace those lost during the diarrhoea.

DIGESTIVE DISORDERS

If the heart, brain, lungs, liver or kidneys cease to function, we die, and it is for this reason that these organs receive the lion's share of people's emotional involvement in health. What most people (including the medical profession) overlook, however, is that there is a far more important set of organs than all of these put together, organs without which none of these would be able to function. These are the stomach and its attached digestive system. Through the mechanism of digestion, the body is able to absorb and use all the proteins, fats, carbohydrates, minerals, vitamins and trace elements that are vital for every cell in the body to survive, and it is problems in this digestive system that are so frequently at the root of many problems.

Details of specific digestive disorders appear under their own headings. Here we shall consider the broad principles of digestive problems.

WE ARE WHAT WE EAT

Apart from the more serious diseases relating directly to deficient nutrition, many of the millions of people throughout the world who rely on the Western diet of refined carbohydrates, processed and junk foods, and high intakes of salt, sugar and animal fats, are condemned to suffer a chronic lack of positive health. Vague feelings of digestive discomfort, lassitude, CONSTIPATION, DIAR-

RHOEA, HEADACHE, general malaise, lack of mental agility, faulty memory and indecision all may be attributed to poor digestion. There is seldom anything fundamentally wrong with the digestive system, only with what is put into it.

THE HAY SYSTEM

Since the turn of the century, a handful of forward thinkers have seen the need for an improvement in society's nutritional habits. They identified the links between food and disease and examined closely the whole question of the digestive process.

Of these early pioneers in food reform, some worked within the framework of orthodox medicine, although most did not. One example is the American doctor, William Howard Hay, who qualified in medicine in 1891. When his own health broke down some 16 years later and his medical colleagues were unable to help him, he took his life in his own hands and decided to treat his body as a whole instead of trying to treat just the symptoms.

He did this by changing his diet drastically: what he called 'fundamental eating' was based on consuming only natural foods in modest quantities, foods that he believed were intended by nature for humans. After making a complete recovery from his supposedly terminal illness, he changed his entire system of practising medicine and devoted his time to treating patients with dietary change.

The Hay system of eating is safe, simple and applicable to anyone at any age. Its benefits are far reaching and frequently dramatic.

Dr Hay's system contains five basic rules:

- Starches and sugars should not be eaten with protein and acid fruits in the same meal.
- Vegetables, salads and fruits should form a major part of the diet.
- Proteins, starches and fats should be eaten in small quantities.
- Only wholegrain and unprocessed starches should be used, and all refined processed foods should be taboo — in particular white flour and sugar and all foods made with them as well as highly processed fats such as margarine.
- An interval of at least 4 to 4½ hours should elapse between meals of a different character.

Although those suffering from overt digestive disease will certainly benefit from this diet, it is the many millions of sufferers of chronic low-grade digestive problems who may be surprised at the immensely beneficial effects of Dr Hay's principles. Even so, the Establishment is hard to shift.

See also **Nutrition** (p. 10); COLIC, COLITIS, CONSTIPATION, CROHN'S DISEASE, DIARRHOEA, DIVERTICULAR DISEASE, FLATULENCE, INDIGESTION, IRRITABLE BOWEL SYNDROME, OBESITY, PILES, ULCERS.

DIVERTICULITIS

Diverticulitis is the development of small pouches — called *diverticula* — in the wall of the colon.

The pouches are caused by CONSTIPATION (itself the result of a low fibre diet). Greatly increased pressure is required to force small portions of hard, dry stool through the bowel, and this rise in pressure can cause pouches to form at weak points in the wall of the colon. The diverticula themselves cause no symptoms, but if waste matter becomes trapped in them, they can become infected and inflamed — a condition called *diverticulitis*.

SYMPTOMS

Diverticulitis causes abdominal pain, sometimes so severe that it is known as 'left-sided appendicitis'. The abdomen itself becomes swollen and tender, and there may be NAUSEA AND VOMITING. Chronic diverticulitis can cause gradual blood loss, as well as alternating DIARRHOEA and constipation — this latter must always be investigated by a doctor as it is also a symptom of other, more serious diseases.

Infected diverticula may also form abscesses, or may burst, spilling the contents of the colon into the abdominal cavity; this is a medical emergency.

Orthodox Treatment
High-fibre diet; fibre tablets.

Acupuncture
Acupuncture treatment can be useful for the relief of discomfort, as can **acupressure**; use the same points described under DIARRHOEA.

Herbal Treatment
Slippery elm gruel, taken twice daily, will be beneficial; follow the manufacturer's instructions. Peppermint and chamomile tea should be drunk alternately before meals.

Naturopathy
Immediately change to a high-fibre, low-fat, low-sugar diet. Eat wholemeal bread, brown rice, wholemeal pasta, potatoes, dried fruits and all types of vegetables. Reduce your intake of dairy products, and exclude red meat, alcohol, coffee, strong tea, and *all* refined carbohydrates (eg sweets, chocolates, confectionary).

Drink vegetable juices, particularly carrot (diluted in an equal amount of apple juice) and cabbage juice, all of which have beneficial effects on the lining of the colon. Fluid intake should be not less than 3 pints (1.7 litres) daily. Add 2 heaped tbsp bran to the daily food intake.

Vitamin and Mineral Treatment
There is no specific therapy, but a high-potency sustained-release vitamin B complex will help to stimulate intestinal bacteria.

DIZZINESS

See *also* ANXIETY; FAINTNESS
Dizziness is a term that people use rather loosely for a range of subjective feelings of disturbed balance. It may merely mean that someone fears that they *might* fall; or it may refer to true vertigo, the actual experience of the room spinning round.

Causes of Dizziness
True vertigo is always the result of a disorder of the ear or brain, and an expert opinion from a neurologist or an ENT (ear, nose and throat) surgeon should be obtained at an early stage, Although they may be able to diagnose the cause, they may not be able to offer effective treatment, and natural health treatment can then be tried.

The commonest causes of true vertigo are
- Ménière's syndrome (a degenerative disorder of the balance mechanism of the ear).
- a viral infection of the balance mechanism.
- reduced blood supply to the balance mechanism due to kinking of the arteries to the brain by arthritis in the bones of the neck.
- ear damage caused by diseases such as mumps.
- effects of certain drugs (quinine, streptomycin) on the middle ear.
- postural hypotension (a fall in BLOOD PRESSURE if one stands up too quickly).

In addition vertigo may simply be the result of spinning around and it is also common in TRAVEL SICKNESS.

Mere fear of falling is usually caused by an ANXIETY state. This may be partly rational, as when a person who has had frequent falls is now afraid of crossing the road — so-called space PHOBIA. In most cases, however, it is a common symptom of agoraphobia.

Symptoms
Sensation of movement can be rotating or a feeling of displacement in one direction only. There is always an accompanying problem of balance. In sudden and severe attacks the patient may fall, break out in a cold sweat, feel nauseous, look pale and sometimes even faint.

Orthodox Treatment
Drugs specific to cause of vertigo;

D

psychotherapy for 'fear of falling'.

ACUPUNCTURE
Sudden dizziness while moving is often evidence of what is referred to as 'movement of wind in the Liver'. Another cause could be an imbalance between Energy and Blood within the heart. Acupuncture treatment may be beneficial to remedy these.

Acupressure The sensation of being about to fall can sometimes be helped by acupressure on the side of the foot at point 40, preferably while sitting, and behind the head at point 41 (see p. 102–3). Both these points are on the pathway of Bladder energy.

ALEXANDER TECHNIQUE
Dizziness may be related to a posture problem in the neck, which is cutting off the blood supply. In these cases, Alexander technique can prove valuable.

HERBAL TREATMENT
An infusion of balm — 25 g/1 oz in 0.5 l/1 pt water — is helpful for dizziness related to anxiety. Take 45–60 ml/3–4 tbsp 2 to 3 times daily.

HOMEOPATHY
For chronic vertigo, consult a homeopath. For temporary episodes:
● *Borax* Associated with fear of downward motion — eg in a lift
● *Bryonia* Dizziness brought on by the slightest movement, even turning the eyes.
● *Calcarea carbonica* Aggravated by looking up.
● *Gelsemium* Accompanied by trembling inside and weakness.

HYPNOTHERAPY
Where dizziness is a result of anxiety, stress or hyperventilation (over-breathing), hypnosis can help sufferers overcome these problems.

MANIPULATIVE THERAPIES
If there is a degenerative change in the neck and accompanying loss of neck movement, manipulative therapy can be extremely effective in the relief of vertigo.

MASSAGE
Sinus drainage by massaging the face, head and neck can relieve dizziness caused by ear problems associated with CATARRH.

NATUROPATHY
If the dizziness is caused by ear problems associated with catarrh, this can be helped by removing dairy products from the diet.

PSYCHOTHERAPIES
Dizziness caused by anxiety responds best to a variety of psychotherapies, particularly **behaviour psychotherapy** (see p. 95).

RELAXATION TECHNIQUES
Any of these can be beneficial.

VITAMIN AND MINERAL TREATMENT
Vertigo may be relieved with nicotinamide (200 mg), nicotinic acid (20 mg) and vitamin B_2 (5 mg), taken 3 times daily.

Drug abuse *see* Addictions

Dysmenorrhoea *see* MENSTRUAL DISORDERS

Dyspepsia *see* INDIGESTION

D
E

E

EARACHE

A common problem especially among young children, this is usually due to an infection of the outer or middle ear. Infection causes pressure to build up in restricted spaces, and this pressure on sensitive nerve endings will cause the pain.

The Eustachian tube can carry bacteria from the throat to the middle ear and an infection may result. In addition, if the adenoids (*see* TONSILS AND ADENOIDS) are infected and swollen, they can block the Eustachian tubes and prevent the ears' natural secretions from draining; this can result in a middle ear infection.

Earache can also be caused by SINUSITIS, infected teeth or even by a BOIL in the ear canal.

SYMPTOMS

High temperature, loss of appetite and general malaise as well as acute pain, especially in children. However, sometimes no pain occurs and the only symptom is a loss of hearing.

Continuing acute earache, especially if accompanied by any discharge from the ear, should not be ignored — medical advice should be sought immediately. No attempt should be made to clean the ear, since an inflamed eardrum is easily perforated, which can result in permanent loss of hearing.

ORTHODOX TREATMENT

Antibiotics; decongestants and antihistamines if adenoids involved.

ACUPUNCTURE

Ear problems may be relieved by treating the pathways that encircle the ear: Small Intestine, Bladder, 'Three Heaters'. When the problem is due to infection, other activities of the body will need to be stimulated.

Acupressure Sometimes earache can be lessened by acupressure on point 42 just behind the tip of the mastoid bone (the knob-like bone behind the ear), and on point 4 in the web between thumb and forefinger (either hand). (See p. 102–3)

HERBAL TREATMENT

Place a few drops of almond oil, warmed to body temperature (check on your wrist first), in the ear with a small dropper. Warm the oil by placing the bottle in a bath of warm water; *do not* heat it on a cooker or over a direct flame.

Hot cotton wool compresses soaked in an infusion of yarrow and placed around the ear can also be very soothing.

HOMEOPATHY
- *Belladonna* Acute throbbing, congested; often with high fever.
- *Chamomilla* For children who scream with pain and anger unless constantly held.
- *Nux vomica* Associated with great irritability and intolerance of noise.
- *Pulsatilla* With thick green catarrh; thirstless; worse in stuffy rooms.
- *Mercurius solubilis* Associated with dribbling of saliva on the pillow at night.

MANIPULATIVE THERAPIES

Where recurrent episodes of earache are associated with chronic sinus infections, osteopathic drainage techniques applied to the sinuses will help.

NATUROPATHY

Treat as for CATARRH.

Eczema *see* DERMATITIS

EMPHYSEMA

Pulmonary emphysema is a gradually progressive, incurable disease of the lungs. The tiny air sacs (alveoli) in the lungs become unnaturally distended with air; this stretches their walls, damages the surfaces and reduces the number of blood vessels there. This in turn interferes with the exchange of oxygen and carbon dioxide.

The heart has to pump much harder to push blood through the lungs. When the person exerts themself the heart has to pump much more blood than normal round the body to deliver enough oxygen to the tissues. There stresses can lead to heart failure.

Emphysema commonly occurs in heavy smokers and in those with chronic BRONCHITIS and ASTHMA; continuous exposure to high levels of pollution and dust can also cause the disease.

SYMPTOMS
The most common symptoms of emphysema are BREATHLESSNESS followed by coughing, even after only the slightest exertion.

ORTHODOX TREATMENT
Treatment of specific symptoms.

SELF-HELP
- Stop smoking.
- Take mild exercise to maintain muscle tone.

HERBAL TREATMENT
Make a decoction of equal quantities comfrey and licorice root, simmered for 15 minutes. Use 25 g/1 oz root mixture to 0.5 ml/1 pt water with a pinch of crushed anise seed. Take 45–60 ml/3–4 tbsp 3 or 4 times a day. See *also* BRONCHITIS

MANIPULATIVE THERAPIES
These will aim to maintain the mobility of the rib cage, improve posture and teach remedial breathing exercises.

NATUROPATHY
A diet that excludes dairy products will help minimize the production of mucus in the lungs.

VITAMIN AND MINERAL TREATMENT
Increase oxygen usage with vitamin E (200 iu, 3 times daily) and toughen up lung tissue with vitamin A (7,500 iu daily). Ensure that copper intake (4 mg daily) is adequate.

EYESTRAIN

See *also* ALLERGY, CONJUNCTIVITIS and HAY FEVER

In this technological age of television, computers and artificial light, more people than ever seem to suffer from eyestrain. Many visual disturbances, together with HEADACHES, neck aches and especially lack of achievement in school, are attributed to eye problems, and glasses are then prescribed, when they are not always necessary.

A particular cause for concern with regard to eyestrain is the now ubiquitous visual display unit (VDU). Visual problems, especially accompanied by headaches and neck and shoulder pains, are a common sequel to their use, and are found not only in professional computer operators but also among the millions of children who use home computers.

SELF-HELP
- Read and work in a good light that ideally should come over the shoulder opposite the writing hand.
- When reading or doing close work, look away and focus on a distant object every half hour.
- If operating a VDU, spend only a maximum of two hours in front of the screen, followed by a minimum of one hour (preferably two) away from it. Pay careful attention to background lighting levels and the relative heights of the operator's chair and the screen (see **Positive Health** pp. 48–50).

ACUPUNCTURE
The acupressure exercises illustrated overleaf can do much to relieve eyestrain. Keep your eyes closed while you do them, and do not use too much pressure. Perform them twice a day—morning and afternoon—and repeat each one eight times.

HERBAL TREATMENT
For sore eyes wash a handful of fresh chickweed. Cover with boiling water, leave to cool, then strain through a paper coffee filter. Apply this to a clean lint or gauze and use as a compress, a fresh one for each eye.

For general eye care add 5 ml/1 tsp eyebright to 1 teacupful of boiling water (if possible, use bottled non-gassy water). Cover and cool; strain through a paper coffee filter. Use as an eyebath, with fresh solution for each eye.

HOMEOPATHY
For sticky, inflamed, watering or burning eyes:
- *Euphrasia Mother Tincture* 3 drops in 4 fl. oz (115 ml) boiled water.
- *Euphrasia 30* Every 2 hours until medical help can be obtained.

MASSAGE
This can relieve the muscular tension, aches and pains that can accompany eyestrain.

NATUROPATHY
In the early years of this century, Dr W.H. Bates, a New York opthal-mologist, came to the conclusion that the prescription of glasses for many visual problems was unwarranted. The 'Bates method of achieving better sight without glasses' (*see* **Positive Health** p. 49) is a routine of specific eye exercises, relaxation aids, visual aids and eye and muscle exercises.

However, while the Bates system may help to improve eyesight it is not suitable for organic diseases of the eye such as glaucoma.

VITAMIN AND MINERAL TREATMENT
Ensure that there is an adequate intake of vitamin A (7,500 iu daily) plus vitamin B_2 (riboflavin; 10 mg daily).

EYE INJURIES
Always wear protective glasses if you

Acupressure points for the relief of eye strain

1 Massage both sides of the top of the nose, using the thumbs. Keep the other fingers slightly curled against the forehead.
2 Massage the bridge of the nose using the thumb and index finger of one hand. Press down, then up.
3 Place the index and middle fingers of both hands on either side of the nose. Remove the middle fingers and massage under the cheekbones using the index fingers. Rest the thumbs on the lower jaw.
4 Place both thumbs on either side of the forehead. Keeping the other fingers curled, rub around the eye sockets, from the beginning of the eyebrow by the nose to the end of the eyebrow, and then round underneath the eye to just under the pupil.

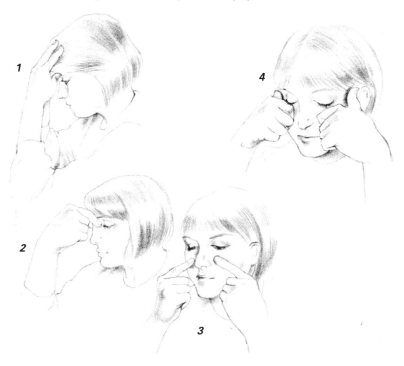

are doing a job or have a hobby that exposes you to flying particles.

All eye injuries are potentially serious. If in any doubt, obtain medical help at once.

- If a foreign particle enters the eye, do not rub it. First, try blinking under water to dislodge the particle. If this does not work, dampen a cotton wool swab or a clean cloth and *very gently* remove the offending particle.
- *Do not* try to dislodge any particle that seems to have become embedded or to have punctured the eye. Go to a hospital casualty department *at once*.
- Irritant chemicals should be flushed out with large quantities of clean water or milk for at least 15 minutes. Make sure that the inside of the eyelids are also flushed out. Take the person to a hospital casualty department.

HOMEOPATHY

- If there is a foreign body in the eye: wash out with *Hypericum Mother Tincture*, 3 drops in 115 ml/4 fl. oz warm boiled water.
- For pain after injury use *Aconite 30*, every 15 minutes as required.

BLACK EYE

To avoid as much swelling and bruising as possible, apply a cold compress to the eye immediately. *See* BRUISES for further treatment.

Taking 1–2 g vitamin C daily for 5–6 days plus Bromelain (300–600 mg), bioflavonoids (600 mg) and zinc (15 mg) will help the bruise to fade quickly. Drink pineapple or papaya juice or eat the fresh fruit.

F

FAINTING

A feeling of faintness or actual fainting is caused by a lack of blood flowing to the brain, leading to a temporary loss of consciousness.

Excessive pain, heat, cold or fear, the sight of blood or any other unpleasant stimulus can cause fainting. A slowing of the heart rate accompanied by dilating of the blood vessels in the outer parts of the body can cause a sudden drop in BLOOD PRESSURE, and since the brain is the highest part of the body, this is the first affected. The faint is actually the body's self-defence mechanism since, once flat on the ground, the head is at the same level as the heart. This encourages a rapid return of blood flow to the brain.

Postural hypotension is a sudden fall in blood pressure caused by a sudden change in position — eg from sitting to standing — and this is perhaps the most common reason why people faint. In addition, if you stand for too long in one position as soldiers on parade do, the blood tends to collect in the veins of the lower part of the body, thus depriving the brain and leading to a blackout.

Lack of oxygen circulating in the blood due to ANAEMIA or a lung disease such as BRONCHITIS or EMPHYSEMA, or a sudden fall in blood sugar levels (*see* DIABETES) can also have the same effect.

Anyone suffering from repeated fainting attacks should consult their doctor.

HOMEOPATHY

- *Aconite* After fright.
- *Arnica* After injury.
- *Opium* After fear, accompanied by great drowsiness.
- *Ignatia* Fainting due to hysteria, resulting from disappointment in love.
- *Arsenicum album* Chilliness, restlessness, exhaustion.
- *Carbo vegetabilis* (Called the 'corpse reviver') chilliness with a desire for air.

VITAMIN AND MINERAL TREATMENT

If due to anaemia, *see* ANAEMIA.

first aid for fainting

If a person feels faint, make them sit down and place their head between their knees until they feel better. Ensure that there is enough fresh air.

If a person actually faints:

- *Lay them on their back* with the legs slightly raised above the level of their heart.
- *Loosen any tight clothing,* especially around their neck.
- *Check that there are no obstructions* in the mouth such as dentures, and that the tongue is not falling back into the throat.
- *If there is difficulty in breathing,* place them in the recovery position as above: lay them on their side, with the upper leg bent and the lower one straight; the upper arm bent at the elbow, the lower one extended behind the back; the head turned to one side.
- *If the person does not recover* within a few minutes, obtain medical help.

Recovery position

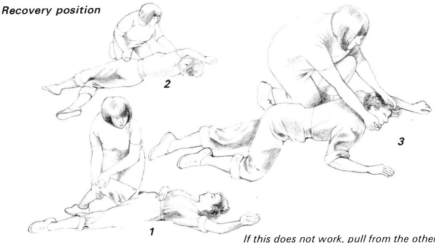

Recovery position
Raise one leg at the knee (1), and push against it to roll patient over gently.

If this does not work, pull from the other side (using patient's clothes) making sure arm does not flop over (2). When the patient is face down, carefully turn the head to one side (3).

FATIGUE

In the abscence of any specific ailment such as ANAEMIA or any explanatory disease state (INFLUENZA for example), generalized fatigue and lethargy is normally associated with poor nutrition, INSOMNIA, or poor quality of sleep, excessive stress (*see* TENSION), ANXIETY or DEPRESSION.

Fatigue can be related to FOOD INTOLERANCE or low blood sugar, although the latter is much less common than many people suppose. *Myalgic encephalomyelitis* (ME) is a disease typified by overwhelming muscle fatigue; it is associated with an infection of the yeast-like *candida albicans* (see THRUSH).

The only sure way to overcome the problem of chronic fatigue is to take an holistic approach. No success can be achieved without consideration for the ecology of the sufferer.

ALEXANDER TECHNIQUE
This can be beneficial.

HERBAL TREATMENT
Mix 5 ml/1 tsp rosemary with 1 teacup boiling water. Cover, allow to stand and drink warm, half a cup on waking and half a cup at bedtime. Peppermint tea 2 or 3 times a day, or an infusion of St John's wort (45–60 ml/3–4 tbsp 3 times a day) are good for occasional fainting.

HOMEOPATHY
Consult a homeopath.

NATUROPATHY
Seek professional advice for possible causes such as anaemia.

Restrict your sugar and refined carbohydrate intake and increase protein with whole grains and pulses.

PSYCHOTHERAPIES
Where fatigue is the result of an underlying psychological problem, psychotherapy will be of enormous value. The repression and anxieties of the depressive patient respond to a clearer understanding of their place in the world and their relationships with those about them. **Psychodrama** (p. 95), **gestalt** (p. 94), **bioenergetics** (p. 95) and basic counselling can all help.

RELAXATION TECHNIQUES
Yoga or **meditation** (pp. 98–9).

VITAMIN AND MINERAL TREATMENT
Take supplements of Vitamin E and the B complex. Extra magnesium (500 mg daily) and potassium (1,500 mg daily) may help.

See also ANAEMIA.

FEVER

A 'normal' body temperature is usually considered to be 98.4°F (37°C), but it can range between 96 and 99°F (35.6–37.2°C). Most infectious illnesses cause a rise in body temperature. However, as well as bacterial and viral infections, other things such as exercise, excitement, hot baths, sensitivities to foods and medicines, plus severe ANAEMIA, circulatory, respiratory and HEART DISEASES and the acute forms of ARTHRITIS can all produce a rise in temperature.

SYMPTOMS
The onset of fever can be gradual or sudden, and temperatures may remain fairly normal during the daytime but rise dramatically at night. As the temperature rises, so do the pulse and respiration rates.

The tongue may become furry and dry, the appetite is poor, and there can be NAUSEA AND VOMITING and CONSTIPATION. The amount of urine passed is reduced, and it becomes very concentrated due to the loss of body fluids through sweating.

Other symptoms such as HEADACHE, lassitude, feelings of hot and cold, shivering and aches and pains in the back and limbs are common factors when the temperature is raised much above normal. If it rises above 103°F (39.4°C), delirium may occur, which can lead to convulsions ('fits') and finally coma if attempts are not made to reduce it. Convulsions are particularly common in children between the ages of one and three (rare after the age of five).

If someone develops a sudden high temperature, has other severe symptoms, becomes delirious or suffers a fit, medical help must be obtained as soon as possible. Mild fevers that are prolonged and/or recurrent should also be investigated.

ORTHODOX TREATMENT
Aspirin or paracetamol.

SELF-HELP
● Tepid sponging is often helpful, particularly with children (see CHILDREN'S ILLNESSES)
● Bed clothes should be kept to a minimum, and the room in which the feverish person is resting should be kept cool and well aired.
● Avoid strenuous exercise.

HERBAL TREATMENT
Take hot herbal teas at frequent intervals to promote perspiration and thus help the body throw off poisons and impurities. After the temperature has returned to normal, the teas may be taken cool for their tonic properties.

The following herbal teas may be useful: elderflower and peppermint in equal quantities; yarrow; boneset herb; elderflower and limeblossom together for feverish colds; lavender flowers for influenza or chesty cold; hyssop to help clear mucus from the lungs; rosemary tips for colds. (Both rosemary and lavender are prepared in weak infusions, half the normal strength.) A combination of lavender, sage and rosemary, half strength, is antiseptic and almost antibiotic in its action.

The herbal teas can be taken every one or two hours, hot, in 45–60 ml/3–4 tbsp doses, until perspiration has taken place, then reduced in frequency. Hyssop should be taken in 15 ml/1 tbsp doses, 4 or 5 times daily.

HOMEOPATHY

- *Aconite* For acute onset, after exposure to cold, dry winds; associated with fear, restlessness.
- *Belladonna* For acute onset, restless with excitement becoming delirious; wide staring eyes, hot red face.
- *Ferrum phosphoricum* For slower onset; less dramatic picture than above two remedies.

NATUROPATHY

Diet: Fast until the temperature is normal and the appetite returns. Drink only pure unsweetened juices or water, 4–5 times daily.
Heat/Cold Treatment: A cold trunk or waist pack may be applied, as well as a cold compress to the forehead.

Fibroids *see* MENSTRUAL DISORDERS

FIBROSITIS

This is an acutely painful inflammation of muscle fibres and may be a long-standing and chronic problem. The most usual site for fibrositis are the large muscles of the neck and shoulders, especially around the shoulder blades, and in the large muscles on either side of the spine. Fibrositis may also occur in the big muscles of the buttocks.

Orthodox medicine does not officially recognize fibrositis as a spec-

ific entity, but any practitioner who spends time with their hands on patients' bodies is not only certain of its existence but can frequently tell the patient exactly where the painful points are, since these will have become fibrositic nodules that can be clearly felt deep within the muscle tissue.

While fibrositis is commonly a result of the way the body is held while performing a particular job, general poor POSTURE, stress and TENSION or a response to other disabling injury, it must never be forgotten that a careful clinical examination must be undertaken before the label *fibrositis* is attached to any ailment. Many diseases produce symptoms affecting the musculo-skeletal system, particularly bone diseases such as OSTEOPOROSIS and some forms of CANCER. Pain and stiffness may also be produced by psychological disorders.

ORTHODOX TREATMENT
Painkillers; muscle relaxants.

SELF-HELP
- Apply a hot water bottle to the affected area, or take a warm bath if the pain is more generalized.
- Avoid going out in cold, damp weather and make sure that your environment inside is warm and dry.
- Rub the aching muscle with liniment, producing a mild irritation that will draw blood to the area, increasing the circulation and making it warmer.

ACUPUNCTURE
Rheumatism, arthritis and fibrositis are characterized by obstructions of Energy and related to excesses of cold or dampness or wind. Individual treatment will depend on the factors involved; cold, for example will require points to be heated by the use of moxibustion.

HERBAL TREATMENT
The anti-inflammatory herbs, such as extract of willow and primula, will be beneficial.

MANIPULATIVE THERAPIES
Fibrositis can be caused by, and can

be the cause of, bad posture, and any attempt to relieve local symptoms without determining the cause is fruitless. A full examination, detailed enquiries as to a sufferer's occupations and hobbies, and an overall assessment of their joint mobility, muscle tone and general psychological attitudes, all form an integral part of the treatment.

MASSAGE
Have both relaxing and pressure-point massage on the shoulders, neck, legs and feet, using essential oils of eucalyptus, thyme, rosemary and lavender, 15 drops to 50 ml/about 3 tbsp vegetable oil.

NATUROPATHY
Diet: Discourage OBESITY. Limit 'acid-forming' foods in the diet (meat, eggs, sugar) and increase fresh fruit, raw vegetables and wholegrain produce.

Aim to increase the circulation in the affected area to help healing. This can be done in a number of ways:
Hydrotherapy:
● hot and cold fomentations: 3 minutes hot and 1 minute cold, for 20–30 minutes;
● contrast (ie hot and cold) bathing: always finish with cold;
● friction rubs using a coarse towel.
Exercise: take exercise in a form appropriate to your ability.

RELAXATION TECHNIQUES
Any one of these will help.

VITAMIN AND MINERAL TREATMENT
High-dose calcium pantothenate (vitamin B_5) should be taken, starting with 2,000 mg daily (in prolonged-release form) until relief is obtained; then reduce the daily dose to one that continues to provide relief. Alternatively, take vitamin B_1 (thiamin), 600 mg daily reducing to 50 mg.

FLATULENCE

This is an accumulation of air or gases produced during digestion, which collect in the stomach and the intestines causing distention and discomfort.

Excessive flatulence, especially when accompanied by abdominal pain, may be a symptom of ULCERS, IRRITABLE BOWEL SYNDROME, DIVERTICULLS, CROHN'S DISEASE or hiatus HERNIA. It is also a common accompaniment to CONSTIPATION, when the gases become 'dammed up' along with the stools.

In the absence of any disease, excessive flatulence is almost certainly a sign of poor dietary habits, and can nearly always be relieved by modification to the diet (see **Nutrition** pp. 10ff).

ORTHODOX TREATMENT
Charcoal tablets.

HERBAL TREATMENT
Relief may be obtained by taking 'seed tea' (*see* COLIC) or peppermint tea, after meals. Drinking hot parsley tea in 3–4 tbsp/45–60 ml doses or chewing a sprig or two of parsley after a meal can be useful. A tea made of equal amounts of balm and chamomile flowers, taken in 3–4 tbsp/45–60 ml doses an hour before each meal, will improve flatulence of nervous origin.

A number of culinary herbs—including thyme, rosemary, sage and marjoram—contain essential oils that aid digestion. If used with moderate generosity in cooking, they should help prevent flatulence.

NATUROPATHY
One main cause of flatulence is meals that contain too great a mixture of foods, making it more difficult for the digestive system to tackle them thoroughly. The solution is to eat simpler meals. The Hay diet (*see* pp. 156–7), which avoids mixing protein and carbohydrate foods at the same meal, has proved helpful to many people. Meals that contain only a little or no fat are also easier to digest.

Some people find that eating plain 'live' yogurt or acidophilus (sold as tablets) helps their digestive systems. Changing to a high fibre diet may

F

occasionally cause flatulence. Introduce more fibre slowly, over a few months.

See *also* ALLERGY

RELAXATION TECHNIQUES
Any one of these can help.

FOOD INTOLERANCE

See *also* ALLERGY

Food intolerance — or 'food allergy', as it is commonly called — is a highly controversial subject, which for many years was the sole preserve of practitioners of complementary medicine. In recent years, however, some orthodox doctors have taken up the cudgels, but sadly they too have been treated largely with scorn by their colleagues.

ALLERGY OR INTOLERANCE?
ALLERGY is a direct response of the body's own auto-immune defence mechanism, and produces very specific reactions. The common test for allergies is the scratch test; if there is no obvious allergic reaction, an immunologist would say that there is no food allergy. However, there are many foods that can cause unwarranted side-effects in some people without producing the classical immunological responses of allergy. Because of this, it is preferable to call this reaction food intolerance.

Despite growing volumes of medical evidence supporting the concept that food intolerance can produce dramatic changes in behaviour and physical well-being, and showing that a gradually increasing proportion of our population is suffering as a result, orthodox medicine has failed to take on board the overall concept of clinical ecology.

While there is little scientific evidence to prove that many food additives are dangerous, but equally there is little to prove that they are absolutely safe. What has been shown is that a large number of chemicals — especially the food colourings as well as many of the synthetic materials

with which we are in daily contact — can produce severe adverse side-effects in some people. Common sense alone must show that it is better to avoid these things when possible than to risk unnecessary exposure.

However, sensitivity to food is not a blanket diagnosis for all the ills that affect us. Food intolerance is currently a 'high-fashion' disease, and while there is no doubt that real food allergies and adverse food reactions exist in many millions of people great care must be taken to establish the existence of any intolerance before committing yourself or your child to extremes of nutritional therapy.

GENERAL SYMPTOMS
General feelings of malaise, lethargy, abdominal pains, HEADACHES and INSOMNIA may be followed by increasing ANXIETY and DEPRESSION as all forms of treatment fail to relieve the symptoms.

TROUBLESOME FOODS AND ADDITIVES
Among foods, milk, eggs, chocolate, fish, soya, wheat and cheese are among the culprits most often identified. among the culprits most often identified.
Among the likely problem additives are:
- E102: tartrazine, an orange dye.
- E210,211: benzoic acids.
- E220,221,223,224: sulphite-based preservatives.
- E250,251: nitrite preservatives.
- E310,320,321: antioxidants.
- E621,622,623: monsodium glutamate and related flavour enhancers.

The sulphite and benzoic acid derivatives are the most implicated in those vulnerable to asthmatic problems.

FOOD-RELATED DISEASES
Infantile dermatitis and COLIC in babies are frequently related to an adverse reaction to cows' milk. This can even occur in

F

breastfed babies when their mothers consume large quantities of cows' milk. In addition, chronic CONSTIPATION and DIARRHOEA can often be attributed to intolerance of milk.

Ear, nose and throat problems are frequently triggered by adverse food reactions. Particularly where there is chronic sinus infection, EARACHE, infected TONSILS AND ADENOIDS and continual runny noses and excessive CATARRH, cows' milk should be suspected, but sometimes wheat and other cereals can also be implicated.

DERMATITIS and ASTHMA are conditions that most often have a component of adverse food reaction. An asthmatic child can have an attack within minutes of consuming food or drink (or even medicine) that contains the food colouring *tartrazine*.

MIGRAINE, IRRITABLE BOWEL SYNDROME, ARTHRITIS, ulcerative COLITIS, hyperactivity, skin diseases and even some gynaecological disorders have all been linked to food sensitivity.

BEHAVIOURAL PROBLEMS

Hyperactivity in children may be caused by food reactions. The most suspect group of products are the salicylates, which are usually found in food colourings and preservatives.

However, it can be very difficult to draw the line between the behaviour of a child that is within the normal limits of high energy and abnormally active behaviour. In addition, hyperactivity can also be the result of a brain disorder, and it and other behaviour problems are also frequently caused by psychological disturbances.

DIAGNOSIS

You must see your practitioner to find out whether your ailment has a relatively simple physical cause.

If not then food intolerance may be involved, or perhaps even a more straightforward allergy. If the orthodox methods of diagnosis do not reveal anything, one of the newer forms of allergy testing may. These include the auricular cardiac reflex (ACR), RAST (radio allergosorbant test), cytotoxic

and sublingual tests, and hair analysis, to check levels of nutritional minerals and trace elements and levels of potentially toxic minerals.

If none of these uncovers any adverse reactions, an exclusion diet may do so (*see* NATUROPATHY *below*).

HOMEOPATHY

This requires individual treatment, so consult a homeopath. However, it is always worth trying.

HYNOTHERAPY

Hypnosis can help overcome anxiety and tension. It is quite effective with children who have less fear of and resistance to hypnosis than do adults.

NATUROPATHY

Identifying foods that cause bad reactions in children can be difficult, as their reactions may be influenced by their own or their parents' expectations, by family relationships (a special diet may improve a child's behaviour just because he or she feels cherished) and by food likes and dislikes.

Because of this, possible non-food causes should be tackled first as they are often easier to change. A diet low in additives should be tried initially, before trying to eliminate particular basic foods. The latter—called an exclusion diet—is best done under supervision. Cutting the diet down to a very limited selection of foods can result in unbalancing a child's nutrition, as well as giving food too powerful an emotional role in the child's life (*see also* ANOREXIA AND BULIMIA NERVOSA).

Many of these same problems are also encountered by adults.

PSYCHOTHERAPIES

Not all hyperactivity in children is caused by adverse food reactions. It may be a mixture of these and psychological disturbances, or it may be totally psychological in origin. In either of these situations, it is important to use psychotherapy appropriate to the child's age.

If drugs are prescribed, they should be made up without colourings or

F

flavourings that might be contributing to the problem.

Vitamin and Mineral Treatment
Hyperactivity may benefit from high doses of vitamins including nicotinamide (1–3 g); vitamin B$_6$ (100–300 mg); vitamin C (1 g); vitamin E (up to 400 iu daily) and the minerals zinc (15 mg) and magnesium (300 mg) daily. Medical monitoring is essential. May also respond to Oil of Evening Primrose (up to 2,000 mg a day). If malabsorbtion is a problem, use vitamins in liquid suspension.

See *also* ALLERGY; **Nutrition** (pp. 23–5).

Frozen Shoulder

The shoulder joint with its complex interrelationships of muscles and tendons and its very wide range of movement make it vulnerable to pain and restriction of movement. What is commonly called 'frozen shoulder' is also known as rotator cuff lesion, capsulitis and bursitis, but there seems little evidence for such fine degree of differentiation.

Torn muscle fibres and inflammation (see FIBROSITIS) are probably the cause, and since movement makes the pain worse, those affected tend to hold their arms to their sides. This lack of use encourages the formation of adhesions and makes movement even more impossible.

Pain is particularly severe when the person tries to lift the arm sideways, and simple tasks such as reaching into a pocket, fastening a bra or brushing the hair at the back of the head become agonizing.

Orthodox Treatment
Painkillers; drugs to reduce muscle spasm and inflammation; physio-therapy; infrared heat treatment; cortisone injections.

Acupuncture
This is one of the few instances when acupuncture treatment is directed to the afflicted part. It is used to relieve the pain and improve the mobility of the joint.

Healing
This is sometimes beneficial.

Herbal Treatment
Extracts of anti-inflammatory herbs such as willow and primula will reduce inflammation.

Manipulative Therapies
A frozen shoulder responds well to manipulative treatment, both to the joint itself and to the vertebrae of the neck, thus ensuring that mobility and the function of all the associated joints and muscles are maintained.

Frequent applications of ice packs (a bag of frozen peas is easy to mould to the shape of the shoulder) and a regime of very gentle but gradually progressing exercises are also necessary. Correct manipulative treatment will shorten the course of this irritating problem by many months.

Where pain in the shoulder arises from calcium deposits in one of the tendons, it is unlikely to be greatly relieved by manipulative treatment. Steroid injections, ultrasound treatment and, sometimes, surgical removal of the deposits are the solution in this case.

Massage
Massaging all the muscles of the shoulder as well as those that extend into the chest, back and neck will help to relieve tension and increase mobility.

Relaxation Techniques
Any of these will help to relax the neck and shoulder muscles.

Vitamin and Mineral Treatment
See FIBROSITIS.

F

G

GALLSTONES

The gall bladder stores bile, which is made by the liver and leaves the latter via a duct. Bile consists of water, salts, bilirubin (a pigment made from the remains of red blood cells) and cholesterol. Sometimes stones made up of various elements of the bile form in the gall bladder, which can then pass into the common bile duct leading to the small intestine.

The typical gallstones candidate:
- Fair
- Fat
- Fertile
- Forty
- Flatulent

Gallstones come in three varieties.
- *Cholesterol stones* are made almost entirely of cholesterol, and usually occur either as one large stone or in pairs.
- *Mixed stones* — a mixture of cholesterol, calcium and bilirubin — are the commonest, and are normally present in very large numbers.
- *Pigment stones* may also occur, although rarely. They are made up almost entirely of bile pigment; there are normally many of them, and they are associated with blood diseases.

SYMPTOMS
Very often the first sign of gallstones is an attack of biliary COLIC, severe pain in the abdomen, which normally moves across to its right side, lasts several hours and can be agonizing. There may also be 'referred' pain to the right side of the body to the back or to the right shoulder blade, and there is nearly always severe vomiting and nausea.

JAUNDICE, in which the dammed up biliburin spills into the bloodstream, is a common sequel to an attack of biliary colic.

ORTHODOX TREATMENT
Removal of the gall bladder.

ACUPUNCTURE
Acupuncture treatment to the Gall Bladder and Liver meridians is helpful in balancing the relative energy levels between these two organs. The Kidney meridians will usually have to be treated as well to ensure an overall balanced eliminative function.

HERBAL TREATMENT
Dandelion leaves added to a daily salad will stimulate the liver and help reduce cholesterol levels. An infusion of 25 g/1 oz each of chopped dandelion leaves and roots should be taken in 90–120 ml/6–8 tbsp doses 15 minutes before eating.

Chamomile tea also has a beneficial effect on the liver.

HOMEOPATHY
Consult a homeopath.

NATUROPATHY
The presence of gallstones obstructs the flow of bile, which is essential for the digestion of fats. A very low-fat diet that excludes all dairy products and animal fats, and includes a high proportion of cereal fibre and raw vegetables, is required. Fish and poultry (excluding the skin) are suitable protein sources, but should be cooked without the use of animal fats.

The globe artichoke has a proven ability to stimulate the flow of bile. It should therefore form a regular part of the diet — say, at least 3 times a week.

VITAMINS AND MINERALS
Increase polyunsaturated fatty acid intake with safflower oil (3,000 mg daily), plus vitamin C (500 mg) and vitamin E (400 iu) daily to reduce the

cholesterol content of the bile.

Gastritis *see* DIGESTIVE DISORDERS

GASTROENTERITIS

This is an inflammation of the lining of both the stomach and the intestines, which produces NAUSEA AND VOMITING and DIARRHOEA, together with abdominal CRAMP and pain and total loss of appetite. In children the commonest cause of gastroenteritis is a virus that is inhaled and spreads rapidly wherever children congregate. It can also be caused by bacteria, most commonly from contaminated foods. In addition it can be a symptom of INFLUENZA (e.g. 'gastric flu') where the infecting organism spreads to the bowel through the bloodstream.

Babies most commonly get gastroenteritis as a result of faulty sterilization of bottles and teats, or through poor hygiene on the part of parents or guardians failing to make sure that their hands are adequately clean before handling sterilized feeding equipment. Gastroenteritis can be extremely serious in children and small babies since the constant vomiting and diarrhoea can lead to dehydration. Any child that has diarrhoea accompanied by vomiting for longer than 6 hours should see a medical practitioner.

Viral gastroenteritis in adults is normally self-limiting, and they recover after a few days with or without treatment. However, poisoning through bacterial infection may be more serious, especially if salmonella is the cause. This can be fatal especially in older people.

SELF-HELP
- Stop all solid foods, and avoid milk and milk based products.
- Take lots of fluid (not ice cold or citrus fruit).
- Take precautions as outlined in DIARRHOEA.

ORTHODOX TREATMENTS AND
NATURAL THERAPIES
See CHILDREN'S ILLNESSES and DIARRHOEA

Genital herpes *see* HERPES

GERMAN MEASLES
(RUBELLA)

See also PREGNANCY AND CHILDBIRTH

This is a mild virus infection that affects the respiratory tract and occurs mostly in children. Those with German measles are infectious from the start of symptoms until at least a week from the appearance of the rash.

SYMPTOMS
German measles starts with a slight cold, slightly sore throat and possibly mild CONJUNCTIVITIS. German measles victims seldom feel unwell. A rash may follow in a day or two, starting on the face and spreading down the trunk. It appears as tiny, flat, pale pink dots and, in a severe infection, may look like mild MEASLES; it disappears within days. However, German measles can be so mild that a rash does not develop; meanwhile, the child is still infectious.

The glands in the back of the neck are usually swollen and tender.

Complications are rare in children, but teenagers may be left with painful, swollen joints for a week or two.

HERBAL TREATMENT
Calamine lotion or calendula lotion applied externally will soothe the irritation.

NATUROPATHY
If the child feels unwell, a light diet and plenty of fluids will suffice. (See CHILDRENS ILLNESSES.)

VITAMIN AND MINERAL TREATMENT
Vitamin C (500 mg, 3 times daily) can be given to assist the body's own anti-viral defences.

German measles and pregnancy.
Although German measles causes
only slight discomfort to the sufferer,
it can have a devastating effect on an
unborn child if a woman contracts it
during the first 3 months of
pregnancy.
  To avoid this:
● All girls between the ages of 11
  and 13 should be vaccinated
  against German measles. (This is
  far more effective than 'German
  measles parties' where children
  are exposed to another with the
  virus; the trouble is that there is no
guarantee that a child will catch
the infection at that particular
time.)
● All children with German measles
  must be kept at home until the
  infectious period has passed in
  order to avoid contact with any
  pregnant woman.
● All women planning to become
  pregnant should have a test to see
  if they are immune. If they are not,
  they should be vaccinated; they
  must then wait for 3 months before
  becoming pregnant.

GINGIVITIS

Gingivitis is a bacterial infection of the
gums. Untreated, it can progress to
peridontal disease — commonly called
'gum disease' — where the gums and
the bone supporting the teeth are
gradually destroyed. In fact, gum
disease, and not tooth decay (see
TOOTHACHE), is the most common
reason why people lose their teeth.
  Gingivitis is caused by inadequate
dental hygiene. Vitamin C deficiency
may contribute.

SYMPTOMS
The gums become swollen and red,
and they bleed easily, especially during
brushing. If untreated, dental plaque
and hard tartar collect in the gum
margin, and pockets of pus develop
around the base of the teeth resulting
in bad breath and, possibly abscesses.
This in turn can lead to severe ulceration of the mouth, and the teeth gradually become loose and fall out.

ORTHODOX TREATMENT
Removal of plaque and tartar; removal
of small section of gum.

SELF-HELP
● Brush firmly and thoroughly, even
  if this temporarily causes more
  bleeding. Brush all parts of the teeth,
but be sure to concentrate on the
area between the tooth and the gum,
where plaque and tartar collect and
set up infections. Using dental floss
may also help (see **Positive Health**
p. 51).
● Use an antiseptic mouthwash after
  every meal until the inflammation
  has subsided (see NATUROPATHY).

HOMEOPATHY
Chronic gingivitis may require the
attention of a homeopath. For the
occasional attack:
● *Mercurius solubilis* For inflamed and
  bleeding gums; bad breath;
  retraction of gums.
● *Nitric acidium* For ulcers on gums;
  sharp, stinging pains.
● *Silica* Chronic disease with
  involvement of bone, or tooth
  fragments not expelled properly.

NATUROPATHY
To make an effective mouthwash, you
will need 10 ml/2 tsp 20 vol hydrogen
peroxide and 230 ml/8 fl oz warm
water and 5 ml/1 tsp Milton fluid and
120 ml/4 fl oz hot water.
  Add the peroxide to the water. Rinse
the mouth thoroughly, using all the
mixture. Squeeze the liquid between
the teeth. DO NOT SWALLOW.
  Then add the Milton to the hot
water. Rinse the mouth out several
times. DO NOT SWALLOW. Do not
rinse out afterwards.
  Follow a low sugar diet, especially
avoiding sugary and sticky foods eaten

between meals. Eat plenty of chewy food. This encourages saliva which protects the mouth from harmful bacteria.

VITAMIN AND MINERAL TREATMENT
Gingivitis has been treated with very high doses of vitamin A (500,000 iu) and vitamin E (30 iu) daily by injection for six days, followed by 50,000 iu vitamin A three times daily, with 200 iu vitamin E twice daily, taken by mouth. These doses require medical supervision as high doses of vitamin can cause severe liver damage.

GLANDULAR FEVER

(INFECTIOUS MONONUCLEOSIS)

An acute viral infectious disease which most commonly affects children and young adults. It is debilitating but seldom serious.

SYMPTOMS
The initial symptoms are similar to INFLUENZA: general tiredness, muscular pains, HEADACHE, FEVER and an enlargement of the lymph GLANDS. SORE THROAT is an early sign, with the swollen glands occurring 3 weeks later. There may also be a skin rash. In severe cases, the spleen may be enlarged but this returns to normal when the infection is over.

Although recovery is complete, some people may be ill for weeks or months with recurrent high fevers, sweats and general weakness. Symptoms may appear for up to 2 years after initial infection. Some people suffer DEPRESSION and should be reassured that this is a result of the infection. All but the mildest cases will need at least four weeks at home to recover fully and should not return to school or work until there is no more fluctuation in temperature. It may be six months until a person is fully fit.

ORTHODOX TREATMENT
Accurate diagnosis must be confirmed by blood tests.

HEALING
This can help to relieve general malaise, aches and pains.

HERBAL TREATMENT
To combat infection and prevent recurrence of FEVER, take garlic oil capsules each night. The glands should be massaged gently with antiseptic herbal oils 2 or 3 times daily, keeping a light, warm scarf around the neck in between. Lavender, eucalyptus, peppermint and bergamot oils are used by aromatherapists; olbas and other proprietary oils can also be employed.

Tea made of equal quantities of yarrow, elderflower, peppermint and clivers—50 g/2 oz to 1 l/1$\frac{3}{4}$ pts water—can be taken in 45–60 ml (3–4 tbsp) doses during periods of fever until profuse sweating occurs and the temperature begins to fall.

HOMEOPATHY
Take *cistus candaensis* 4 times a day for up to 3 days. If there is no improvement, consult a homeopath.

VITAMIN AND MINERAL TREATMENT
Supplements should include a high intake of vitamin C (up to 1,500 mg daily), and high-potency B complex and amino acid L-lysine (1,500 mg daily).

Gout *see* ARTHRITIS

Grazes *see* CUTS AND GRAZES

Gripe *see* COLIC AND STOMACH ACHE

Gum disease *see* GINGIVITIS

H

Haemorrhage *see* BLEEDING

Haemorrhoids *see* PILES

HAIR AND SCALP PROBLEMS

Hair is a very early barometer of general health. Frequently, a hairdresser will detect changes in quality and quantity of hair only for the person to develop the symptoms of an illness a short time later. Hair analysis (*see* FOOD INTOLERANCE) can also be a useful guide to the general well-being of the body. A measurement of essential trace elements and minerals, as well as the presence of any excess amounts of toxic minerals, can be established by this process. There are a number of common disorders affecting the hair and scalp.

GREASY HAIR AND SCALP
This is caused by overactivity of the sebaceous glands; if these glands are underactive, the hair will become dry and brittle, and the scalp may develop dandruff (*see below*). Frequent shampooing does not increase the amount of sebum, but it can dry out the scalp.

DAMAGED HAIR
Nearly all cosmetic procedures that are applied to hair can be damaging. Bleaching, drying, perming, straightening, even heated rollers, curling tongs and blow-drying can all cause the hair to become dry, break and split. In addition, many of the chemicals used can be irritant and cause contact DERMATITIS.

HAIR LOSS
Male-pattern baldness runs in families: this is due to changes in the levels of male sex hormones. Hair loss from the temples may start soon after puberty.

All women lose some hair with age, and occasionally the hair may also become very sparse and fine, especially on the front of the scalp. Again, this is due to changes in the levels of sex hormones, and often occurs after the MENOPAUSE. In addition, most women lose some hair two or three months after having a baby; this is because hormonal changes during pregnancy prevent normal hair loss.

Temporary baldness is quite common after serious illness or surgery, and particularly after radiotherapy. There may also be a sudden appearance of circular areas of baldness on the scalp or in the beard in men, and these can sometimes join up to form one large patch. This condition—called *alopecia areata*—usually occurs for no known reason, although sometimes it is preceded by an emotional shock. Time is the healer: hair growth normally returns within six to twelve months.

None of the proprietary preparations that claim to restore hair have any effect other than to cause irritation and even contact dermatitis on the scalp.

ANAEMIA can also be a factor in hair loss, and extra iron taken on a regular basis may help, especially in women who suffer heavy periods.

DANDRUFF
When the shedding of the skin of the scalp becomes excessive and obvious, this is termed *dandruff*. It is normally the result of too little or too much sebum being secreted by the sebaceous glands in the skin. Dry, white flakes are produced when there is too little sebum, and yellowish, oily, sticky flakes are a result of too much sebum.

SEBORRHOEIC DERMATITIS
This is also a common complaint. In infants — when it is called 'cradle cap'. It first appears as a rash and then as greasy yellow scales on the scalp. It usually disappears before the age of one year. In adults, it affects the scalp, eyebrows and eyelashes, as well as the beard and pubic hair, and is most common in men between 20 and 30 years old. It can be very difficult to clear up and can easily become inflamed.

A number of other conditions can also affect the hair and scalp: *see* LICE, PSORIASIS, TINEA.

ORTHODOX TREATMENT

See DERMATITIS for the treatment for seborrhoeic dermatitis. Coal tar ointments and shampoos may be prescribed for dandruff.

SELF-HELP

- Avoid harsh shampoos and other treatments, as well as hair products containing perfume.
- Use a conditioner to make it easier to comb out hair after washing and to reduce the static that can cause 'flyaway' hair.
- Don't use tight hair grips and slides or elastic bands.
- Avoid handling the hair: pulling it as a nervous tic can break it, and fiddling with it will help the sebum to travel down the shafts and make it greasy.
- If possible, wash your hair only once or twice a week—any more and it may dry the scalp.
- Avoid exposing the hair to harsh winds and salt spray.

HERBAL TREATMENT

General conditioning: An infusion of rosemary rubbed into the scalp is a general hair tonic. An infusion of comfrey should be used on dry hair, and lavender on oily hair; rub this in daily, but do not rinse it off. Brunettes might try massaging sage tea well into the scalp daily. It is also good as a final rinse after shampooing and will also mask up to 5 per cent of grey hairs. (Blondes should use chamomile tea).

Before shampooing, rub a little almond oil into the scalp to prevent drying. You could also rub aloe vera gel into the scalp; leave this on overnight and then shampoo. This is a general tonic, but it may also reduce excess sebum.

- *For hair loss* Drink an infusion of clivers herb — 25 g/1 oz to 0.5 l/1 pt water—in 45–60 ml/3–4 tbsp doses, 3 times daily. Also try the aloe vera gel (*see above*).
- *For dandruff* An infusion of sage, clivers or nettles should be massaged thoroughly into the scalp each day, and be used warm as a final rinse when shampooing. The aloe vera gel (*see above*) may also be used.

HOMEOPATHY

Hair problems generally reflect the condition of the rest of the body. Consult a homeopath who may offer the following:

- *Kali carbonicum* For dry hair.
- *Bryonia* For greasy hair.
- *Phosphoric acid* When hair loss follows a period of stress or a death of a close friend or relative.
- *Sepia* When hair loss is associated with pre-menstrual depression or tension, and there is chilliness, weeping and irritability.

MASSAGE

Massage the scalp daily to increase the blood supply to the hair follicles, thus improving nutrition and removing impurities. Once a week, massage with olive or coconut oil or homemade mayonnaise to condition the hair.

NATUROPATHY

Hair and scalp problems may reflect underlying imbalances of function and nutritional deficiencies; seek professional advice. Adopt a wholefood diet excluding refined carbohydrates, dairy products and animal fats, and take an adequate amount of exercise.

For dandruff: apply plain 'live' yoghurt as a conditioner: leave it on for at least 10 minutes and then rinse out and wash the hair in the normal way. As a final rinse, use a strong infusion of nettle, thyme or sage plus 30 ml/2 tbsp vinegar or Listerine.

VITAMIN AND MINERAL TREATMENT

For healthy hair and to prevent or retard hair loss, multivitamin/multimineral preparations containing adequate vitamin B complex, vitamin E, iron, copper, manganese and zinc should be taken. Eggs can supply useful cysteine and methionine. The scalp requires the same nutrients plus vitamin A and polyunsaturated fatty acids. Scalp problems should be treated with these plus evening primrose, safflower or wheat germ oil.

Hay Fever

(ALLERGIC RHINITIS)

Hay fever is an ALLERGY to pollens, specifically those from trees, grasses and flowering plants. An allergic reaction normally occurs when these plants flower—from late spring through to late summer, depending on the specific plant to which the sufferer is reacting. Many people have multiple allergies to different pollens and may be affected throughout the flowering season.

Frequently, those who suffer from hay fever are *atopic* — that is, they also suffer from ASTHMA and DERMATITIS (*see also* FOOD INTOLERANCE).

Those who suffer hay fever-like symptoms all through the year are described as having *perennial rhinitis*.

SYMPTOMS
Inflammation of the mucous membranes of the nose, watering of the eyes, fits of sneezing, runny nose and chronic CATARRH.

ORTHODOX TREATMENT
See ALLERGY.

SELF-HELP
See ALLERGY.

ACUPUNCTURE
An allergic response can be reduced by the acupuncturist's attention to the energies of the Lungs, Colon and Liver.

HOMEOPATHY
Consult a homeopath. Treatment is best given at the end of the year, before the flowering season, and repeated in February/March if required. It can take up to two to three seasons before control is fully established. In obstinate cases, homeopathic desensitizing can be used — eg *Mixed Pollens 30.*

The following can be taken to treat existing symptoms:

- *Allium cepa* For burning discharge from nose; eyes water profusely.
- *Arsenicum album* For burning discharges from nose and eyes.
- *Euphrasia* For burning discharges from eyes; bland discharges from nose.
- *Sabadilla* For sneezing and itching; frontal headache; sore throat.

NATUROPATHY
A reduction in the intake of dairy products and the avoidance of refined carbohydrates (especially sugars) can reduce the amount of mucus that the body produces.

Instant but temporary relief can be obtained by thoroughly irrigating the eyes with cool distilled water using an eyebath (change the water for each eye), and by sniffing water through the nose to wash away any allergenic pollens.

Some clinical ecologists believe that a food exclusion diet (see p. 104) can help to relieve hay fever symptoms, although this has yet to be proved.

VITAMIN AND MINERAL TREATMENT
Take 500 mg of vitamin C every 6 hours; this has a recognized antihistamine effect.

It has been claimed that, in some cases, hay fever may be prevented with high doses of vitamin B complex, plus extra calcium pantothenate (100 mg) and pyridoxine (vitamin B₆; 100 mg). Some people may find relief with daily doses of vitamin E (300 iu) and bioflavonoids (300 mg).

H

Headaches

Headaches are rarely a symptom of a serious underlying disease, although meningitis, brain tumours and excessively high BLOOD PRESSURE can be causes. Most commonly, however, they are the result of TENSION, stress and ANXIETY.

Emotional stress and anxiety can lead to an increase in tension in the large muscles of the neck and shoulders; this can, in turn, cause a headache.

On a purely physical level, poor posture can also lead to tension in the same muscles. The damage caused by a WHIPLASH injury can also result in a nagging ache in the neck and the back of the head.

EYESTRAIN can also create headaches. An early visit to the optician is always recommended for someone who is suffering from recurrent headaches, to see if there has been any deterioration in vision. A headache may also be a symptom of an infection (*see* FEVER), SINUSITIS, nerve damage in the face (*see* NEURALGIA) and tooth and gum infection (*see* GINGIVITIS and TOOTHACHE).

Eating and drinking chocolate, caffeine and red wine as well as adverse food reactions — especially to some food additives such as monosodium glutamate and nitrates—can all cause headaches in susceptible people, and of course they are also a significant part of hangover, lack of sleep, MENSTRUAL DISORDERS, some prescribed drugs and overdoses of vitamin A. Environmental factors such as air conditioning, poor lighting (particularly fluorescent) and fumes are also known triggers. Drastic changes in eating patterns (very low calorie diets, fasting and insufficient fluid intake) also cause headaches.

Many sufferers from recurrent tension headaches believe that they have MIGRAINE, since this is a more socially acceptable diagnosis than admitting to being under stress. However, migraine is a very specific condition and is quite different from the headaches that afflict so many people.

However, a headache is a cause for concern if it comes on suddenly for no apparent reason *and* is accompanied by weakness in an arm or leg, numbness or pins-and-needles, a reduction in or loss of consciousness, a high fever, a very stiff neck, a drooping eyelid and/or an epileptic seizure. In such cases, obtain professional advice as soon as possible.

ORTHODOX TREATMENT
Painkillers.

ACUPUNCTURE
The site of the headache often indicates the pathway(s) that require investigation and treatment. Most organ systems can be involved. It is not wise, therefore, merely to *suppress* the pain as this would leave untreated an imbalance that could spread deeper into the meridian system.

Acupressure to point 41 at the base of the occiput (the bone at the back of the skull) will give relief. For a frontal headache, add points 45 and 46; for one in the temples, add 47; and for one in the occiput, add 42. For any head problem, it is worth adding points 4 and 18 and, to clear the brain, point 48. (See p. 102–3)

ALEXANDER TECHNIQUE
This can be beneficial in reducing stress in the neck and shoulders.

HERBAL TREATMENT
The following may be useful in relieving pain:
- *Limeblossom, rosemary and lavender tips* Infusions (a weak one of the lavender) will relieve headaches caused by stress and nervous tension. Take a teacupful as required, and 3–4 tbsp (45–60 ml) twice daily to soothe the nerves.
- *Melilot* A good remedy for a throbbing headache associated with cold extremities.
- *Peppermint* For headaches of liver or gall bladder origin; the leaves can be used as a poultice over painful migraine or neuralgia.
- *Rue* Tablespoon doses will relieve headaches due to eyestrain; the infusion can also be applied to a compress and placed over the eyes; diluted with an equal quantity of pure water, it can be used as an eyebath.
- *Antispasmodic tincture* Contains skullcap and valerian and is a good standby; teaspoon doses in warm, sweetened water will give relief; undiluted tincture can be massaged

over the forehead, temples and back of the neck.

HOMEOPATHY
- *Arnica* For headaches after injury.
- *Belladonna* For bursting headaches with hot face; aggravated by light, noise and jarring.
- *Glanoine* For throbbing headache after too much heat, as in sunstroke.
- *Bryonia* For sharp, severe headache; aggravated by the slightest movement, even turning the eyes; thirsty.
- *Nux vomica* For after overindulgence, with constipation; irritable.
- *Pulsatilla* With weepiness, indigestion; worse in stuffy rooms.

HYPNOTHERAPY
When headaches are due to acquired habitual responses—eg raised blood pressure in response to stressful situations—hypnosis can be used to alter the person's response to the stimuli.

MANIPULATIVE THERAPIES
This is by far the most effective treatment for the relief of headaches, especially those caused by stress and muscular tension combined with postural problems. Massage, mobilization and manipulation to relieve the cycle of tension, muscular contraction, headache or tension is the first step, followed by exercises, postural correction and, if necessary, changes in the person's occupational posture. For example, changing the height of an office worker's chair can remove postural stresses that might otherwise cause headache.

MASSAGE
This can reduce tension in the neck and back, and will relax generally.

NATUROPATHY
Heat/cold Treatment: Head pain may be relieved by cold compresses to the forehead. Hot and cold fomentations to the neck and shoulders will relieve muscular tension.
Diet: Adopt a wholefood diet, restricting refined carbohydrates and increasing protein intake.

PSYCHOTHERAPIES
Initially, attention should be paid to diet and lifestyle. Planning ahead to avoid unnecessary tension, rush or anxiety can be helpful. Some people—overachievers, competitive, highly motivated people, type As (*see* p. 44)—are certainly more prone to develop headaches than others, and need to be particularly careful.

RELAXATION TECHNIQUES
These can be extremely helpful.

VITAMIN AND MINERAL TREATMENT
Take high-potency vitamin B complex of the prolonged-release type, plus 7,500 iu vitamin A in one dose.
See also FEVER, EYESTRAIN, MIGRAINE

H

HEARING PROBLEMS

Deafness may occur in one ear or both, and may be partial or total.

There are many causes of hearing loss, ranging from congenital deformity to tumours, but all of these fall within two main divisions. conductive deafness and nerve deafness.

CONDUCTIVE DEAFNESS
In this, the sound waves are prevented from reaching the inner ear.
- *Earwax* may be blocking the ear canal. This is simply dealt with by removing the wax, either by syringing or the more modern techniques of suction. A few drops of almond oil and lemon juice, heated to body temperature (*see* EARACHE), can help soften wax; otherwise seek professional help. *Never* poke into the ear with hair grips, matches, cotton wool buds or similarly sharp instruments: this can result in perforation of the eardrum and permanent deafness.

- *Foreign objects* Small children often put beads, nuts, sweets etc into their ears, which prevent sound waves from reaching the eardrum. NO ATTEMPT WHATSOEVER SHOULD BE MADE TO REMOVE ANY FOREIGN OBJECT FROM THE EAR: more often than not, the object is pushed further into the ear canal. The removal of these should be left to skilled medical practitioners.
- *Middle ear blockage* occurs in some children. The chamber behind the eardrum is filled with fluid (called 'glue') when they are born. If the fluid does not drain away, they experience a hearing loss. This is usually detected at the routine child clinic check ups.
- *Ear infections* (*see* EARACHE) can cause fluid and pus to block the ear canal or the chamber behind the eardrum, both of which can lead to a reduction in hearing. Chronic SINUSITIS and infections of the TONSILS AND ADENOIDS can also result in infection travelling up the Eustachian tube from the back of the throat to the tube's other end in the middle ear.
- *Fusion of the tiny bones* in the middle ear (*otosclerosis*) also prevents transmission of vibrations to the inner ear. This can be treated by surgical replacement with synthetic parts.

NERVE (OR PERCEPTIVE) DEAFNESS
Damage to the auditory nerve leading to the brain or to the hearing centres of the brain itself may cause a loss of hearing.
- *Viral infections* such as MEASLES, MUMPS and meningitis can (rarely) cause deafness, and congenital damage to the auditory nerve is a common problem in babies whose mothers have suffered GERMAN MEASLES during the first three months of pregnancy.
- *Ménière's disease* in which the pressure inside part of the inner ear is abnormally raised, can cause gradual deafness (*see also* DIZZINESS and TINNITUS).

- *Senile deafness* is the uncharitable name for nerve deafness in older people. It begins with the gradual inability to hear high-pitched sounds, but can progress to affect the full range of sound.
- *Sudden loud noises or long exposure to a high-level of noise* can also cause nerve deafness. Gunfire and industrial noise such as machinery, aircraft, pneumatic drills, chain saws, etc can all cause a loss of hearing at specific wave lengths.
- *Personal stereos* are another worrying factor: many young people listen to these at very high volumes, which can rapidly cause irreversible hearing loss.

ORTHODOX TREATMENT
Drainage (middle ear blockage); hearing aids.

ACUPUNCTURE
If deafness is the result of obstructed flow of Chi, there is a good chance of restoring hearing. Between visits to the acupuncturist, tiny needles may be left in selected points near the ear and in the arm to augment the effect.

Massage of the back of the arm from elbow to wrist may be helpful in stumulating a number of points on the main meridians concerned with deafness.

HERBAL TREATMENT
If the deafness is due to CATARRH, treat as for this condition.

HOMEOPATHY
- *Pulsatilla* For catarrhal deafness, with thick, green catarrh from ear or nose; better in the open air.
- *Mercurius solubilus* Where there is increased sweating and salivation at night and intolerance of extremes of temperature.
- *Nitric acid* If hearing improves in noisy surroundings.
- *China officinalis* Deafness associated with ringing in the ears, especially in weakened old people.
- *Phosphorus* When deaf to human voice.

H

- *Salicyclic acid* For Ménière's disease.
- *Silica* For great sensitivity to noise to the point of pain.

MANIPULATIVE THERAPIES
In cases of conductive deafness, manipulative therapy can be a help, especially the techniques for drainage of the sinuses.

NATUROPATHY
Conductive deafness caused by chronic sinusitis or obstruction of the Eustachian tube with mucus should be treated by a diet that excludes dairy products, to reduce the body's production of mucus. Deep-breathing techniques and the avoidance of obvious nasal irritants (eg tobacco smoke, exhaust fumes, dust) will also help.

VITAMIN AND MINERAL TREATMENT
An adequate intake of vitamin A throughout life (at least 2,500 iu daily) may prevent senile deafness.

Heartburn *see* INDIGESTION

HEART DISEASE

Heart disease in all its various guises is the single largest factor in premature death affecting the Western world. It includes coronary artery disease, diseases of the heart muscle and those of its valves, as well as those two well-known symptoms of heart disease — ANGINA *and heart attacks.*

By far the greatest cause of heart disease is the development of ATHEROSCLEROSIS. *Raised blood levels of a naturally produced substance — cholesterol — have been implicated in extensive studies, especially in the USA.*

In addition, consistently high levels of BLOOD PRESSURE, *a sedentary lifestyle,* OBESITY, *stress (see* TENSION*), smoking and alcohol abuse (see* ADDICTIONS*) are other precursors of early heart disease.*

ORTHODOX TREATMENT
See ANGINA, ATHEROSCLEROSIS, BLOOD PRESSURE, OBESITY.

ACUPUNCTURE
Acupuncture is helpful in dealing with some aspects of heart disease—eg muscular spasms, wheezing and coughing. Its traditional aim is to 'calm the heart and the spirit'.

Acupressure on the inner side of the forearm, especially any sensitive areas along its midline, will be helpful if done on a daily basis.

ALEXANDER TECHNIQUE
This can be beneficial, especially in the reduction of stress.

HEALING
Healing can be used to deal with problems of stress; it is also valuable as a treatment for people suffering from heart disease. It is effective in the reduction of high blood pressure.

HERBAL TREATMENT
Two remedies can be taken with perfect safety. Hawthorn is antispasmodic and sedative, will strengthen heart action, gently regulate the rate of the heartbeat, will be beneficial in atherosclerosis and will contribute to lowering raised blood pressure. It can be taken over a long period of time without any cumulative effect. A decoction of the berries or an infusion of the flowers, taken in 45–60 ml/3–4 tbsp doses 2–3 times daily, will be sufficient; it also comes in tablet form.

Lily-of-the-valley also regulates and strengthens heart action, and will correct an irregular beat. Its action has been claimed to be similar to that of digoxin, a standard drug used in the treatment of heart disease, but without any of the latter's cumulative effects. Take an infusion of the leaves 1–2 times daily in 45–60 ml/3–4 tbsp doses.

See a herbal practitioner for other heart disease remedies.

HYPNOTHERAPY
While not directly affecting heart disease, hypnosis can help to reduce

PAIN, blood pressure and anxiety.

Remember that pain is a warning signal, and elimination before its cause is diagnosed is not recommended.

MANIPULATIVE THERAPIES
This can make the middle part of the back more mobile, improve breathing and can have a beneficial effect on the nerve supply to the heart.

MASSAGE
Massage as a relaxing therapy is always helpful in the reduction of stress.

PSYCHOTHERAPIES
Many of those likely to suffer heart disease — eg the type As (*see* p. 44) — will have high blood pressure, which may be related to deeply repressed anger, resentment or fear, and may hide inner hostility with an outer show of restraint and nonchalance. Psychotherapy, particularly those forms that encourage the release of aggression (eg **bioenergetics, psychodrama** (p. 95), **Gestalt** (p. 94) can be very beneficial in both the prevention and the treatment of this type of high blood pressure.

Extreme dissatisfaction with lifestyle (eg wrong job, marriage, friends) also produces frustration, the cause of which may be unrecognized. This can be resolved by exploratory psychotherapy in which discussion of the problem forms the basis of treatment (eg professional counselling).

RELAXATION
Meditation, yoga, biofeedback and **autogenics** (pp. 97–9) are all extremely safe techniques through which it is possible to control your own blood pressure. Having learned the techniques, diligent application of them can play a vital role in the self-help treatment of all forms of heart disease.

VITAMIN AND MINERAL TREATMENT
Regular vitamin B complex plus high-potency vitamin E (400–1,200 iu daily), vitamin C (500–1,000 mg daily), vitamin B_6 (100 mg daily), potassium, magnesium aspartate (1,200 mg daily) and lecithin (15–45 g daily), as well as

How to stay good-hearted
To keep your heart healthy and to promote more rapid recovery after problems, follow these simple rules:

- Maintain recommended height/weight ratios. *See* p.21.
- Eliminate animal and other fats, especially hidden fats in sausages, patés, meat pies, potato crisps, etc.
- Eat more wholegrain cereals and 'good' carbohydrates — wholemeal bread and pasta, brown rice, jacket potatoes etc.
- Eat more fish and poultry.
- Eat more fresh fruits, vegetables and salads: aim to have one-third of your daily intake as raw, fresh produce.
- Reduce intake of all sugars and salt: watch out for carbonated drinks and unlikely hiding places for sugar and salts — baked beans, tomato ketchup, canned vegetables.
- Reduce alcohol consumption. One drink a day is good for you — a glass of wine, a pint of beer, a measure of spirits — but two drinks is not so good and three or more is bad.
- Substitute herbal teas and decaffeinated coffee for some drinks, and use skimmed milk, not non-dairy creamers.
- Make time for regular exercise. Use the stairs, not the lift. Don't take the car for short distances: ride a bicycle or walk instead. Take up any active sport that you enjoy and that is appropriate to your age and health. Aim for three one-hour sessions of gentle exercise (or three half-hour sessions of strenuous exercise) per week, preferably in the open air.
- Make time for relaxation. Yoga, meditation, relaxation exercises are all useful.
- Use your time well. Plan your day and avoid overcommitment and its ensuing stress.

If you are over 40, undergoing medical treatment for any heart condition (or other disorder) and/or have recently recovered from a heart attack or heart surgery, consult your doctor before taking up any vigorous activity programme.

H

replacement of saturated animal fats in the diet by PUFA (vitamin F) and a regular intake of fish oil containing EPA and DHA may help to reduce the chances of heart disease and decrease the possibility of further problems in those who have already developed it.

See *also* ATHEROSCLEROSIS

HERNIA

There are three common types of hernia — often called 'ruptures' — which are all protrusions of the digestive tract through weaknesses in the muscular walls of the abdomen.

HIATUS HERNIA
This is a weakness in the part of the diaphragm where the gullet passes through the stomach. The lower end of the gullet and the upper part of the stomach bulge up through the diaphragm into the chest cavity, and acid, normally restricted to the stomach, can then wash into the gullet where it irritates and burns.

This occurs more commonly in women than in men, and normally in middle age or later. It can be aggravated by PREGNANCY and OBESITY. It produces symptoms of chronic HEARTBURN and great discomfort behind the breastbone.

INGUINAL HERNIA
This is more common in men and occurs in the groin. Usually part of the intestines protrudes through the inguinal canal containing the blood vessels supplying the testicles, and this may even enter the scrotum; however, a hernia may also protrude through the weaker muscles of the groin wall without passing through the inguinal canal.

FEMORAL HERNIA
This occurs mostly in women and is a protrusion of the abdominal contents through the femoral canal (which carries the large blood vessels to the thigh), producing a swelling at the top of the leg.

ORTHODOX TREATMENT
Surgery (inguinal and femoral); antacid drugs (hiatus hernia).

H

Stomach Strengthener
The following will strengthen the abdominal muscles: lie flat on your back; bend knees with feet flat; raise your buttocks so that you are holding the weight of your body with your feet and shoulders while, at the same time, pulling in your abdominal muscles; lower yourself and repeat 6–10 times. This should be carried out twice daily.

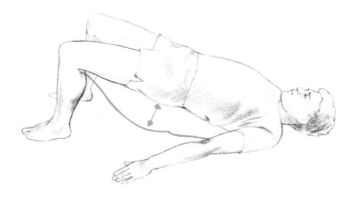

Inguinal and femoral hernias:
- Avoid obesity.
- Follow a regular programme of abdominal exercise (*see below*).
- Learn to lift correctly and avoid lifting excessive weights unaided (see **Back Pack** pp. 53–9).

Hiatus hernias:
- Avoid obesity and large meals, fatty fried foods, spices, very acidic foods and large quantities of alcohol.
- Check your posture; bend at the knees and not the hips, don't sit in chairs that are too low and avoid a hunched-up position.
- Raise the head of the bed or use extra pillows to minimize discomfort at night.

NATUROPATHY
Ensure a proper body weight and regular bowel function with a wholefood diet.

HERPES

See *also* PREGNANCY AND CHILDBIRTH

There are two types of herpes virus: *herpes simplex*, two strains of which cause cold sores and genital herpes; and *herpes zoster*, which causes CHICKENPOX, shingles and facial herpes.

HERPES SIMPLEX
Cold sores are very infectious, and most children have acquired the *herpes simplex* virus from someone else by the time they are five years old. The virus remains forever dormant in nerve tissue in the lips until something triggers off an attack. In this, a group of small blisters appears on the lips, a crust forms and, within about 10 days, this dries up. Cold sores are infectious as long as the blisters are still moist.

Cold sores can be triggered off by illness, a very high FEVER and COLDS and SORE THROATS. Exposure to cold weather and to sunshine can also be precipitating factors.

Genital herpes are caused by a separate strain of the *herpes simplex* virus, but about 10 per cent of cases are acquired through oral sex with someone who has cold sores.

Genital herpes are particularly common in young people. Small, painful, tender and highly infectious blisters appear on the genital region, thighs and buttocks. The first attack is always the worst, and is accompanied by a fever and swollen glands; sometimes the blisters can rupture to form open sores that are extremely painful. Usually, however, the blisters crust over after about 10 days and then disappear; nonetheless, the virus still lies dormant in nerve tissue and can never be eliminated. Some people have recurrent attacks, while others have only one mild attack.

An attack of genital herpes during pregnancy can be extremely serious. The affected woman is liable to pass on the virus to her baby, either in the womb or as the baby passes through the birth canal. In addition, women who have been infected with this strain of the *herpes simplex* virus run a slightly increased risk of developing cervical cancer; they should therefore have a cervical smear performed at least once a year.

In both these forms of herpes infection, any factors that lower the body's normal resistance are liable to trigger an attack. Bad eating habits, ANXIETY, TENSION, lack of sleep, menstruation, a low level of general health or DEPRESSION can all be aggravating factors, and sexual intercourse can bring on an attack of genital herpes.

ORTHODOX TREATMENT
Anti-viral lotions and creams; antiseptic lotions or surgical spirit to dry up cold sore blisters.

HERPES ZOSTER
Shingles is caused by the same virus that causes chickenpox. A person with shingles can give someone else a case of chickenpox and vice versa.

An attack of shingles is often preceded by 3 or 4 days of intense pain in the affected area and by some malaise. Then numerous small and excruciating painful blisters develop very quickly. These normally last between 7 and 14 days, and finally form crusty scabs and drop off.

Sometimes an outbreak of *herpes zoster* can affect the trigeminal nerve of the face — a condition called *facial herpes*.

After an attack of shingles or facial herpes, the pain may continue even after the blisters have disappeared, and this can sometimes last for months or years. This *post-herpetic syndrome* can be even more painful than the original infection, and it can cause the sufferer to become extremely depressed (*see also* NEURALGIA).

ORTHODOX TREATMENT
Painkillers; anti-depressants; tranquillizers.

SELF-HELP
● Avoid physical contact as both forms of herpes are highly contagious.
● If you have recurrent cold sores, sun block creams will help.
● If you have genital herpes, a warm salt bath may reduce the discomfort.

ACUPUNCTURE
This can be extremely effective in dealing with the pain of all forms of herpes infection and, especially, with the pain of post-herpetic syndrome.

HERBAL TREATMENT
For cold sores, apply distilled witch hazel and tincture of myrrh (combined in equal quantities); tincture of St John's wort, calendula or wild indigo can also be used if available. Both myrrh and St John's wort are antiseptic; wild indigo even more so. A good eau-de-Cologne can also be very effective.

Aloe vera gel may help; apply twice a day.

HOMEOPATHY
For cold sores
● *Natrum muriaticum* Cold sores

associated with a deep crack in the middle of the lower lip.
● *Rhus tox* Sores associated with a coated tongue except for a red patch at the tip.
● *Arsenicum album* Sores associated with burning pains.
If cold sores are recurrent, see a homeopath.

NATUROPATHY
When you feel the itchy sensation heralding the arrival of a cold sore, cut a lemon and rub the area with fresh lemon juice.

VITAMIN AND MINERAL TREATMENT
All types of herpes infection may respond to daily intakes of the essential amino acid L-lysine (0.5–1.5 g). In addition, high-potency vitamin B complex of the prolonged-release type and extra vitamin B_{12} (10 μg daily) are needed.

HICCUPS

A hiccup is the sudden spasm of the diaphragm, caused by the irritation of the nerves that supply it. As the diaphragm contracts, air is involuntarily and rapidly breathed in and the vocal cords snap shut—and it is the sound of this quick breath and of the vocal cords that is known as a hiccup.

Hiccups usually occur in repetitive groups and may be triggered off by INDIGESTION or excessive gas in the stomach, or to the excessive consumption of fizzy drinks.

ORTHODOX TREATMENT
Sedative drugs; specific drug for underlying cause; surgery.

SELF-HELP
The following exercise may help: lie on your back on the floor and bring your knees up to your chest; hold them there for a count of 3; then relax. This puts

pressure on the diaphragm and may stop the spasms.

ACUPUNCTURE
Hiccups can develop if the energy of the Stomach is 'rebellious', ascending in the body instead of descending as it ought to. Acupuncture treatment will aim to correct the direction of Chi energy.

Acupressure on point 27 on the abdomen and point 43 on the ring finger can be useful as a first aid measure (see pp. 104–5).

HERBAL TREATMENT
- Chew fresh mint leaves or dill seeds.
- Gripe water for babies contains dill as one of its main components; this can be tried.
- Take small sips of hot catmint tea.
- Place 5 ml/1 tsp crushed dill seeds in a little hot water; stir and infuse for a few minutes; strain, add cold water and drink.

High blood pressure *see* BLOOD PRESSURE

Hives *see* NETTLE RASH

Hoarseness *see* SORE THROAT

Hyperactivity *see* FOOD INTOLERANCE

Hypertension *see* BLOOD PRESSURE

Hyperventilation *see* BREATHLESSNESS

Hypotension *see* BLOOD PRESSURE

I

INDIGESTION

(DYSPEPSIA)

See *also* DIGESTIVE DISORDERS

Indigestion is usually caused by over-eating or eating the wrong foods. Spicy or very rich foods are commonly responsible, but individual items such as cucumbers and pickled onions can also cause discomfort. In general, these take longer than usual for the stomach to digest and cause it to produce an excess amount of acid. This acid may also escape from the stomach into the gullet where it causes heartburn. Sometimes gas produced by the food becomes trapped in the stomach, resulting in pressure, pain and FLATULENCE. If food or drink irritates the stomach lining, gastritis may occur, with inflammation, pain and sickness (*see also* GASTROENTERITIS).

Food is not the only cause of indigestion. Smoking, alcohol and common drugs such as aspirin can all have powerful effects on the ability of the stomach to cope. Stress and TENSION in general can have adverse effects on digestion ('nervous dyspepsia'). (*See also* COLIC, CONSTIPATION, DIARRHOEA, NAUSEA AND VOMITING.

Most bouts of indigestion are temporary and their causes are obvious. However, if the indigestion is chronic and/or the pain is severe and persistent, a more serious disorder may be the cause and must be investigated. Some examples are: GALLSTONES, HEART DISEASE, hiatus HERNIA, ULCERS and stomach CANCER.

ORTHODOX TREATMENT
Antacids.

SELF-HELP
Modify your lifestyle if it is rushed and stressful. Avoid those foods that obviously cause this condition.
- Avoid eating too much at one time.
- Simplify meals so that the digestion does not have to cope with too many ingredients or too much fat. Try the **Hay Diet** (p. 157)
- Chew well and avoid drinking with meals, which dilutes the digestive acids.

ACUPUNCTURE
The Spleen and Stomach function together as a reciprocating unit in energy

terms, and indigestion is often associated with a deficiency of Spleen energy. This can be treated with acupuncture, and the efficiency of the digestive organs will also be investigated.

Acupressure on point 23, augmented by pressure on points 28 and 27 often encourages peristalsis and relieves nausea (see pp. 104–5).

HERBAL TREATMENT

For simple indigestion: Take an infusion of centaury — 115 ml/4 fl oz 3 times a day between meals — plus a few fresh dandelion leaves daily; alternatively, drink peppermint tea. The gel made from the pulp inside an aloe vera leaf, mixed with milk, will aid digestion and soothe the stomach. Chewing coriander seeds before meals may prevent indigestion and chewing them afterwards may ease any discomfort.

Many culinary herbs are aids to digestion when included in food: caraway and fennel seeds, marjoram, bay leaves, thyme and rosemary are especially good.

For chronic indigestion: Mix 5 ml/1 tsp powdered slippery elm bark with a little water to form a paste. Gradually add 230 ml/8 fl oz boiling water (or half milk and half water). Take 2–3 times daily.

For nervous dyspepsia: This is eased by 45–60 ml/3–4 tbsp cold catmint tea or cool rosemary tea.

For hyperacidity: Drink a teacupful of meadowsweet infusion, 3 times daily.

For gastritis: Take 45–60 ml/3–4 tbsp of an infusion of marshmallow leaves, 3 times daily; alternatively, try an infusion of avens. The slippery elm gruel as described above may also help.

HOMEOPATHY

Those with chronic indigestion should consult a homeopath. For the occasional bout:

- *Arsenicum album* Diarrhoea and vomiting at the same time; thirsty for small sips, cold, exhausted and restless.
- *Argentum nitricum* Loud belching, butterflies in the stomach, apprehension; craving for sugar and tendency towards diarrhoea.

- *Lycopodium* Large amounts of wind, feeling of fullness after eating only a small amount of food, constipation.
- *Nux vomica* Upsets from overindulgence.
- *Pulsatilla* Stomach upsets after eating rich, fatty foods.
- *Sulphur* Much offensive wind smelling like bad eggs.

NATUROPATHY

Diet: Withhold all solid food for 24–48 hours, taking only apple or pineapple juice 4–5 times daily. Gradually reintroduce food over a period of 2–3 days, starting with plain goats' milk yogurt and finely grated or puréed apple and, later, vegetable stew or lightly cooked vegetables. Avoid all fried food, coffee and sugar.

Heat/Cold Treatment: Hot fomentations on the abdomen will help to relieve pain or colic.

VITAMIN AND MINERAL TREATMENT

Digestive disorders are best treated with high-potency vitamin B complex (preferably of the prolonged-release variety), to stimulate gastric and intestinal juices and normal mobility of the gut. These vitamins will also encourage a good growth of intestinal bacteria.

INFERTILITY

Failure to conceive may be due to problems with the woman, problems with the man or problems with both.

In women, there may be obstructions in the Fallopian tubes that prevent eggs from reaching the womb, she may not be producing viable eggs or there may be physical defects in the structure of her womb. (See *also* MENSTRUAL DISORDERS, MISCARRIAGE.)

In men, there may be impotence, lack of sperm or the sperm may be abnormal or too few in number.

The physical reasons for infertility are varied and complex, but all to often it is a simple matter of ANXIETY, timing and technique. Many couples who adopt a child soon find they are expecting their own. Removal of the pressure to conceive allows a much more relaxed attitude towards sexual intercourse, and this on its own may lead to conception.

The medical profession almost totally ignores nutritional deficiencies as a possible cause of infertility. While a lot of attention is given to nutritional advice for the pregnant woman, virtually none is available to couples trying to conceive.

ORTHODOX TREATMENT
Sperm count; hormone treatment; fertility drugs; artificial insemination; surgery on blocked or damaged Fallopian tubes.

HOMEOPATHY
Consult a homeopath. The following remedies may be tried:
- *Sepia* For loss of sex drive, irritability, weepiness, hair loss.
- *Conium* For painful, swollen breasts after suppression of sexual instincts.
- *Iodum* For heat intolerance, great hunger but loss of weight.
- *Natrum muriaticum* For emotionally upset, often following bereavement; cries alone, does not show feelings.

HYPNOTHERAPY
Hypnosis may help by removing barriers to sexual enjoyment, which in turn enables better lubrication of the vagina, more enjoyable sex, better penetration and a higher probability of achieving a fertilized egg.

PSYCHOTHERAPIES
Persistent infertility usually has a predominantly physical cause. It is often believed that desires and attitudes can affect fertility adversely at a deep level, but while this can happen (especially in the short term), it can cause unnecessary anguish to hold exclusively to this belief.

However, in the absence of any evidence to suggest physical reasons for infertility, psychotherapy can be a helpful technique.

How to encourage conception
FOR HER
- Get the timing right: be sure to make love when you are most likely to conceive—ie halfway between periods (usually around the 14th day after a period in a 28-day cycle).
- Get plenty of rest, eat well, take vitamin and mineral supplements.
- Don't smoke or drink.
- Make time for making love.
- After making love, stay where you are with your legs and feet up for at least half an hour.
- If you have problems with vaginal dryness, use a suitable odourless, water-soluble lubricant (eg KY jelly), a little of which should also be applied to your partner's penis.

FOR HIM
- Avoid tight jeans and underpants.
- Avoid hot baths before intercourse.
- Gentle warm and cold splashing to the genital area will help stimulate circulation.
- Take 200 iu vitamin E daily.
- Cut down on alcohol, cigarettes and caffeine.
- Take regular exercise.
- Eat a healthy diet.
- Get plenty of sleep.

RELAXATION TECHNIQUES
Autogenics (p. 97).

VITAMIN AND MINERAL TREATMENT
There is some evidence from animal studies that vitamins A, B_{12} and E are needed for normal sperm production. Vitamin B_{12} may also help some women unable to conceive. Vitamin C and zinc may also help.

INFLUENZA

Influenza ('flu')—is an acute viral illness that spreads very rapidly via coughing or sneezing wherever people congregate.

There are three types of influenza virus:

Influenza A is responsible for worldwide epidemics the Asian strain of the A virus has caused several severe outbreaks during the past 20 years.

Influenza B is normally associated with smaller and less virulent epidemics.

Influenza C is fairly rare.

Once you have had one type of flu, this confers lifelong immunity against it. However, within the three broad categories of influenza viruses, individual strains are constantly changing, so a different sort of virus will usually cause each epidemic. This is why immunization against influenza is only about 60 per cent effective.

SYMPTOMS

The virus incubates in the body for one to three days, and then the illness starts suddenly with HEADACHE, aching back and limbs, APPETITE LOSS, sometimes NAUSEA AND VOMITING and chronic malaise. A FEVER of up to 102°F (39°C) is common, accompanied by chills and shivering. The pulse becomes rapid, and there is frequently a harsh, dry COUGH. In the majority of cases, people recover within three to five days.

However, there can also be secondary bacterial infections that can lead to SORE THROAT, BRONCHITIS and PNEUMONIA, especially in the elderly and those with chronic heart and lung conditions. If someone with the flu develops a severe illness, brings up green or yellow sputum, has chest pains and/or is breathless, a doctor should be consulted; medical advice should also be sought if the person is already in ill health.

ORTHODOX TREATMENT

Painkillers; anti-flu vaccine.

SELF-HELP

See CHILDREN'S ILLNESSES for general care for both adults and children. Allow at least 3 to 4 days after all the symptoms have gone before returning to normal activities and then be prepared to feel low and depressed for up to 2 weeks.

HERBAL TREATMENT

Catmint tea is very good for fevers. If there is sore throat, an infusion of sage can be used as a gargle, or 45–60 ml/3–4 tbsp can be taken warm with honey as required. Vervain tea (3 cups daily) can be taken as a tonic during recovery.

NATUROPATHY

During the early stage, when there are aching limbs and back, sore throat and chills, withhold all food and take an Epsom Salts bath: soak for 20 minutes in hot water to which 45 ml/3 tbsp commercial Epsom Salts have been added. Then rest in bed.

During the feverish and sweaty stage, when respiratory symptoms have developed, give juices only and apply cold trunk packs and throat compresses. Gradually reintroduce starch-free, dairy-free foods only — fruit, salads, vegetables, wholegrains.

VITAMIN AND MINERAL TREATMENT

Increase the vitamin A intake to 7,500 iu daily during the period of illness. Take 1 g vitamin C every 4 hours until relief is obtained; then gradually reduce the dosage over one week to 1 g daily, then to a maintenance dose of 500 mg daily. Vitamin B complex can be taken as a tonic during convalescence.

INSOMNIA

'Insomnia' technically means habitual sleeplessness, a lack of sleep that is repeated night after night and seems endless. However, more often what is commonly referred to as 'insomnia' is really a long-term dissatisfaction with the duration and/or quality of sleep. Half the population claim to suffer from 'insomnia' at some time in their lives.

For many people, sleep becomes an obsession: the idea that they must have their 'eight hours' can become consuming, and anything that deprives them of even half an hour's sleep is a catastrophe. However, if you really need only six hours, and you wake up re-

I

freshed and active, your body is sending all the right messages to your brain.

INSOMNIA AND THE ELDERLY
Since most people need rather less sleep as they get older, there are many who can be described as 'phoney insomniacs', who believe that they are being deprived of what is rightfully theirs when, in fact, their bodies simply require less sleep than they think. In addition, sleep patterns frequently change in old age. The elderly tend to doze on and off throughout the day and be awake more during the night. This is not an illness that needs treatment, just a fact that needs accepting.

CAUSES OF INSOMNIA
Insomnia is seldom related to any specific physical cause, although any illness that is producing PAIN, discomfort or a high FEVER will cause at least one bad night's sleep. Insomnia can almost always be linked to TENSION, ANXIETY, work problems, financial difficulties, an unsatisfactory sex life, domestic crises — any aspect of life that is a source of worry. A severe bout of DEPRESSION can cause early-morning waking or difficulty in getting to sleep.

ORTHODOX TREATMENT
Sleeping pills.

SELF-HELP
- Take a hot milky drink with honey or a bowl of cereal before bed time
- Get plenty of exercise and fresh air, and be sure to sleep in a well-ventilated room.
- Avoid stimulants such as coffee, tea and cola as well as heavy meals late at night.
- Get up earlier in the morning; you may find it easier to get to sleep at night.

See *also* **Stress and how to deal with it** (p. 45).

HERBAL TREATMENT
A warm bath containing an infusion of hops taken just before getting into a warm bed will promote drowsiness. A bath containing essential oils such as hops, meadowsweet and orange blossom can also be relaxing.

Infusions of sedative herbs such as limeblossom, chamomile flowers, catmint, passion flower and melilot will all calm the nerves and reduce mental and emotional excitability. Sweeten with a little honey and take warm in teacupful quantities before bedtime. Taking 45–60 ml/3–4 tbsp once or twice during the day will reinforce the sedative action, but will not cause you to feel dopey or drugged during waking hours.

HOMEOPATHY
- *Aconite* When sleep is restless and associated with fear.
- *Arnica* When you are overtired and the bed feels too hard.
- *Coffea* When you find it impossible to switch off your mind and it keeps racing as if you had drunk a very strong cup of coffee.
- *Ignatia* When there is a lot of yawning and sighing, and a feeling that you will never ever get to sleep again.
- *Nux vomica* When you get off to sleep but wake at 4 a.m. and cannot get back to sleep again until about 7 a.m., especially after having had alcohol.
- *Phosphorus* If you feel very tense and fearful and are having nightmares.

HYPNOTHERAPY
Hypnosis can certainly help.

MANIPULATIVE THERAPIES
When insomnia is a direct result of musculo-skeletal pain or physical tension, manipulative therapy can be extremely helpful.

MASSAGE
Massage the whole back with repetitive, rhythmic, soothing strokes. To ensure that the massage ends in sleep, stroke slowly and rhythmically down the back, one hand lightly and gently following the other down.

NATUROPATHY
Large meals in the evening mean that

the digestive system is working overtime when you are trying to sleep. Fatty foods especially put a greater strain on the system, so avoid cheeses and other dairy products. A general, healthy wholefood diet will also help.

Psychotherapies

Behavioural therapies are often very effective in relieving the vicious cycle of sleeplessness and worry about it. Insomnia can be the result of significant depression and anxiety, and the appropriate remedies for these should be sought.

Relaxation Techniques

Autogenics (p. 97).

Vitamin and Mineral Treatment

Insomnia can be treated by taking 500 or 1,000 mg of the essential amino acid L-tryptophane and 25 mg vitamin B_6 just before sleep. In addition, dolomite tablets (containing calcium and magnesium) should be taken at bedtime with a hot milk or sweetened herbal drink.

Irritable Bowel Syndrome

Irritable bowel syndrome (IBS) is the medical term for what is commonly known as 'spastic colon' — a distressing and often painful condition affecting the large intestine. IBS is very common, but twice as many women as men suffer from it.

IBS can develop for no reason at all, but it may occur after a bout of GASTROENTERITIS or after repeated courses of antibiotics.

Blood tests, special X-rays and other investigations seldom produce any positive results, although they may rule out other digestive disorders such as COLITIS, DIVERTICULAR DISEASE and bowel CANCER. Consequently, many doctors believe that IBS is a psychosomatic problem. This is not true, but what is evident is that most people who suffer severe abdominal pain and disturbance of the digestive function over prolonged periods do become very stressed and frequently depressed. This is an effect of the condition rather than its cause.

Those interested in clinical ecology have long believed that, for many sufferers, IBS is a problem of FOOD INTOLERANCE.

Symptoms

Those with IBS suffer varying degrees of abdominal pain and DIARRHOEA, or alternating diarrhoea and CONSTIPATION. The abdomen is usually bloated, the pain is felt all over or only in one area, is often only relieved by passing a bowel movement or FLATULENCE ('wind') and is normally aggravated by food.

Orthodox Treatment

Sedatives; tranquillizers; high fibre diet.

Herbal Treatment

To help control spasms, mix together 25 g/1 oz each of meadowsweet, marshmallow root, plantain leaves and bayberry powder, and 12 g/$\frac{1}{2}$ oz each of hops, chamomile flowers and prickly ash bark. Add 50 g/2 oz of this mixture to 1 l/1$\frac{3}{4}$ pts boiling water. Simmer, covered, for 15 minutes; cool and strain. Take 45–60 ml/3–4 tbsp before each meal.

Manipulative Therapies

As with all digestive and bowel problems, manipulation of the spine can have a very positive effect as a beneficial adjunct to treatment.

Naturopathy

The first requisite for any bowel problem is a well-balanced, high-fibre, wholefood diet. Wholegrain cereals, fresh and dried fruits, raw vegetables and salads should be the normal pattern once an exclusion diet (see p. 104–5) has identified any items that may cause trouble. Fluid intake must be 1–1.5 l/2–3 pt daily. Avoid alcohol, strong spices,

I

curries, coffee, food additives and strong tea. Be sure to take exercise, especially to strengthen abdominal muscles (see **Fit for Life** p. 37).

RELAXATION TECHNIQUES
Any of these, especially **yoga** (p. 99).

VITAMIN AND MINERAL TREATMENT
IBS will occasionally respond to up to 1,000 mg daily of calcium pantothenate of the prolonged-release variety.

J

Jaundice *see* LIVER PROBLEMS

K

KIDNEY DISORDERS

Several things can go wrong with the kidneys. **Serious illnesses** such as high BLOOD PRESSURE, lupus erythematosus (*see* ARTHRITIS), tuberculosis and genetic diseases can all prevent the kidneys from performing their proper function.

Infections of the bladder (*see* CYSTITIS) and prostate gland (*see* PROSTATE PROBLEMS) can spread up into the kidneys, causing secondary infections.

Kidney stones are a common problem. They consist of calcium phosphate, calcium oxalate or, more rarely, uric acid (*see* 'Gout' under ARTHRITIS). A reduced intake of fluid or excessive sweating as found in such occupations as baking and steelworking or in the overuse of saunas can lead to concentration of the urine, which makes it more likely that calcium salts will be precipitated out and form kidney stones. Kidney infection can also cause stones to form, and since women are more likely to develop cystitis, they are also more likely to develop stones.

There are three types of stones: very small ones which can pass unfelt from the kidney; medium-sized ones; and very large stones (often caused by infection) that fill the collecting area in the centre of the kidney and thus take on peculiar shapes – hence the name 'staghorn stones'. The medium-sized stones often become stuck in the ureter, where they obstruct the flow of urine and can cause waves of excruciating pain called *renal colic*. The staghorn stones often cause no pain or any other symptoms, but eventually they may so damage the kidney tissue that the kidney will have to be removed.

Sudden kidney failure is usually caused by a stone obstructing the flow of urine. Tumours or strictures can also do this as can severe injury to the spinal cord. A number of diseases usually grouped under the heading 'nephritis' (inflammation of the kidney) can also damage the organ so badly that failure occurs. In all cases of urinary retention, urgent medical attention must be sought.

With advancing age, there is usually a reduction in the efficiency of the kidneys in eliminating waste products. This can also affect the body's ability to remove drugs from the system, and can be a worrying problem for the older segment of the population who are more likely to be treated by drugs for such chronic conditions as ARTHRITIS.

You should seek medical advice if:
● you pass blood in your urine, or if it is in any way abnormally coloured.
● you feel pain in your loins or abdomen.
● if pain on passing urine persists for more than 24 hours.
● you are urinating more frequently than usual.
● your ankles are swollen.

ORTHODOX TREATMENT
Antibiotics; dialysis; transplant; removal of kidney stone by surgery.

ACUPUNCTURE
The terrible pain of renal colic is effectively relieved by acupuncture analgesia. General treatment of the Kidney and Bladder meridans can be used to deal with infections and loss of function.

Herbal Treatment

Parsley piert (related to the common lady's mantle) is also known as 'parsley breakstone' and has been used for many years to dissolve kidney stones. Clivers, wild carrot, horsetail and pellitory-of-the-wall taken together are soothing when inflammation is present, have a diuretic action and will also gradually dissolve stones. Buchu herb is antiseptic and, when combined with marshmallow leaves, can relieve infection; couchgrass and meadowsweet can be added if the condition does not respond quickly.

Dandelion is a gentle diuretic: young leaves can be added to the daily salad, which should also include parsley, radish and finely chopped young leeks, each of which will benefit kidney complaints. Drink 3–4 tbsp (45–60 ml) leek cooking water each morning.

Aloe vera gel mixed with milk will relieve kidney infections.

Homeopathy

To relieve renal colic
- *Berberis* Sticking pains from the kidneys radiating round the abdomen and then into the hip and groin; worse on standing.
- *Magnesia phosphorica* For colicky pains causing doubling up; relieved by heat.
- *Calcarea carbonica* For severe cramping pains and vomiting; relieved by heat.

Naturopathy

The following may help those prone to kidney stones. Ensure adequate fluid intake, and prevent fluid loss by avoiding profuse sweating in direct sunlight, sauna baths, etc. Regulate the bowel function by the adoption of a wholefood diet and the avoidance of purgatives.

Avoid spinach, beetroot, rhubarb and chocolate, which contain large quantities of oxalic acid, and restrict calcium-rich dairy products. Drink mineral water containing magnesium, but steer clear of alkaline mineral water and fluoridated water. Take a dessertspoonful of apple cider vinegar, mixed in warm water with a little honey, each day.

Vitamin and Mineral Treatment

Kidney stones may be treated—and prevented—by taking vitamin B_6 (25 mg) and magnesium (100 mg), 3 times daily. Potassium citrate may prevent recurrence.

Kyphosis *see* POSTURAL PROBLEMS

L

Laryngitis *see* SORE THROAT

LICE

Lice are blood-sucking parasites that affect all mammals. They are very host-specific—that is, human lice cannot live on any other animal and vice versa—and the three different varieties of human lice cannot live in different places on the body. Humans are liable to be infested by head lice, body lice and pubic (or crab) lice.

Head Lice

The head louse is currently enjoying a great revival among schoolchildren, who catch it by head-to-head contact. Lice cause severe irritation of the scalp by injecting chemical substances into the skin every time they feed, and if a child is greatly infested with the parasite, they may become irritable, dull, listless and unwell.

Lice are usually discovered by this itching or by the presence of their white egg cases — called 'nits' — attached to the bases of hairs. Removing these will, however, not remove the lice.

Treatment

The most effective treatment is a special insecticidal lotion (available from chemists) applied to the hair and scalp. Lice may be prevented from getting hold if you regularly comb your child's hair thoroughly with a fine-toothed comb.

ALL the family should be treated if one member is infested.

BODY LICE

Body lice are normally the lice of abject poverty, living in the clothes (especially the seams) of down-and-outs, refugees and chronic alcoholics, as well as in those of troops in wartime. Body lice require constant warmth to thrive, and if clothes are not changed often or washed in hot temperatures, they will continue to multiply. In fact, they are further encouraged in these energy-conscious times by the use of low-temperature washing powders, and the risk of their spread has grown with the installation of washing machines with low-temperature programmes in launderettes. They can be treated by using an insecticide on the clothes; alternatively, the infested clothing can be washed in hot water, and then the seams ironed.

PUBIC LICE

Pubic lice ('crabs'—because they look like miniscule crabs) act much as head lice do, but these are attracted to the skin beneath the pubic hair and also sometimes to that under the hair of the chest, armpits, eyebrows and eyelashes.

TREATMENT

Pubic lice are always spread through sexual contact. They can produce intense irritation, which as a result of scratching can then develop into unpleasant, weeping sores. Soak in disinfected baths and apply specific lotion to get rid of them. All sexual partners must be checked to see if they will also need treatment.

LIVER PROBLEMS

Since the liver is one of the most important organs in the body, anything that affects it can have dramatic repercussions on general health.

Minor dysfunctions of the liver can be caused by general over-indulgence, a diet too rich in saturated fats or isolated instances of excessive alcohol intake.

There are also a number of serious illnesses and conditions that can affect the liver and consequently are potentially life-threatening. Virus infections such as hepatitis, parasites such as the liver fluke or the excessive consumption of alcohol resulting in cirrhosis are all damaging. The liver can be severely affected by poisons and by some drugs, the most common of which is paracetamol in overdose. CANCER can also occur in the liver, and it is often the site for secondary cancers, most frequently when the primary cancer is in the breast or lungs. (See also GALLSTONES.)

SYMPTOMS

One of the first indications of liver malfunction is jaundice. This can be followed by APPETITE LOSS, nausea and vomiting. In chronic liver problems, the organ itself becomes enlarged and can be felt under the rib cage on the right side of the body.

ORTHODOX TREATMENT

Medical treatment of severe liver disease is essential and complex, and may result finally in a liver transplant.

ACUPUNCTURE

The functions of the liver include the regulation of Chi and the storage of blood when the body is at rest. It is therefore a nourisher as well as a detoxifier of the tissues. In conjunction with the Gall Bladder, it is associated with the colour green, the season of spring, the wind, the eyes, nails and sinews and the sound of shouting that typifies the emotion of anger.

Acupuncture treatment of any liver disturbance will take account of deficient or excessive energy of the Kidney (chief nourisher of the liver) or the Lungs (controller of the liver).

Acupressure in the web between the big and second toes is useful for recharging the liver.

HERBAL TREATMENT

If constipation is not a problem, a good

Cirrhosis

The liver has an amazing capacity for rapid regeneration, but if damage occurs to this vital organ too quickly and repair cannot take place, scarring may occur, and if this is extensive, cirrhosis—the hardening and shrinking of the liver—may result.

In mild cirrhosis, there are usually no symptoms, but if a large area of the liver has suffered damage, poisonous chemicals will accumulate in the blood and affect the brain, jaundice will appear and there may be internal bleeding because the liver cannot make clotting factors.

The commonest cause of cirrhosis is excessive alcohol consumption, and women may be more susceptible to this than men. Cirrhosis is also a relatively infrequent consequence of viral hepatitis.

After a certain point, a cirrhotic liver will continue to deteriorate even if the cause (usually alcoholism) is eliminated. However, those with mild cirrhosis will often improve by total abstinence and a careful dietary regime.

---

combination for a herbal tea is agrimony, balmony and centaury, taken in 45–60 ml/3–4 tbsp doses 2–3 times daily. A decoction of gentian root and black root in equal quantities will stimulate the liver and improve appetite and digestion. Herbs such as rosemary, peppermint and chamomile exert a gentle influence on liver function and improve the assimilation of food.

Combining Aloe vera gel with milk will stimulate a sluggish liver and increase its secretion of bile, which will also aid digestion.

HOMEOPATHY

- *Podophyllum* When you suddenly turn pale, start vomiting bile and have constipation with the passage of light-coloured stools.
- *Iris versicolor* When there is bilious vomiting and diarrhoea, especially associated with flashing lights and headache.
- *Chelidonium* When there is tenderness and pain in the region of the liver and this passes to the right shoulder.
- *Bryonia* When there is a sharp pain in the liver that goes between the shoulders, a frontal headache and you are worse after the slightest movement.

NATUROPATHY

Excess alcohol and excess fat are prime causes of liver problems. Avoiding these, coupled with eating more fresh fruit and vegetables and simply eating less, will resolve most minor disorders (*See* **Nutrition** pp. 14–15). Drinking vegetable juices (a small glass, 3 times daily), especially cabbage, celery and celeriac, will also aid liver function.

Abdominal cold packs, drinking at least 1 l/2¼ pts non-fizzy mineral water daily and abdominal exercise (including **yoga** *see* p. 99) will all stimulate the liver.

VITAMIN AND MINERAL TREATMENT

High-potency multivitamin complex is needed to restore vitamins lost from the liver both during and after an attack of hepatitis and because of chirrhosis.

Liver problems due to hepatitis can be relieved by very high doses of vitamin C (25–30 g) for a few days, preferably by intravenous injection, but also by mouth, when you should take 5 g every 4 hours. Medical supervision is recommended for this.

Fatty liver should be treated with calcium orotate (1,200 mg daily) and choline and inositol in the form of lecithin, 15 ml/1 tbsp of granules with each meal.

Lordosis *see* POSTURAL PROBLEMS

Low blood pressure *see* BLOOD PRESSURE and FAINTING

Lumbago *see* BACK PAIN

Lupus erythematosus *see* ARTHRITIS

L

195

M

Mastitis *see* PREGNANCY AND CHILDBIRTH

MEASLES

See *also* GERMAN MEASLES

This is a viral infection that attacks the respiratory system and causes a rash. It is normally an illness of childhood, but can affect adults. It is very infectious and spread by coughs and sneezes.

SYMPTOMS

Cold and cough symptoms at first, then the child gradually becomes more feverish and feels unwell. During the first few days, bright lights may be uncomfortable and the eyes may be sore. A day or two later, small white spots rather like grains of salt appear on the inside of the cheeks level with the back teeth. These are certain sign of measles.

The rash begins to appear on the child's face around the third or fourth day. Red, slightly raised spots may join together making the skin look blotchy. The child is now very unhappy and unwell, with a disturbing COUGH and a FEVER of up to about 102°F (38.9°C). During the next few days, the rash spreads to the lower limbs, and by now the child is probably starting to feel better. In another couple of days, the rash fades and a brownish stain persists for another few days. The rash is usually not itchy.

Complications Middle-ear infection (*see* EARACHE) as a result of severe measles is quite common, especially if the child has a history of repeated ear infections. If the cough develops into a sharp barking sound together with loud and noisy breathing and hoarseness, this is probably a sign of BRONCHITIS or CROUP. If the child shows signs of getting worse within two or three days of the rash developing, PNEUMONIA is a possibility. Always seek medical advice if your child has measles, as the complications may be worse than the original illness.

SELF-HELP

See CHILDREN'S ILLNESSES for general home care.

You can have your child vaccinated against measles after the age of 1 year, but this is not 100 per cent effective.

HERBAL TREATMENT

Mix together equal amounts of clivers, meadowsweet and elderflowers. Add 25 g/1 oz of this mixture 0.5 l/1 pt boiling water; stand, then strain. Give every 3 hours: 20–30 ml/1½–2 tbsp to children under 10; 45–60 ml/3–4 tbsp to older children. This will help stimulate the body's own defence mechanisms.

You can also bathe the rash with an infusion of elderflowers.

Naturopathy
Feed the child a light diet, excluding all dairy products. Ensure that plenty of fluids are drunk: fruit (especially pineapple, pawpaw and pears for certain enzymes) and vegetable juices are soothing.

Vitamin and Mineral Treatment
Give 500 mg of vitamin C, 3 times daily, to increase the body's anti-viral resistance. You can also give a multivitamin/mineral tablet or drops.

Menopause

The menopause — commonly called 'the change of life' — is the point at which women stop ovulating. The time leading up to this, when the ovaries are beginning to fail, is called the climacteric, and it may last for several years. It usually occurs between the ages of 45 and 55, but is extremely variable.

The menopause can pass virtually unnoticed for many women, but others suffer considerable discomfort. Night sweats, hot flushes and a loss of the lubricating secretions in the vagina are all common side-effects of the menopause. There may also be a gradual depletion of calcium in the bones leading to OSTEOPOROSIS, which makes fractures of the long bones far more likely to occur. These symptoms are linked to the reduction of hormones oestrogen and progesterone. Other symptoms commonly experienced by women — FATIGUE, HEADACHES, INSOMNIA, DEPRESSION, irritability, etc — do not have such a close connection to the loss of these hormones, and there may well by a psychological element to them, which does not, however, mean that they should be taken any less seriously.

Heavy or very frequent regular periods are *not* normal during the climacteric; nor is any sort of vaginal bleeding after the menopause. Any bleeding of this type must be investigated as soon as possible.

Orthodox Treatment
Hormone replacement therapy.

Self-help
● Use a lubricating gel such as KY jelly which may help to prevent vaginal dryness interfering with lovemaking.
● Avoid hot curries and other spicy foods to make hot flushes less likely and/or uncomfortable.
● Don't wear synthetic fibres.

Herbal Treatment
Mix together equal amounts of hops, centaury, agrimony, wormwood and bog-beans. Add 50 g/2 oz of this mixture to 1 l/1¾ pts cold water, bring to the boil, simmer for 15 minutes, then strain. Drink ½ teacupful before meals. This is a useful tonic.

A good relaxant is an infusion made up of equal quantities of raspberry leaves, limeblossom and pulsatilla. Add 5 ml/1 tsp of this mixture to 1 teacup boiling water; let stand 5 minutes. Add honey to taste.

Naturopathy
Nutrition can play an important part in the treatment of menopausal problems. Follow a balanced wholefood diet as this will improve vitality, energy and general well-being, and will enable you to handle any unpleasant side-effects with greater ease.

Relaxation Techniques
Any of these will help to relieve the stress that can be an accompaniment of the climacteric and menopause. **Yoga** (p. 99) in particular will also help maintain flexibility and muscle tone.

Vitamins and Minerals
Vitamin E (100 iu with each meal) is claimed to relieve hot flushes, headaches and nervousness. Pyridoxine — vitamin B_6 — may help to relieve depression if 50–100 mg are taken

M

daily. Calcium loss from bones can be eased by taking 800 mg calcium, 15 minutes of sunlight daily and 6.25 μg vitamin D daily.

MENSTRUAL DISORDERS

See *also* ANOREXIA NERVOSA

The menstrual cycle is controlled directly by the hypothalamus and pituitary gland and by the ovaries; it can be affected by upsets in the thyroid gland and liver, as well as by less specific problems such as stress and weight gain or loss.

- *Painful periods (dysmenorrhoea)* may be caused by the overproduction of some of the naturally occurring substances, the prostaglandins, one of which cause muscles to contract; by high hormone levels late in the cycle that increase body fluid and blood flow to the pelvic area; or to a lack of the hormone progesterone or vitamin B$_6$ (pyridoxine). *NB* an IUD ('coil') should not cause pain during a period: if it does, seek medical help immediately.
- *Lack of periods (amenorrhoea)* may be caused by serious conditions such as diabetes and thyroid disease. Extreme weight loss (especially ANOREXIA NERVOSA) and gain, excessive exercise and emotional stress may also halt the menstrual cycle. A change in the type of contraceptive pill you use may also stop periods temporarily.
- *Irregular periods* can herald the beginning of the MENOPAUSE; they can also be caused by emotional upset and certain diseases.
- *Heavy periods (menorrhagia)* can be caused by underactive thyroid, fibroids (non-malignant fibrous growths in the womb that require medical attention), and pelvic infection. They can result in ANAEMIA.

- *Overly long, infrequent periods* may mean the woman is not ovulating due to some disorder of the hypothalamus.

ORTHODOX TREATMENT
Hormone therapy.

SELF-HELP
Exercise may speed up menstrual flow and shorten a period, and the relaxation of the muscles it provides will alleviate period pains. Some women find the exercises designed to help you through the first stages of labour can be helpful.

ACUPUNCTURE
A number of meridans are involved in menstrual disorders, and climatic factors of cold or heat may be the cause of or may aggravate disturbances of Energy flow. Treatment would be concerned with dispersing blockages of Energy or Blood, removing stagnation and neutralizing the ill-effects of excessive heat or cold.

Acupressure on point 44 on the lower abdomen and on point 34 on the inside of the leg above the ankle relieves period pain (see p. 104–5).

HERBAL TREATMENT
Melilot, chamomile flowers, balm and rosemary can each be taken in warm infusions to relieve pain just before or during a period. Melilot is specifically good for spasmodic pain, balm will ease cramp-like pains and rosemary will relieve an accompanying tension headache and irritability. An infusion of wild yam will help low abdominal pain, and one of pulsatilla can be taken when nervous problems are a feature. Peppermint tea (available in teabags) is also very good.

Motherwort has a tonic and sedative effect, gently assisting normal function and relieving a dull ache at the top of the head. Headaches before or during a period, and associated with some irregularity of periods, can often be resolved by taking an infusion of feverfew: take 45–60 ml/3–4 tbsp, 2–3 times daily, for a few days before the period is due; and 15 ml/1 tbsp, 3 times daily, for the rest of the month.

M

Teas made of couch grass, wild carrot or dandelion leaf and root, taken 4 or 5 times daily during the few days before a period, will relieve fluid retention.

An infusion of aloe vera leaf is said to promote suppressed menstruation and relieve period pain.

HOMEOPATHY

For chronic disorders, consult a homeopath. For the occasional problem:

- *Magnesia phosphorica* Colicky pains relieved by curling up with a hot water bottle.
- *Belladonna* Face red and congested; cutting pains; blood feels hot.
- *Pulsatilla* Cutting pains with chilliness and diarrhoea; periods easily suppressed by emotional upset.
- *Chamomilla* Severe pains associated with anger.
- *Cimicifuga* For stout, red-faced women with premenstrual headache and labour-like pains.
- *Aconite* Lack of periods after exposure to cold, dry winds or after fright.
- *Colocynth* Lack of periods after anger.
- *Natrum muriaticum* Lack of periods from grief or emotional upset.
- *Ignatia* Lack of periods after disappointment in love.

MANIPULATIVE THERAPIES

These can help when the presence of fibroids cause pressure resulting in backache, or problems with the lower part of the spine cause 'referred' pain to occur in the womb.

MASSAGE

Abdominal massage can be of assistance, for by relaxing tension there, menstruation can become less painful and more regular.

NATUROPATHY

Diet: Ensure adequate nutrition with a wholefood diet, supplementing protein intake with nuts, seeds, grains and pulses. A general feeling of well-being can make it easier to handle period pains and/or PMS symptoms. Eat plenty of dietary fibre to avoid the constipation that can accompany painful periods, and reduce salt, sugar and dairy products. A raw food diet for the 7 days preceding a period may also be of great benefit.

Heat/cold treatment: Apply hot and cold fomentations to the abdominal area and low back — 3 minutes hot and 1 minutes cold, for a total of 20–30 minutes — to relieve period pains.

RELAXATION TECHNIQUES

Any of these will help.

M

Premenstrual Syndrome (PMS)

Commonly called 'premenstrual tension' or 'PMT', this is a much-ignored but very troublesome problem for many women. As well as intense and changeable moods, the following physical symptoms may also appear: headache and migraine, back pain, swelling of hands and feet (*see* oedema), breast tenderness, painful periods, weight gain. PMS most commonly develops in women after the age of 30 and occurs in the latter half of the menstrual cycle.

PMS has been successfully treated with natural progesterone or with synthetic progesterone, called progestogen. Sadly, PMS is also frequently treated with tranquillizers and little understanding, all of which can make the situation worse.

Self-help is the only answer to PMS. Learning to spot the onset (usually round about 10 days before period is due to start) is a great help. Then you can take some positive action to minimize the effects. Natural therapies can help here. Herbalists recommend agnus castus tablets, supported by nerve remedies if necessary.

Vitamin B_6 (ie pyridoxine) up to 100 mg daily) plus magnesium (300 mg daily) for the 10 days preceding menstruation may help, or 2,000 mg evening primrose oil daily over the same period, or both. Sometimes a lower dose of vitamin B_6 (25–50 mg daily) over the whole month will suffice.

VITAMIN AND MINERAL TREATMENT

Painful periods: Take 500–1000 mg calcium daily during the week preceding menstruation until it finishes, plus 100 iu vitamin E, 3 times daily. Alternatively or in addition, take 2,000 mg evening primrose oil daily for the 10 days preceding menstruation.

Lack of periods may be a feature of malnutrition. Take a high-potency multivitamin/multimineral preparation of the prolonged-release type. Alternatively, to relieve the condition take 100 iu vitamin E, 3 times daily, or a mixture of vitamin B_{12} (10 μg) and folic acid (500 μg).

Heavy periods see ANAEMIA.

See *also* ANOREXIA NERVOSA

MIGRAINE

Migraine is often confused with HEADACHES caused by TENSION, DEPRESSION and other things, but migraine is very much a separate disorder.

Attacks usually start after puberty and continue until middle age (in women, they often disappear after the MENOPAUSE), but they can occur at any time in a person's life. It is quite common for migraine to run in families, and for a child who suffers from TRAVEL SICKNESS to develop migraine as an adult.

CAUSES OF MIGRAINE

There is uncertainty over the exact cause, but it is believed to be due to disturbances in the blood supply to the brain and scalp. These disturbances can be triggered by a wide range of things:
- additives.
- emotional stress.
- certain foods, especially cheese, chocolate, citrus fruit, red wine, sherry, port and coffee.
- lack of food.
- stuffy, smoky rooms.
- hot, dry winds.
- bright and/or flickering lights.

- hormonal changes before and during periods, and the hormones contained in the contraceptive pill.
- high BLOOD PRESSURE.
- head or neck injury.
- fluid retention in the body.

Food and stress seem to be the most common triggers. Many practitioners regard nutritional causes of migraine as food allergy. However, this is a questionable theory since there is no evidence of the normal immune responses that occur in true allergic reactions. A more correct description is FOOD INTOLERANCE, or adverse food reactions. This is often linked to the chemical substance *tyramine*, which affects the diameter of the blood vessels in the brain (and thus the blood flow through them) and is found in many of the 'trigger' foods.

SYMPTOMS

Simple migraine involves a throbbing headache that is usually centred above or behind one eye, or begins at the back of the head and then spreads to all of one side of the head. This is often accompanied by NAUSEA AND VOMITING. In what is called 'classical' migraine, the headache is frequently preceded by an 'aura', an exaggerated sense of well-being, as well as by disturbances in vision and touch; the latter can continue during the attack itself.

ORTHODOX TREATMENT

Drugs which affect the blood vessels of the brain and scalp; drugs to reduce vomiting; tranquillizers.

AVOIDING MIGRAINE ATTACKS

The following list of 'do's and don'ts' may help:

DO
- Try to identify situations that trigger attacks.
- Keep a detailed diary of your food intake and any attacks you may have for a two-week (or longer) period—is there a pattern?
- Try an elimination diet (*see* pp. 104–5) and keep and accurate record of what happens.
- Increase your fluid intake to 1.5l/3 pints daily.

- Learn some form of relaxation (*see below*).
- Learn to exercise your neck and shoulder muscles (*see* pp. 32–3).
- Plan your life to avoid over-commitment.
- Avoid extremes of heat and cold.

DO NOT
- Eat or drink items on your own 'trigger' list.
- Leave emotional problems unresolved—this can lead to unsupportable stress levels and migraine (*see* pp. 44–5).
- Go for long periods without food.
- Get overtired to the point of exhaustion.

Coping with a migraine attack
These suggestions may alleviate an attack:
- Rest in a darkened, well-ventilated room; do not use a pillow.
- Try to sleep.
- Apply acupressure to sensitive areas (*see below*).
- Apply a cold compress to the part of the head that hurts.
- Drink two or three glasses of cold water.

Acupuncture
It is rare for a case of migraine not to involve the Gall Bladder energy and, by association, that of the Liver and perhaps the Stomach. Nutrition is therefore implicated as well as stress response and structural integrity. An acupuncturist will balance Energies between attacks, and can sometimes help to stop or minimize an acute attack.

Acupressure on points 4 and 1 (both on the line of the Large Intestine) will encourage the waste disposal functions of the body. During an attack, it is worth trying the same points, as well as point 41 at the base of the skull and any sensitive points around the eyes or the temples.

Herbal Treatment
During an attack: Take an infusion of lavender flowers, leaves and stalks. Massage 2 drops of lavender oil into the temples. Peppermint tea may relieve the headache and nausea. A few mint leaves, moistened and bandaged on to the forehead, may ease the pain. *To prevent at attack:* Try feverfew leaves: 3 small leaves — $1\frac{1}{2} \times 1\frac{1}{4}$ in (3.8×3.2 cm) — or one large leaf daily. These can either be eaten on their own or in a sandwich. (A small number of people get mouth ulcers from this herb, so use with care.)

The following may also help: mix together equal amounts of motherwort, vervain, finely chopped dandelion root, centaury and wild carrot; add 25 g/1 oz to 0.5 l/1 pt water to make an infusion; take 45–60 ml/3–4 tbsp, 3 times daily.

Homeopathy
If you have chronic migraine, consult a homeopath. For acute attacks:
- *Silica* For right-sided attack; pain begins at back of head and neck and shoots through to behind the eye.
- *Spigelia* For left-sided attack; often associated with PALPITATIONS and pressing pain on the eye, which feels too large.
- *Natrum muriaticum* For blinding headache like 1,000 little hammers knocking on the brain from sunrise to sunset; worse with menstrual periods.
- *Lycopodium* For right-sided attack; worse between 4 and 8 p.m. and brought on by irregular eating.

Hypnotherapy
This can be extremely useful in eliminating the stress that may trigger attacks.

Manipulative therapies
Migraine sufferers commonly have excessive muscular contractions in the large muscles of the neck and shoulders. There can also be some narrowing of the spaces between the vertebrae in the neck and some loss of mobility of these neck joints. All these factors can cause irritation to the nerves that supply the muscles and thus increase muscular tension, which can itself be a trigger of attacks. Neuromuscular massage to the affected muscles, mobility exercises and

M

mobilization and manipulation of the neck joints are all of great benefit.

Sometimes a faulty bite can produce uneven stresses in the joints of the jaw, which can in turn lead to severe muscular tension and/or pressure on nerves. A combination of manipulative treatment to these joints and dental treatment to improve the mechanics of the bite will help prevent migraine. (*See also* TEETH GRINDING.)

MASSAGE
Perform a gentle, lifting massage on the face and around the eyes, and a pressure-point massage around the neck and back of the head.

NATUROPATHY
Carry out a naturopathic regime of balanced eating, with a preponderance of raw fresh food—at least one-third of daily intake—and drink at least 1.7 l/3 pt, of liquid daily. Avoid tea, coffee, alcohol, citrus fruit and red meat and keep an eye on the common daily foods known to sometimes precipitate a migraine attack (eg cow's milk, eggs, wheat, cheese, tomato, rye and fish).

RELAXATION TECHNIQUES
Yoga (p. 99).

VITAMIN AND MINERAL TREATMENT
Take the following 3 times daily: whole vitamin B complex (10 mg potency, nicotinamide (100 mg), calcium pantothenate (100 mg) and pyridoxine (vitamin B₆; 50 mg). If this regime prevents attacks, reduce the dosages gradually to levels that maintain relief.

Mineral deficiencies *see* VITAMIN AND MINERAL DEFICIENCIES

MISCARRIAGE

Miscarriage is the expulsion of the foetus from the womb before the 28th week of pregnancy. No one can be sure just how many pregnancies end in miscarriage. Estimates are as high as one third of all pregnancies.

The greatest number of miscarriages occur during the first 12 weeks of pregnancy. Most of these are due to abnormal defects in the foetus, or in the placenta, or in the way the placenta attaches to the uterus wall. Very occasionally, the miscarriage may be due to illness in the mother.

Miscarriages after 12 weeks may be caused by an 'incompetent cervix'. The cervix softens, as it should just before birth, but far too early in the pregnancy. It can be caused by surgery to the cervix, a previous termination or miscarriage, or a previous forceps delivery. It can be remedied by inserting a tape around the top of the cervix—the Shirodkar stitch—under general anaesthetic at 14 weeks of pregnancy. The stitch is removed two weeks before the anticipated delivery date. This technique is very successful.

Women with a history of more than one miscarriage should consult a gynaecologist. Various causes for recurrent miscarriage are put forward: hormone deficiency or imbalance, virus, infections and even ALLERGY to the partner's sperm. If a woman has carried one baby successfully to term and given birth without too much difficulty, there is no reason why she should not do it again. Most women have an 80 per cent chance of successful pregnancy next time round.

SELF-HELP
The best thing is to make sure you are in optimum health *before* you conceive (*see* PREGNANCY AND CHILDBIRTH).

NATUROPATHY
Nutrition is paramount. If there is a history of miscarriage, gentle exercise, plenty of rest and a diet of one third raw food, particularly green leafy vegetables, plus whole grain cereals will ensure optimum vitamin and mineral intake.

PSYCHOTHERAPIES
A miscarriage, especially in later pregnancy, is a sad experience for both partners. Women may suffer periods of depression. It is essential to allow time

for grief and mourning and to allow the couple to talk through their experience. Where feelings of anger and repressed aggression dominate, **bioenergetics** (*see* p. 95) will be helpful.

VITAMIN AND MINERAL TREATMENT
Take 100 iu vitamin E twice daily for 3 months before conception and 100 iu daily during pregnancy. Sometimes the partner should also take 100 iu vitamin E daily before conception.

Morning sickness *see* PREGNANCY AND CHILDBIRTH

MOUTH ULCERS

These painful, raw sores can be caused by injury, as when you bite the inside of your cheeks or by ill-fitting dentures wearing away some of the tissue lining the cheeks and gums. They may also be related to the cold sores caused by the HERPES virus or to thrush (*see* YEAST INFECTION), and cracks or ulcers at the corners of the mouth may be a sign of vitamin B₂ deficiency.

Mouth ulcers can reflect a rundown state of health, which may include poor eating habits. Little orthodox medical attention has been paid to the question of ALLERGY or diet as a cause of these ulcers.

Stress, too, can play an important part in their onset.

Ulcers can also develop in the mouth if acid from the stomach reaches it (*see* INDIGESTION). Vomiting can also bring up acid, and mouth ulcers caused by this are very commonly seen in sufferers of ANOREXIA AND BULIMIA NERVOSA.

ORTHODOX TREATMENT
Local anaesthetic lozenges; steroid ointments or tablets.

HERBAL TREATMENT
Apply undiluted tincture of myrrh several times daily; it will smart but is effective. You can also try a mouthwash made either from blackberry leaves or,

to reduce inflammation, agrimony herb. Marshmallow root is soothing.

Rinse the mouth with extract of red sage — 2.5 ml/½ tsp in a cup of warm water — several times daily.

Rub aloe vera gel on to mouth ulcers and onto areas of the gum rubbed by dentures.

NATUROPATHY
Try a cleansing programme of fruit juices, fruit and vegetables for two or three days, being sure to avoid those foods that can make mouth ulcers worse. If vitamin B₂ deficiency is suspected, eat such rich sources as wheatgerm, meat, vegetables, fruit and brewer's yeast.

VITAMIN AND MINERAL TREATMENT
Mouth ulcers can be prevented or treated with daily doses of vitamin A (7,500 iu), vitamin E (250 mg; open the capsule and apply locally to the ulcer), and vitamin B₂ (10 mg). Vitamin C with supplements of zinc may also be helpful.

M

MUMPS

Mumps is a viral infection spread by droplets of saliva. It normally affects children between the ages of 5 and 14, but a very small percentage of adults contract it as well.

SYMPTOMS
Not all children are obviously unwell with mumps.

Pain around the ear or when eating, a slight FEVER and a general feeling of being unwell are the first symptoms. The next day, one of the parotid glands — salivary glands covering the angles either side of the jaw — will become swollen and painful; the other gland usually (but not always) becomes affected within five days. At this point, the fever may rise. The swelling and the temperature gradually subside, generally returning to normal within 10 days.

A bout usually gives lifelong immunity, even if only one gland has become swollen.

Complications In about 1 in 4 males, the infection will spread to the testicles (where it is known as *orchitis*) but usually only affects one of them. Orchitis most commonly occurs after the swelling in the jaw is beginning to subside, when HEADACHE, BACK PAIN, chills, sweats and severe pain in one or both testicles are followed by gross swelling. When only one testicle has been affected, this is likely to be reduced in size after the illness, but this does not affect fertility. It is only when both testicles are severely infected that there is a risk of subsequent sterility, but the fear of this has been greatly exaggerated.

Mumps will eventually resolve itself. However, see your doctor if:
● the pain in the jaw is very severe.
● the sufferer is complaining of headaches or EARACHE.
● if there is any pain in the abdomen or testicles.
● if you are worried.

SELF-HELP
See CHILDREN'S ILLNESSES for general care. Because of the pain in the jaws, there may be difficulty in eating if the child is hungry; give soft nutritious foods, liquidized if necessary and plenty of fluids. If the mouth is dry, rinse it out often to keep it moist and clean.

NATUROPATHY
Diet: A high fluid intake (but avoid acidic fruit juices as they stimulate the flow of saliva and aggravate the pain), when the child is willing a diet of raw vegetables, fruit and salads will help to resolve the problem.
Heat/cold treatment: Cold compresses will help relieve pain and reduce swelling.

VITAMINS AND MINERALS
Give 500 mg vitamin C, 3 times daily, and a high dose multi-vitamin and mineral tablet to supplement the body's own anti-viral defences.

N

NAPPY RASH

Nappy rash occurs when the contact between an infant's bottom and a urine-soaked nappy is too prolonged, and can be made much worse if the baby also has frequent and/or loose bowel movements — the organisms from the bowel break down the urine into even more irritating substances (*see* DERMATITIS).

SYMPTOMS
Small red pimples and areas of rough skin first develop on the baby's buttocks and thighs; if severe, these areas can break open and ulcerate. Frequently, THRUSH is associated with this condition, and red circular patches of it may appear around the edges of the affected area.

SELF-HELP
Keep your child as dry as possible until the nappy rash goes away. Exposing the baby's bottom to the open air is the best (if messiest) method; otherwise, change nappies as frequently as possible, and do not use plastic pants as these create an environment that encourages harmful bacteria to grow.

HERBAL TREATMENT
A mild infusion of chickweed or one of chamomile flowers can be applied as a lotion, dabbing it on at intervals during the day, or as a compress on lint. Comfrey or chickweed ointment or calendula cream can be rubbed on two or three times a day. Aloe vera gel greatly aids healing.

HOMEOPATHY
If the nappy rash is severe, try:
● *Sulphur* When the rash is aggravated by heat and hot baths.
● *Rhus tox* When the rash is red, swollen with itching; blistering may be present.

The quality of the baby's urine during breastfeeding is directly related to the mother's food intake. Avoiding citrus juices, highly spiced food, alcohol and excessive quantities of coffee, tea and all acidic drinks and foods may help.

VITAMIN AND MINERAL TREATMENT

Nappy rash can be treated by directly applying vitamin E cream (*not* the oil) on to the affected area.

NAUSEA AND VOMITING

Nausea is a feeling of sickness that may be followed by vomiting, the violent expulsion of the stomach contents through the mouth.

In adults, nausea and vomiting may be the result of gastric irritation due to bacterial infection or excessive intake of alcohol, as well as infectious diseases that cause FEVER, peptic ULCER, hiatus HERNIA, appendicitis, MIGRAINE, TRAVEL SICKNESS and PREGNANCY, especially during the first three months. Self-induced vomiting is a common feature of ANOREXIA AND BULIMIA NERVOSA, especially the latter. In addition, both nausea and vomiting can occur because of ANXIETY and TENSION. Attacks of vomiting for no obvious reason may be associated with LIVER PROBLEMS or other disorders. Consult a practitioner.

Any of the common childhood infectious diseases may cause vomiting, as can ear infections (*see* EARACHE), a high temperature or even the common cold, especially if the child swallows large quantities of mucus. It may follow a severe bout of coughing, especially during WHOOPING COUGH, and accompanies severe DIARRHOEA in GASTROENTERITIS. In small babies, pyloric stenosis (a congenital condition that prevents the stomach contents passing into the intestines) may cause severe vomiting — called 'projectile vomiting' because of the forceful way the food is ejected. This usually occurs a few weeks after birth and needs urgent surgical attention.

Children may become severly dehydrated as a result of continual vomiting, and it is important to maintain body fluids (*see* CHILDREN'S ILLNESSES).

ORTHODOX TREATMENT

Anti-emetic drugs (except during pregnancy).

HERBAL TREATMENT

Until the stomach is clear, its natural response to infection or alien substances must not be suppressed.

Antispasmodic tincture, taken as 5 ml/1 tsp doses in a teacup of warm water every 2 hours, will assist the stomach when vomiting is due to dietary errors or some infection.

For vomiting with a nervous origin, balm or chamomile tea, taken regularly with other remedies for the nerves (*see* ANXIETY), should help.

HOMEOPATHY

- *Ipecachuana* For persistent nausea, usually with diarrhoea.
- *Arsenicum album* When associated with collapse, diarrhoea, restlessness and chilliness.
- *Cuprum metallicum* With associated severe cramps in the abdomen.
- *Nux vomica* After overindulgence.
- *Pulsatilla* After rich, fatty foods.

HYPNOTHERAPY

Hypnosis can be employed to overcome the impulse to vomit under stress.

NATUROPATHY

Maintain fluid intake, but avoid dairy products. As the vomiting abates, introduce a light diet (still avoiding dairy products). The first solid food should be plain, toasted wholemeal bread and a little clear vegetable soup. Plain, boiled brown rice with some steamed vegetables, especially carrots or other root vegetables, are the next step, and the diet should return to normal over a period or two or three days.

N

These can be used to relieve anxiety states that lead to nausea and vomiting.

RELAXATION TECHNIQUES
Yoga (p. 99), **relaxation exercises** and **autogenics** (p. 97).

VITAMIN AND MINERAL TREATMENT
This may respond to vitamin B$_6$, taken in 25 mg doses 3 times daily.

Nerves *see* ANXIETY

NETTLE RASH

(URTICARIA)

Nettle rash, or 'hives' is a term used to describe an allergic skin reaction resulting in a rash of pale, irritating weals. It is caused by stinging nettles or other substances to which the body is sensitive (allergens). The rash may appear only in areas of skin that have been in contact with an allergen or it can appear all over the body after the person has consumed a food to which they are highly allergic. The most common factors are shellfish, chocolates, strawberries, eggs, wheat, nuts, food additives and milk. Sunlight may also trigger off a reaction, and nettle rash can also arise after insect stings or even vaccination. Heat, cold and pressures may also result in a rash, and it can develop during or after a period of emotional stress (*see* ANXIETY and TENSION).

The only long-term treatment is the identification and avoidance of the allergenic substances; an exclusion diet may help here (*see* p. 103). Desensitization therapy (*see* ALLERGY) may also be an answer.

SELF-HELP
Attacks of hives are normally short lived, although extremely uncomfortable. Cool baths, cotton clothing and the use of calomine lotion all provide a measure of symptomatic relief.

HERBAL TREATMENT
An infusion of equal quantities of burdock root, yellow dock root, fumitory and clivers can be taken 3 times daily, as well as 2 echinacea tablets each day. An infusion of calendula flowers should be applied to relieve inflammation, but the weals should not be handled. A decoction of burdock root can also be used as a lotion or, alternatively, an infusion of clivers.

Aloe vera gel applied twice a day will reduce the rash.

HOMEOPATHY
- *Aconite* When the attack is acute and severe, accompanied by FEVER, agitation and anxiety.
- *Apis* When the weals are swollen and stinging.
- *Sulphur* For chronic cases, where there is swelling, itching, redness and maybe ulceration and infection.
- *Urtica urens* When the stinging and itching are made worse by touch and water.

VITAMIN AND MINERAL TREATMENT
Nettle rash can be prevented or relieved by taking 500 mg vitamin C, 3 times daily. Direct application of vitamin E cream will alleviate the irritation.

NEURALGIA

Neuralgia is pain that arises in a nerve. Initially, it is usually severe and lancing, after which a continual and extremely painful ache may persist for a considerable period.

Neuralgia may be the result of an infection along or near a nerve, such as the pain that people suffer during and after shingles caused by a HERPES virus, or in addition to a dental abscess. It can also follow injury to a nerve or, commonly, occur for no apparent reason.

Neuralgia may also arise through attacks of MIGRAINE, and from pressure on the nerve roots at the lower part of the spine, which causes sciatica (*see* SLIPPED DISC).

Trigeminal, or facial, neuralgia (in the past, known as *tic douloureux*) is a condition that frequently affects older people. One of the trigeminal nerves on either side of the face is involved, and through its branches, severe pain can occur in the jaw, cheek, forehead, lips and around one eye. 'Trigger zones' develop on the affected side of the face, and touching these or even a cold draught, chewing or talking can be enough to start an attack. The pain is agonizing and frequently intractable.

A frequently overlooked cause of trigeminal neuralgia is a fault in the bite mechanism of sufferers' teeth (the way their teeth come together when eating).

ORTHODOX TREATMENT
Painkillers; injections into the nerve to block the pain pathway; surgery.

SELF-HELP
See PAIN AND PAINKILLERS.

ACUPUNCTURE
In neuralgia, there will inevitably be pathways of Energy involved, and the selection of treatment will depend on the site of the neuralgia/Energy meridian. For example, neuralgia occurring around the ribs, common in shingles, could relate to an imbalance in the Liver and its co-worker, the Gall Bladder; in addition, the emotion linked to these organs — anger — often spills out as this type of neuralgia.

MANIPULATIVE THERAPIES
Sciatica is best treated by osteopathy or chiropractic. Trigeminal neuralgia seldom responds to manipulation.

NATUROPATHY
Applying hot and cold fomentations to the affected area — alternating 3 minutes hot and 1 minute cold for a total of 20 minutes — may relieve pain.

RELAXATION TECHNIQUES
Any of these may help someone with chronic neuralgia.

VITAMIN AND MINERAL TREATMENT
Neuralgia can be treated with high doses of vitamin B_1, B_6 and B_{12}, starting with 600 mg daily and reducing gradually as the pain is relieved.

Nocturnal enuresis *see* BEDWETTING

O

OBESITY

Of all the nutritional disorders in infants, children and adults, obesity is the commonest in our affluent society. Obesity is indisputedly linked with premature death and also predisposes the sufferer to a range of other problems: degenerative joint disease, BACK PAIN, HAEMORRHOIDS, VARICOSE VEINS, *high* BLOOD PRESSURE, *raised cholesterol levels and coronary* HEART DISEASE *and stroke. Socially it prevents people from taking part in sporting activities and reduces their overall efficiency. The underlying psychological and emotional problems which both cause and are caused by obesity can be extremely disruptive.*

CAUSES OF OBESITY
Obesity is defined as an excess of body fat. Anyone whose weight is 20 per cent more than the norm for their age, build and height is described as obese.

One of the key factors determining weight problems is the basal metabolic rate, that is the efficiency with which the body at rest burns up fuel which is consumed as food. This explains why two members of the same family eating the same diet can be totally different in body shape, one slim the other fat. Brown fat is also thought to play an important role in obesity.

Brown fat (so called because its connective tissue is brown) can store great amounts of energy without causing obesity. Newborn babies have a cushion of brown fat down their back to protect them from the cold outside the womb. People who have less of this fat tend to convert their surplus energy into normal white fat.

Many people believe that overweight is the result of some glandular disturbance in the body. While it is true that this may be a reason for obesity it is in fact extremely rare.

Some drugs, particularly steroids, oral contraceptive and insulin may also cause obesity. However, the vast majority of obese people are obese because they eat too much.

ORTHODOX TREATMENT
Extreme cases, or sufferers whose obesity is threatening their health because of other diseases (HEART DISEASE, ARTHRITIS, DIABETES) may be taken into hospital for an enforced fast.

SELF-HELP
See **Nutrition/Obesity** (pp. 20–3).

ACUPUNCTURE
Overeating is an addiction and can be successfully treated with acupuncture when used in conjunction with a regime of exercise and sound nutrition. Small needles are inserted in the ears and left there. They can then be stimulated by the wearer when a compulsion to eat assails them. This may help to override the compulsion.

HYPNOTHERAPY
Hypnosis is valuable for those who wish to lose weight. It can also be used to build in aversions to food (this must be done with care to avoid ANOREXIA NERVOSA).

MASSAGE
Massage can improve skin tone and minimize stretch marks. *No form of manual or mechanical massage can remove any body weight at all.*

PSYCHOTHERAPY
Food is often used as emotional support: 'it will make me feel better', and some people become fat through overeating out of unhappiness. Psychotherapy can be valuable for them, and can improve low self esteem and poor self image. Cognitive therapy helps a person to a better understanding of the image they have of themselves, and

allows the superimposition of a more positive one. An active therapy such as **bioenergetics** (*see* p. 95) can help. Self-help groups like Weight Watchers are supportive and helpful.

VITAMIN AND MINERAL TREATMENT
While on a calorie-reduced diet, take a general multivitamin/multimineral supplement daily.

OEDEMA

Oedema is a swelling of the body tissues caused by fluid retention. This occurs for a number of reasons:
- sluggish circulation due to heart inefficiency.
- mechanical blockage of the veins and capillaries by VARICOSE VEINS, or external factors such as elastic topped socks impedes blood flow.
- damage to the capillary blood vessels (this can happen after bruising or scalding).
- fluid not being efficiently excreted by the kidneys.
- too much salt retained in the body, either because kidneys are not functioning well, or because the hormonal balance of the adrenal glands (which regulate the kidneys) is unbalanced.

Oedema may be generalized over the whole body or affect only local areas, usually the ankles or belly.
- *Generalized oedema* is not usually detectable unless the total fluid retained increases by 15 per cent above normal.
- *Localized oedema* is a frequent symptom of CIRRHOSIS, KIDNEY DISORDERS and HEART DISEASE. Heart failure, for instance, reduces the heart's ability to cope with the full volume of blood circulating the body. The ankles swell as surplus blood collects in the leg veins and water in the blood seeps out into surrounding tissue.

Gross malnutrition, vitamin B deficiency and steroid drugs can also cause oedema before menstruation and it frequently occurs during pregnancy (due to hormonal changes, or varicose veins).

ORTHODOX TREATMENT
Diuretics.

ACUPUNCTURE
Treatment to the meridians of the Kidneys and Bladder is sometimes effective.

HERBAL TREATMENT
Dandelion extract is a natural diuretic and does not upset the body's potassium level. Dandelion leaves can be brewed to make tea, or used in salads.

MASSAGE
Effleurage to the affected area and specific lymph drainage techniques of massage are both beneficial.

NATUROPATHY
Eliminate salt from the diet, since excessive sodium encourages fluid retention.

Reduce weight when required and exercise to stimulate the circulatory flow.

Osteoarthritis *see* ARTHRITIS

OSTEOPOROSIS

This is a reduction in the density of bones, caused by a loss of calcium. Osteoporosis is normal with advancing age, but deficiencies of calcium and vitamin D will exacerbate the problem. More women than men develop the disease, particularly after the MENOPAUSE when hormonal changes have an adverse effect on calcium metabolism. Recent research show that young girls and women who suffer from ANOREXIA NERVOSA may also develop osteoporosis due to lack of oestrogen which affects the body's efficient use of collagen, the main ingredient in connective tissue.

Any bone that is immobilized is at risk of osteoporosis and corticosteroid drugs (anti-inflammatory drugs) can also encourage it.

SELF-HELP
Increase your calcium intake and let your limbs bathe in the sun for as long as is compatible with your skin type (see SUNBURN).

HOMEOPATHY
Usually, you must consult a homeopath, but in addition *calc. fluor.* and *calc. phos.* can be taken over long periods as a tissue salt preparation (*see* **Homeopathy** p. 79). After one month take a week's break in the treatment.

NATUROPATHY
Diet: Maintain a wholefood diet. Use nuts, seeds, grains and pulses to supplement your protein intake.
Exercise: Ensure weightbearing exercise.

VITAMIN AND MINERAL TREATMENT
A typical supplementary regime is 1,000–1,500 mg calcium daily, preferably with 400 iu vitamin D; this is safe for self treatment; 45 mg per day sodium fluoride may also be taken, but since this is a toxic substance, it must only be taken under medical supervision.
See *also* MENOPAUSE

P

PAIN AND PAINKILLERS

Pain is an experience that everyone will go through at some point in their lives. For the most part, pain is a warning that something is wrong with the body — either because of a disease within it or because of an injury to it — and in this sense, it can be seen as beneficial. This is also true of what is known as 'referred' pain — that is, pain felt at sites distance from the actual cause — for instance, the pain in the leg and foot (sciatica) caused by pressure on the nerve roots in the back (see SLIPPED DISC*), or the pain in the shoulder that arises from certain* LIVER PROBLEMS. *However, sometimes pain outlives its usefulness, yet continues for weeks, months or even years and this becomes chronic, as can be seen in* ARTHRITIS, MIGRAINE *and chronic* BACK PAIN.

Almost all people have the same pain threshold *— that is, they all feel pain at the about the same time during any sort of stimulus. However,* pain tolerance *— the level of intensity at which pain becomes unpleasant — can vary considerably from person to person: a level of discomfort that, for one person, would be merely irritating, can, for another, be intolerable.*

For most people, this signifies a difference in mental attitude. We feel pain more when we are feeling under the weather, tense or anxious. Our expectations can also have a big impact on how we actually 'feel' pain. The debilitating effects of pain are seen much more strongly in those who can see no end to it — those with cancer, neuralgia and arthritis. Chronic pain can, in turn, have devastating psychological effects, causing DEPRESSION, *irritability, withdrawal and even suicidal feelings.*

THE RELIEF OF PAIN

The holistic therapist approaches the task of pain relief with rather more caution than the orthodox practitioner, since the former will be less willing to remove this symptom without first establishing the underlying cause of, say, recurrent HEADACHE.

There are certain conditions for which the alleviation of pain is the only solution: the phantom pain following amputation of a limb, the residual pain after SHINGLES, the excruciating pain of trigeminal NEURALGIA. Chronic conditions also greatly benefit from pain relief, and in all these cases, the alternative practitioner can often offer safer and more effective relief than an orthodox one.

PAINKILLERS

The most widely used painkiller is aspirin, derived originally from the white willow tree *Salix alba* and used for many hundreds of years. It is still the drug of choice for the relief of many everyday pains. Its irritating effect on the stomach can be minimized by using soluble aspirin and not taking it on an empty stomach. Natural extracts of willow, however, do not have such adverse effects on the stomach lining. Paracetamol has similar effects to aspirin (except that it does not relieve inflammation), but while it does not irritate the stomach lining, it can cause severe liver damage if taken in even a small overdose.

Modern painkillers are divided into two categories: *non-narcotic drugs* for mild pain; and *narcotic drugs* (often derived from opium) for severe pain. All narcotic drugs can be addictive (*see* ADDICTIONS), including codeine.

Anti-inflammatory drugs are frequently used to relieve the pain of arthritis and rheumatism. Whether these are aspirin, steroids or what are called NSAIDs (non-steroidal anti-inflammatory) drugs, none is without side-effects, which can include stomach irritation, CONSTIPATION, NAUSEA, DIZZINESS, PALPITATIONS and kidney and liver damage.

The natural painkillers, while with few or no side-effects, do not produce the dramatic results sometimes associated with the more powerful drugs.

ACUPUNCTURE

Pain relief will be as permanent as the dispersal of its cause. Sometimes this is not possible, in which case repeated treatments may be required to maintain a degree of comfort. The general approach is to treat the meridian(s) passing through the painful area.

Acupressure on point 17 on the outside of the foot just below the ankle bone is sometimes helpful (see p. 104).

HEALING

Healers will try to discover the cause of pain and then heal it. Chronic pain is more difficult because it tends to

P

change people both physically and emotionally. The latter, therefore, usually need self-healing more than a laying-on of hands to help them. However, with self-motivation, pain will usually be alleviated by healing.

HYPNOTHERAPY

Hypnosis has been used extensively and been found to be very effective in pain relief. Learning auto-hypnosis is a very good way to achieve quick relaxation.

MASSAGE

The relaxing effect of massage can help in the relief of chronic pain by relieving local muscle spasm, which can aggravate already sensitive nerve endings. The use of essential oils (especially lavender) further enhances the benefits.

PSYCHOTHERAPIES

The depression that chronic pain can cause can be treated by psychotherapy. In addition, many of those with chronic pain find themselves falling into the trap of becoming 'painful patients' — when they discover that a groan of pain will elicit sympathy from others, that others will fetch and carry for them because they are in pain, and thus the pain begins to have 'rewards'. Such sufferers tend to hang on to their pain rather than taking measures to deal with it.

Group counselling with other chronic pain sufferers is often a good way to force such a 'painful patient' to come to terms with the pain and cope with it. In certain cases, behaviour therapy either on an outpatient basis or in a hospital setting can also be tried: in this, patients are ignored if they moan but rewarded if they cope, and their painkillers are either greatly reduced or withdrawn altogether. This treatment is used in conjunction with counselling, acupuncture, relaxation techniques and training in auto-hypnosis.

RELAXATION TECHNIQUES

Autogenics, biofeedback (p. 97), and if you have no physical disability, **yoga** (p. 99).

PALPITATIONS

Palpitations are a conscious awareness of the heartbeat, most commonly the result of ANXIETY and stress. The awareness may be due either to the individual focusing attention on the heartbeat, or to an increase in the strength of the pulse. They are common, normal and transient, but obsessive awareness can lead to fear, panic and even FAINTING.

Palpitations can be caused by excessive use of stimulants, especially nicotine and caffeine, alcohol abuse and overexertion. Some prescribed drugs can cause them.

ORTHODOX TREATMENT

Tranquillizers may be prescribed.

SELF-HELP

Avoid stimulants such as coffee and alcohol; cut down on cigarettes.

ACUPUNCTURE

Treatment of the Heart meridian removes excessive energy.

HERBAL TREATMENT

An infusion of hawthorn leaves and flowers — 5 ml/1 tsp to a cup of boiling water — can be taken morning and evening; it has a mild sedative effect on the heart muscles.

HYPNOTHERAPY

Hypnotherapy helps where the cause is emotional.

MASSAGE

Massage promotes relaxation, and therefore aids the relief of palpitations.

RELAXATION TECHNIQUES

By far the most effective treatment, especially **biofeedback** (see p. 97).

VITAMIN AND MINERAL TREATMENT

See ANXIETY.

Period pain *see* MENSTRUAL DISORDERS

P

Pertussis *see* WHOOPING COUGH

Pharyngitis *see* SORE THROAT

PHOBIAS

See *also* ANXIETY

A phobia is an exaggerated fear of a commonly encountered object or situation. It will produce the normal fear symptoms — rapid breathing and sweating.

There are three kinds of phobias, specific, social and agoraphobia. They each have a different cause and treatment, and it is important to keep them separate.

SPECIFIC PHOBIAS

These are caused by overgeneralizing from one unfortunate incident. The most common triggers are cats, dogs, spiders, snakes, needles, flying, heights and lifts, but there are many unusual ones. They can usually be traced back to an unfortunate encounter with the feared object in childhood — a fierce dog, a faulty lift, an unsympathetic nurse. Sometimes, phobia develops by association: the grief consequent to the death of a family member becomes attached to the family cat, and you cannot bear to see cats again.

Specific phobias respond best to **behaviour psychotherapy** (see p. 95).

AGORAPHOBIA

This is 'fear of the market place' (NOT fear of open places), fear of crowded places away from the safety of home. The cause is hard to pinpoint but it often develops gradually in adolescence. *Claustrophobia* is a refinement of agoraphobia in which fear and panic are brought on by confined spaces.

Agoraphobia needs a behavioural approach which encourages the gradual increase of outdoor activity combined with explorative psychotherapy for both sufferer and spouse or family members. It can be regarded as an anxiety neurosis.

SOCIAL PHOBIA

This is an exaggerated case of shyness, and rarely develops in an extrovert.

Sufferers will avoid eating with strangers, avoid meeting new people and dread the most casual encounter.

Social phobics can be treated by

Visualization therapy
One of the most useful ways to help yourself escape from a phobia is to think yourself through the feared situation in the safety of your own home. For example, people who fear shopping might picture a scene in which they successfully enter a shop, choose an item, pay for it and come home. After several such mental 'rehearsals' the real thing will not be so frightening.

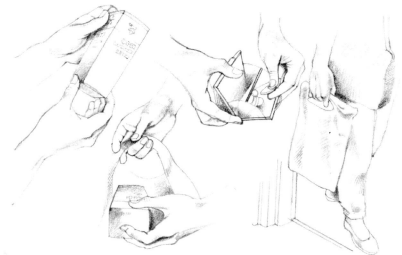

behavioural therapy or exploratory psychotherapy.

HEALING
Agoraphobia responds readily to visualization. If for example you have difficulty going into shops, sit down at home and start by imagining yourself going through the shop doors and browsing around in a peaceful and relaxed state. Set yourself the mental target of buying a specific item and see yourself selecting the one you want from the imagined display. Think of yourself taking it to the cash desk, paying, having it wrapped then walking out of the shop and home with the item. When you have visualized this several times successfully, try it for real and see how much easier it is.

HYPNOTHERAPY
Hypnosis can desensitize phobic reactions very successfully. For many patients it works faster than conventional psychotherapy. It is particularly effective with specific phobias.

VITAMIN AND MINERAL TREATMENT
See ANXIETY

PILES

(HAEMORRHOIDS)

Piles are varicosed veins (see VARICOSE VEINS) in the lower bowel and anus wall. When external they appear as painful and irritating brown swellings around the anus. They may bleed, which in chronic cases leads to ANAEMIA. Piles are normally caused by CONSTIPATION. The raised abdominal pressure needed to pass a hard stool dilates small blood vessels and leads to the formation of piles. OBESITY, inactivity, habitual use of laxatives, and anal intercourse can also cause piles. Pregnant women occasionally develop them because the foetus increases abdominal pressure as well as body weight. They usually go away after childbirth.

ORTHODOX TREATMENT
Local anaesthetic creams; injections to shrink them; surgery.

SELF-HELP
Sensible eating habits providing enough dietary fibre will alleviate and normally prevent piles. Scrupulous personal hygiene, to prevent infection, is important if they occur. Wash the anus carefully after passing stool.

HERBAL TREATMENT
A good specific remedy is the herb pilewort (lesser celandine) available as an ointment. Apply 2 or 3 times daily, certainly after each bowel movement to relieve pain, ease inflammation and reduce the piles.

Distilled witch hazel may also be applied frequently. An infusion of yarrow herb may be useful for its astringency and its influence on blood vessels. Take it cold in dosage of 45–60 ml/3–4 tbsp 2 or 3 times daily. It can also be applied as a compress.

P

HOMEOPATHY
For chronic cases, consult a homeopath. Acute cases use hamamelis or paeony ointment or suppositories. The following remedies are helpful:
- *Aloes* Where piles look like a bunch of grapes and there is explosive diarrhoea.
- *Hamamelis* For bruised feeling with bleeding.
- *Nux vomica* For itching and constipation.
- *Aesculus* With backache and where there is dry itching and burning.
- *Pulsatilla* Often required in pregnancy; helps with indigestion from fatty foods.

NATUROPATHY
Diet: The main step in prevention is to avoid constipation and obesity to prevent pressure on the lower bowel. Foods which result in more motions may not appeal; gelling fibres, such as linseed and porridge made from coarse oatmeal will help soften stools.

Exercise: Improve circulation in the area of the piles by exercise and good posture. Exercise also helps with constipation.

Heat/Cold Treatment: Local contrast hot and cold bathing and the use of ice packs will relieve intense discomfort.

Both diet and exercise measures are important in pregnancy to avoid piles.

VITAMIN AND MINERAL TREATMENT

Piles have been known to respond to vitamin B_6 (25 mg daily). If there is loss of blood, take iron, folic acid and vitamin B_{12} to restore red blood cells.

'Pink Eye' *see* CONJUNCTIVITIS

PNEUMONIA

Pneumonia is an acute inflammation of the lungs caused by bacterial or viral infection. The infection causes the tiny air pockets (alveoli) at the ends of the air passages to become waterlogged. There are two main kinds of pneumonia, depending on where the affected alveoli are distributed: *lobar pneumonia*, where the whole lobe of the lung can become solid, and *bronchopneumonia*, where only patches of the lung are inflamed. Pneumonia can develop as a sequel to other respiratory diseases such as COLDS and INFLUENZA, and sometimes in children as a complication of ASTHMA, WHOOPING COUGH, and MEASLES.

Hypostatic pneumonia develops in the lowest parts of the lungs of people who have been ill and bedridden for a long time. Because of immobility and poor circulation, fluid stagnates at the bottom of the lungs, becoming a breeding ground for bacteria. This type of pneumonia is entirely a result of immobility, which is why too much bed rest is discouraged wherever possible. Elderly bed-ridden patients often die of pneumonia, not the disease that confined them to bed.

SYMPTOMS

The chest hurts and breathing is painful and difficult, the effort of breathing producing grunting sounds. Temperature is high, up to 39°C or 102°F, normally with a dry cough.

Any upper respiratory infection which fails to respond quickly to treatment, especially if accompanied by breathing difficulties and a dry cough, could be developing into pneumonia. Pneumonia is *always* a serious illness and must be referred to a medical practitioner immediately.

ORTHODOX TREATMENT

Antibiotics if the cause is bacterial.

SELF-HELP

See CHILDREN'S ILLNESSES for general care. Dehydration can occur rapidly during an attack of pneumonia, so take care to ensure an adequate fluid intake during the course of the disease.

ACUPUNCTURE

Local secondary techniques to relieve chest pain should be used in conjunction with moxibustion to the Lung meridian and treatment of the Kidney and Bladder meridians to improve fluid elimination.

NATUROPATHY

Diet: Give only fruit and vegetable juices for the first 48 hours, then introduce lightly cooked vegetables and fruits, cereals, and finally proteins. Exclude dairy products for the first 4 days of solid food.

Heat/cold treatment: Cold packs to the neck and chest (*see* CHILDREN'S ILLNESSES) and tepid sponging will make the patient more comfortable. Avoid a hot dry atmosphere in the sick room.

VITAMIN AND MINERAL TREATMENT

Extra vitamin A (7,500 iu daily) plus vitamin C (500 mg every 4 hours, reducing to 500 mg every 8 hours) should be taken in addition to any other medical therapy.

Postnatal Depression *see* PREGNANCY AND CHILDBIRTH

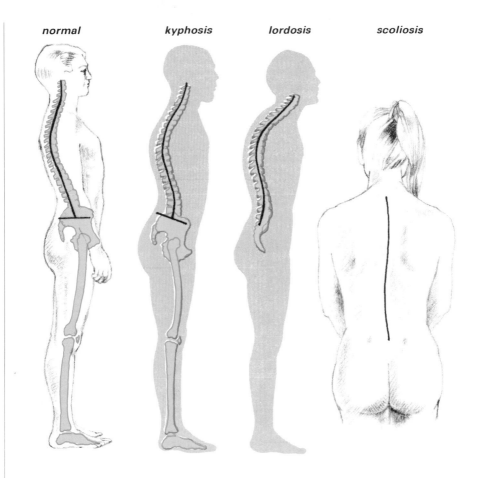

normal   kyphosis   lordosis   scoliosis

POSTURAL PROBLEMS

See *also* BACK PAIN

Good posture should be an effortless and non-fatiguing stance which can be maintained without discomfort for long periods of time. It is remarkably rare.

The major factors influencing bad posture are:

- Hereditary postures and hereditary variation in muscle tone and ligament strength.
- Structural abnormalities: They may be congenital or the result of ARTHRITIS, multiple sclerosis or polio. Structural problems also arise as a result of injury—for example, a

badly fractured leg may be slightly shorter than the other leg.
- Habit and training: Children mimicking parents, too little attention paid to school desks and chairs, occupations which involve the asymmetrical use of the body or parts of the body, or postures adopted for psychological reasons. This largely ignored source of postural deformities is the easiest to correct in theory, and the most difficult in practice.

COMMON POSTURAL FAULTS
The three most common postural fault are exaggerated lordosis, exaggerated kyphosis and scoliosis.

- *Lordosis* and *kyphosis*. Viewed from the side the spine should have three basic curves: going in at the neck, out at the shoulders and in again at the bottom. The neck and lower

Common causes of postural problems
Bad habits and thoughtless fashions can ruin your back.

CAUSE	PROBLEM
High heeled shoes	Exaggerated lordo-kyphosis
Shoulder bags, heavy briefcases	Scoliosis
Wrong relationship between chair and work station (office workers, draughtsmen, VDU operators, telephonists)	Loss of/exaggeration of normal curve of spine
Wrong position of VDU screen machines, switchboards	Scoliosis
Sitting with crossed legs	Rotation of the pelvis; loss of lumbar lordosis; varicose veins; lumbar scoliosis
Driving with poorly aligned pedals, bad seat designed, insufficient height and rake adjustment, bad ergonomics	Change in normal spinal curve; scoliosis

inward curves are called lordosis; the outward curve is called kyphosis. If these curves are exaggerated or diminished you have a postural problem.

● *Scoliosis.* Viewed from behind, your head should be exactly above your tail, with the shoulders and pelvis parallel to the floor. If there is any deviation from the normal symmetry, if the pelvis is tilted to accommodate an injured leg for example, the spine develops an S-shaped curve in order to keep the head above the centre of the pelvis. This is called scoliosis.

Bad posture produces a wide range of problems including back ache, HEAD-ACHE, bad feet, lack of mobility, breathing and digestive difficulties. Bad posture can also predispose you to a SLIPPED DISC.

ALEXANDER TECHNIQUE
Practise of the technique can both prevent and correct postural problems.

Where postural faults are solely the result of bad habits, they are reversible under the guidance of a skilled manipulative therapist or teacher of Alexander Technique, but success depends on 10 per cent of instruction by the therapist and 90 per cent application by the sufferer.

MANIPULATIVE THERAPIES
Osteopathy and chiropractic are usually very successful at correcting problems, as long as the exercises are regularly practised.

MASSAGE
Used in conjunction with the other therapies, massage will help to relieve the muscular tension set up by postural faults and break the cycle of bad posture–muscle tension–pain–worse posture.

RELAXATION TECHNIQUES
Yoga (p. 99).

PREGNANCY AND CHILDBIRTH

'A place to give birth should be more like a place to make love in than a hospital room.'
Dr Michel Odent

The mechanics of pregnancy and childbirth are the same as they have been for millions of years. What has changed is the impact of the Western lifestyle and of Western

P

orthodox medicine on the pregnant woman and mother, in particular, the technological development of the Western way of birth and attitudes towards infant feeding and care.

However, in the past few decades women and their partners have begun to take a new interest — and responsibility — in the management of pregnancy and birth. While not deriding the beneficial advances that science and medicine have brought, there has been a return to some of the techniques used by our ancestors, and a trend towards more gentle births.

Pregnancy

Your baby will be born approximately 266 days from the time of fertilization, or 280 days (about 40 weeks) after the first day of your last menstrual period.

However, only 15 per cent of babies are born within the predicted 40th week; the vast majority are born during the two weeks before that date or the two weeks after.

Fitness During Pregnancy

Throughout the nine months of pregnancy, it is essential that the woman takes special care of herself, both for the benefit of the baby growing in her womb and herself.

- **General exercise** If you have always been involved in sports, there is no need to give up your physical activities. Many pregnant women continue to enjoy sensible sport almost up to the time of labour; however, you should avoid horse-riding, climbing, and skiing

---

Pre-conceptual care.

The best possible way to enhance fertility and produce a healthy baby is to pay attention to a few basic rules. Once you have decided that it is time for a baby, give yourselves a three-month period in which both of you can achieve ultra health.

For the Mother

- Check that you are immune to GERMAN MEASLES. If you are not, have a vaccination, remembering that you must then wait at least three months before you begin to try to conceive.
- If you are on the contraceptive pill, change to some other method at least three months before trying to get pregnant.
- Try to get your weight as near to its ideal level as possible. Once you are pregnant is not the time to start slimming.
- If you are not already taking regular exercise, now is the time to start. Swimming, walking, exercise classes or any moderate sport that you enjoy will help to tone up your muscles, improve your circulation and your breathing.

For Both Parents

- Good nutrition is the foundation of fertility, a good pregnancy and a healthy baby. Make sure that you are eating a balanced diet.
- Reduce your intake of nicotine and alcohol drastically. Try to stop smoking entirely, and cut down your alcohol intake to a maximum of three alcoholic drinks a week.
- The presence of genital HERPES gonorrhoea, syphilis and other sexually transmitted diseases in either partner can cause serious problems with the baby. If you suspect any of these, you must consult your doctor. Babies have already been born suffering from AIDS (acquired-immune deficiency syndrome), and if you or your partner are in a high-risk group for this disease, again it is essential to seek specialist advice.
- Many drugs — both prescribed and over-the-counter medicines as well as illegal habituating drugs — can affect the ease of conception and the health of the growing foetus. Take only those drugs that are absolutely necessary — none at all if possible.

P

because of the risk of falls as well as sub-aqua diving because of the pressure found in deep water. Regular walking, swimming and cycling are perfectly safe and extremely beneficial for the non-athletic pregnant woman. If you have never been a regular sports enthusiast, this is *not* the time to take up such vigorous sports as squash, tennis or jogging.

● **Relaxation** Learning to relax is also a great aid to a comfortable pregnancy and childbirth. Practising regular relaxation exercises will encourage the establishment of a conditioned reflex pattern that will enable you to relax more easily (see p. 97).

Gentle massage throughout pregnancy, during labour and after the birth is a great aid to muscular relaxation and the maintenance of food muscle and skin tone. It also helps to relieve some of the TENSION and ANXIETY of pregnancy.

● **Posture** Correct posture and the proper use of your body while performing household chores such as lifting, gardening, shopping, cleaning, etc are also vital (see **Positive Health/Back Pack** pp. 53–9).

NUTRITION

The baby will draw nutrients from the pregnant woman's body, so the key feature of healthy eating in pregnancy is to choose food rich in nutrients so that the expectant mother's own nutritional status is maintained. (*See also* 'Weight gain' *below*.) The nutrients most likely to be reduced by the baby's needs are:

● *Calcium* found in cereals, pulses, green leafy vegetables, almonds, sardines.
● *Iron* found in offal, black pudding, leafy green vegetables, cereals, dried apricots.
● *Vitamin A* found in oily fish, fish liver oil, margine, orange vegetables and fruit—eg carrots, yellow melons, peaches, tomatoes.
● *Vitamin C* (will aid absorption of iron) found in leafy green vegetables, most other vegetables and fruit, especially green peppers, strawberries, blackcurrants, guavas and citrus fruit.
● *Vitamin D* found in oily fish, fish liver oil, margarine, sunlight on the skin.
● *Folic acid* found in leafy green vegetables, liver, wheatgerm.

Although cows' milk is a good source of calcium, some research has indicated that if a pregnant woman drinks it (or eats dairy products containing it), her baby may be more likely to develop DERMATITIS (see *also* 'Breastfeeding').

It is also a good idea to take an all-round low-potency multi-vitamin/multimineral preparation. Iron-deficiency ANAEMIA may be averted by taking the homeopathic tissue salts *Ferr. phos.* and *Calc. phos.* and an organic form of iron such as iron chelate.

COMMON PROBLEMS IN PREGNANCY

'Morning sickness' More than 50 per cent of all pregnant women experience NAUSEA AND VOMITING during the first three months of pregnancy. However,

---

Pelvic Floor Exercises

Specific exercises to increase the elasticity and strength of the pelvic floor muscles help you during actual birth. They also minimize problems of urinary incontinence that can occur both before and after labour, and help ensure that your sex life returns to normal as soon as possible after delivery.

It is particularly important to practise contracting and relaxing the muscles of the vagina, anus and urethra. This can be done by tightly clenching your buttocks, imagining that you are holding a coin between them. Or practise while you are actually urinating: make yourself stop in midstream for a count of 5; then allow the flow to start again; repeat several times whenever you go to the lavatory.

These invisible exercises should be done regularly and can be carried out anywhere. If you do have problems of incontinance brought on by sneezing, a homeopathic remedy is *caustricum canthavis.*

although this commonly occurs in the morning, it can just as well happen at any other time of the day or night. The risk to the foetus of taking drugs for this condition far outweighs any benefit to the expectant mother. However, some of the herbal or homeopathic treatments (*see below*) may help.

Very occasionally, pregnant women develop a condition (*hyperemisis gravidarum*) in which vomiting is severe and persistent. They usually have to stay in hospital so that the fluids lost can be replaced by intravenous drip to prevent dehydration.

Normally, if the mother is well nourished, morning sickness will not deprive the baby of any nutrients.

If you are suffering from morning sickness, try eating frequent, small meals. A cup of tea with some dry toast or unsweetened wholemeal biscuits on waking often helps the initial early morning nausea. Avoiding fatty, greasy foods, coffee, strong tea and alcohol and ensuring a well-balanced diet with increased protein (eg nuts, seeds, grains, pulses) will also be beneficial.

As for **herbal treatments**, chamomile tea is the first remedy to try: drink warm, a 45–60 ml/3–4 tbsp at bedtime and a cup (sipped) first thing in the morning. Some woman find raspberry leaf tea helpful; others prefer peppermint.

There are also a number of **homeopathic remedies**:

- *Nux vomica* For irritability, constipation and brown tongue.
- *Pulsatilla* For weepiness, thirstlessness and white tongue.
- *Tabacum* For constant nausea all day without vomiting.
- *Sepia* For nausea on smelling food, associated with chilliness, irritability, low dragging abdominal pain.
- *Argentum nitricum* For craving for sweets and excessive flatulence; great apprehension and tendency to panic.
- *Ipecachuana* For continual nausea, vomiting of bile, diarrhoea; thirstlessness and irritability.

Morning sickness may also be relieved by vitamin B_6 (up to 100 mg daily for a short period), preferably in conjunction with magnesium (300 mg daily). However, check with your gynaecologist first.

Back pain During pregnancy, many women suffer from recurrent and persistent BACK PAIN. There are a number of possible causes for this:
- The foetus presses on the nerves in the floor of the pelvis.
- The curve of the spine in the lumbar region becomes exaggerated — a condition rather majestically known as the 'pride of pregnancy' — because correct posture is not maintained while the weight of the developing baby increases and tends to tip the woman forwards.
- The pelvic ligaments stretch in the later stages of pregnancy as a preparation for childbirth.

Manipulative treatment for back pain in pregnancy is extremely beneficial.

The following **homeopathic remedies** may help:
- *Kali carbonicum* For weakness and dragging in the loins.
- *Arnica* Pain associated with a bruised sensation.

However, prevention of back pain is far the best. Correct posture must be maintained. No pregnant woman should wear high-heeled shoes. Continuing with your normal sports and other physical activities is important to maintain muscle tone and strength.

Alexander technique (*see* p. 69) and **yoga** (*see* p. 99) are ideal therapies, and swimming the ideal exercise, even in the latest stages of pregnancy, since the water supports the body and allows free movement without imposing strain on the weight-bearing joints.

Weight gain weight gain is an important factor during pregnancy and must not be allowed to creep beyond normal limits. You should aim to put on no more than 9.5 kg/21 lb: 3.2 kg/7 lb for the baby; 3.2 kg/7 lb for the uterus, placenta and the fluid surrounding the baby; and 3.2 kg/7 lb for an increased volume of blood and breast size.

P

At the first sign of unusual weight gain, take matters in hand immediately, as the more you gain, the more difficult it will be to get your weight back under control. Sensible eating and an increase in gentle exercise is all that is required.

Several conditions common in pregnancy can be aggravated by excessive weight gain, particularly VARICOSE VEINS, PILES and raised blood pressure. Taking extra vitamin E (200 iu daily) will help strengthen the circulatory system, and preventing CONSTIPATION with a healthy high-fibre diet, avoiding standing for long periods or sitting with crossed legs and sensible amounts of rest will all help with these problems.

Stretch marks These wavy stripes that can occur on the abdomen, buttocks, breasts and thighs are the result of relatively rapid and excessive weight gain and frequently occur in pregnancy. They appear when the skin becomes over-stretched and the fibres in the deep layers break. This results in reddish marks that gradually fade to white. Unfortunately, they are permanent.

Gentle massage of the skin of the abdomen, thighs, buttocks and breasts, using a good quality oil enriched with vitamin E, helps to maintain the suppleness of the skin. And, of course, avoiding excessive weight gain is also important. If you do develop stretch marks, applying expensive lotions (especially those containing collagen) will do no good.

Other problems   *See* BREATHLESSNESS, FAINTING, HEARTBURN, OEDEMA.

PREPARING FOR CHILDBIRTH

Most hospitals run antenatal classes, which teach simple methods of relaxation (both for pregnancy and labour) as well as the mechanics of childbirth; in addition, you will usually be able to tour the labour and delivery rooms.

There are also antenatal classes run by various organizations that will teach more complicated breathing and relaxation exercises.

Perhaps the best advice is to follow your body's messages rather than those given by outsiders. Although it may have a time and a place, the modern gadgetry of the delivery room can weaken a woman's confidence in her own body to do what it is designed to do: give birth.

Antenatal Check Ups

Regular visits to your family doctor or to an antenatal clinic are vital and no attempt should be made to treat your pregnancy only totally with alternative methods. The most important check is on your BLOOD PRESSURE.

At each visit, a sample of urine will be tested, your blood pressure will be measured and you will be weighed. All three checks are intended to discover whether or not you are developing a condition called *pre-eclampsia* (Formerly known as 'toxaemia of pregnancy'), in which blood pressure rises dangerously, the ankles swell and there is protein in the urine, and which, if left untreated, can result in the death of the woman and her baby. In addition, testing the urine will detect whether DIABETES is developing.

Your abdomen will be examined to check that the baby is growing properly and in the correct position, the baby's heart will be monitored and you may be given a blood test to make sure that you are not anaemic.

ACUPUNCTURE

Childbirth is obviously not a disease, but the mechanisms involved sometimes need encouragement. For efficient and safe use of acupuncture in childbirth, it is preferable that the mother-to-be consults the acupuncturist as early on in the pregnancy as possible. The aim is to ensure nutritional and general health so that the minimum amount of interference with natural birth processes will be required.

HOMEOPATHY

To promote delivery, try *caulophyllum 30*. Take one weekly from 36–38 weeks term, one daily from 38 to 40 weeks and one 3 times a day when you are over 40 weeks.

P

Episiotomy—the unkindest cut

An episiotomy is a diagonal cut made from the rear end of the vaginal opening towards the anus. This is performed to make the passage of the baby's head to the outside easier when the skin in the area does not stretch sufficiently. After delivery, the cut is closed with self-dissolving stitches. The wound may be acutely painful until healing is complete, and the scars left behind can also be painful. Some women still experience pain on sexual intercourse after three months.

Unfortunately, episiotomy has become routine in most Western hospitals: between 65 and 90 per cent of all women delivering vaginally will have them, especially if it is a first birth. However, advocates of natural childbirth claim that correct preparation for birth by the mother and gentler methods of delivery totally avoid the necessity for routine episiotomy. In addition, although the medical fraternity has always said that this surgical procedure prevents large ragged tears in the skin and will prevent prolapse of the uterus, a recent study carried out in London has shown that the tears in the skin are usually much less extensive than the cuts, that they heal better and that episiotomies do not prevent prolapse.

If you do have to have an episiotomy, the following will all help promote rapid healing: soaking in warm sea-salt baths; scrupulous attention to personal hygiene; wearing only pure cotton underwear; preventing constipation, avoiding excessive quantities of citrus fruits and other acidic foods so that the passing of urine does not cause additional discomfort. Regular application of calendula cream to the scar will relieve discomfort and aid healing.

PAIN RELIEF IN CHILDBIRTH

Every labour and delivery is different, and how much pain you will be able to handle will depend on your level of pain tolerance (see PAIN AND PAIN-KILLERS), how prepared you are for what is to come, how you are treated by medical staff and the length and course of your labour.

Antenatal training has benefited many women, and this may be because the breathing techniques are as much a distraction to the pain as they are a help. Acupuncture (see below) has proved effective with others.

Remember that there is no point in suffering terribly if none of these methods works for you, and you shouldn't feel guilty if you ask for ortho-dox pain relief (gas-and-air, local or epidural anaesthesia) even if you planned not to.

EATING BEFORE AND AFTER CHILDBIRTH

During early labour, light, non-fatty snacks such as toast and honey can be eaten, and if the labour is long, the woman may take glucose or honey to build up her energy.

Following childbirth, two areas that require prompt attention are blood-building nutrients and fibre. Loss of blood requires adequate amounts of iron, folic acid and vitamin B_{12} for res-toration — all found in leafy greens, offal, black pudding, apricots and other dried fruits. Vitamin C is also necessary, for iron absorption.

The first bowel movement after child-birth should not be expected for a few days. As the area will be very sore and also fatigued after the effort of labour, evacuation should be made easy by eating stool-softening foods such as dried fruit and wholegrain cereals.

BREASTFEEDING

Breastmilk is tailor-made to meet all a baby's nutritional needs and, in addi-tion, the first watery milk — the colo-strum — contains important antibodies that protect against infections such as GASTROENTERITIS. Because breastmilk does not contain 'foreign' constituents as does, say, cows' milk, breastfed

P

221

babies are less likely to suffer from ALLERGY, and because the baby is controlling its own food intake, there is some evidence that breastfed babies grow up to be less obese adults than those who have been bottlefed. The psychological bonding that occurs while a baby is held close and cuddled during breastfeeding can dramatically affect its relationship with its mother and its ability to thrive.

For successful breastfeeding, you need a well-nourished mother who is keen to breastfeed, and a supportive partner and family group. However, our society has very ambivalent attitudes towards breastfeeding, and certainly there is often very little provision away from home for a mother to breastfeed her child in comfort, privacy and with a minimum of fuss (from others). Because a woman's ability to produce breastmilk is intimately involved with her mental attitude towards breastfeeding, it is vitally important that she receive as much sympathetic encouragement as possible.

If a mother is unable to breastfeed her baby it is still possible to achieve the closeness that is so important: cuddle the baby while bottlefeeding, talk to it and play with it frequently. Bottlefeeding also has the advantage that the baby's father can take an equal part.

Breastfeeding does have its pitfalls, and some of these are listed below:

- *'Insufficient milk'* This is the reason often given, even by medical staff, for a woman to stop trying to breastfeed. The milk supply declines (for physical or psychological reasons) and then the mother begins to worry about it, which in turn leads to less milk production — a vicious circle that is difficult to break.

  In addition, it may be that the baby is not sucking hard enough from the start (milk is produced and 'let down' by the trigger of this sucking), or the mother may not be feeding the baby often enough: the undrunk milk distends the milk glands, preventing further milk production. This last is one of

the reasons why 'demand feeding' is preferable for both mother and baby.

- *Sore/cracked nipples* To avoid this, prepare the nipple, before the baby is born: during the last few months of pregnancy, rub breasts and nipples firmly with a towel, rolling the nipples between her fingers; then apply lanolin. This slightly abrasive technique will serve to toughen the skin.

  If the nipples do become cracked and sore, this may be due to the baby sucking and biting the nipple rather than taking the whole areola (the brown area around the nipple) into its mouth. It might help to express the milk manually for a few days until the nipples are healed.

- *Sore breasts* This can be due to engorgement, when the breast becomes overly full of milk, because the baby is not feeding often enough or feeding too long from one breast: a baby can empty a breast in under seven minutes, and no breast should be sucked for longer than 12 minutes. Feed the baby from both breasts equally at each feed.

- *Mastitis* This occurs when infection enters the breast, often through a cracked nipple. The breast becomes engorged, hard, red, tender and painful. If the condition is caught early enough, it is possible to avoid it becoming worse by having the baby feed more often from the affected breast: unless the breast is leaking pus (very rare), the baby will come to no harm. Doctors will often prescribe a form of penicillin to treat this. It is important not to stop using that breast: if necessary, express the milk manually.

(See *also* COLIC.)

The following therapies can be of great value.

HERBAL TREATMENT

Acute *mastitis* can be treated with soothing poultices of a mixture of chopped comfrey leaves and some crushed linseeds: pound them into a paste with hot water, put them in a muslin bag and apply this to the affected area. Tincture of calendula and garlic capsules taken internally are also useful. For some local relief, gently apply distilled witch hazel to the sore breast, or bathe with an infusion of marshmallow flowers and leaves.

MASSAGE

A good general massage will relieve tension and fatigue. If engorgement develops, the affected breast can be gently massaged in a bath of warm soapy water.

HOMEOPATHY

- *Ignatia* When the milk flow is unsatisfactory because the mother is emotionally distressed.
- *Calcarea carbonica* When the milk is plentiful but watery, the infant does not thrive and the mother is chilly, worse for cold air and tends to sweat on the back of the head at night.
- *Lac defloratum* Where the milk flow is slow, the breasts are growing smaller and the mother is very depressed and despondent and feels thirsty.
- *Pulsatilla* Where the milk supply is poor, it becomes painful to breast-feed and the mother feels weepy and worse in a hot room. (NB this is also helpful after the baby is weaned and the breasts feel stretched and sore).
- *Bryonia* Where there is a painful lump in the breast and the possible start of mastitis. This should be taken in the 30c potency (see **Homeopathy** p. 78) every 2 hours; if there is no improvement after 3 doses, call your medical practitioner.

NATUROPATHY

Unless a woman is very under-nourished, she is likely to produce milk that is ample both in quantity and quality. Breastfeeding uses 300–500 calories a day, much of which comes from fat reserves built up during pregnancy; it is *not* necessary to 'eat for two'. To maintain supply later and to preserve the mother's nutritional status, a balanced diet similar to that eaten during pregnancy is important.

Some babies can develop FOOD INTOLERANCE to some constituents of the foods their mothers eat, causing intestinal gas ('wind'), colic, dermatitis and other symptoms. Chocolate, cabbage, Brussels sprouts, broccoli and garlic are often culprits, and cow's milk in a breastfeeding mother's diet has been found in some studies to increase the chances of a breasfed baby developing dermatitis.

Liquid is naturally needed for milk production, but huge amounts are unnecessary: drinking enough to satisfy thirst is the best guide

Engorgement and *mastitis* may be helped by applying, alternately, hot and cold compresses to the affected breast.

P

MANIPULATIVE THERAPIES

While breastfeeding, you should sit in a chair with a low seat and high back, so that the baby's weight is supported on the knees; if necessary, the baby can be placed on a pillow. This will avoid undue strain in the neck and shoulder muscles, and will support the mother's lower back.

However, if there is neck and shoulder tension and backache, occasional, gentle manipulative treatment can relieve this discomfort without recourse to drugs, which can pass via the mother's milk to the baby.

PSYCHOTHERAPIES

Breastfeeding problems are often (but by no means always) a reflection of ambivalent feelings—sometimes about the sexual element of breastfeeding, sometimes about the extreme dependency of the baby. A quiet and sensitive therapy such as Rogerian counselling (or just a talk with a trusted and experienced friend) are probably the best approaches. Take advice from a midwife, or breastfeeding counsellor first, to exclude practical problems of technique, or just plain tiredness.

To relieve stress and fatigue, any one of these therapies may prove invaluable.

VITAMIN AND MINERAL TREATMENT
Low or moderate potency multi-vitamin/multimineral supplement daily when nursing.

POSTNATAL DEPRESSION
This term is used loosely to cover any short or long-term psychological or psychiatric ill-health in the months after childbirth.

There are four main conditions: *puerperal psychosis, true postnatal depressive illness, postpartum ('baby') blues* and *general lack of coping.*

- *Puerperal psychosis* is the most severe occuring after about 1 in 1,000 childbirths. It is caused by hormonal change, in susceptible women, and causes bizarre ideas and behaviour, starting in the second week after the birth. It always gets better, but the mother should be in hospital during the illness, because she is so out of touch with reality and may damage herself or the baby. It is commonest in first pregnancies and may not recur, but a specialist opinion should be obtained before starting further pregnancies. It has nothing to do with schizophrenia or other sorts or madness.
- *Postnatal Depressive Illness* occurs in about 10% of women after childbirth and is exactly similar in form to common depressive illness (see DEPRESSION). It usually begins several months after giving birth and is thought to be more common in women who, for various reasons, did not 'bond'—fall in love—with their baby at or soon after birth. Drug treatment is usually effective. Supportive psychotherapy and natural health treatments will reduce the severity of the depression.
- *Postpartum Blues* affect at least half of all mothers. They appear on the 5th or 6th day after the birth of the child when the mother becomes weepy and pessimistic for no reason. Baby blues do not last long and are due to a brief upset in hormone levels. No treatment is required other than support and reassurance from relatives and hospital staff that this is a normal consequence of childbirth.
- *Lack of Coping* Many new mothers find the aftermath of childbirth less exhilerating than they had been led to expect. The process of giving birth is exhausting, instruction in aftercare may have been sketchy, new fathers are often ill-prepared for supporting and helping the mother. The marital relationship is altered by the arrival of a new member of the family and this may result in sexual, emotional and social difficulties. It is important to seek some support from partners, or friends, other mothers, health visitor.

HOMEOPATHY
Consult a homopath. For specific remedies try:

Loss of sexual desire
Lack of sexual desire and arousal is a very common occurrence following childbirth. Apart from hormonal changes, other factors involved are tiredness, vaginal discomfort, loss of privacy, depression, altered body image and lack of time. However, as life slowly returns to normal and both partners adapt to the presence of the baby, sexual desire usually becomes normal again.

Men frequently feel rejected, excluded and isolated from the new mother/baby relationship. Consequently, they suffer their own loss of self-esteem and importance, and this may lead to impotence. A widely neglected but simple solution to these problems is to make the man an integral part of the new family unit, encouraging him to participate fully before the birth by accompanying his partner to antenatal classes and being present during labour and birth, and later by bathing, feeding, changing and, most importantly, enjoying the presence of the baby.

- *Sepia* For falling hair, nausea at the smell of food, irritability weepiness, aversion to sex, feelings of chilliness.
- *Natrum mur* When feelings are so bottled up that nothing seems to be fun and where the mother is weepy but averse to consolation.
- *Aconite* Where there are feelings of fear.
- *Arnica* When the labour was very long or difficult.

HYPNOTHERAPY
Hypnosis can help, as in any depressive state.

VITAMIN AND MINERAL TREATMENT
Take vitamin B$_6$ (up to 100 mg daily) magnesium (300 mg daily) and zinc (15 mg daily) immediately after birth. Evening primrose oil (1,500 mg daily) may help as an alternative or in addition to this regime.

Premenstrual Syndrome *see* MENSTRUAL DISORDERS

Prolapsed intervertebral disc *see* SLIPPED DISC

PROSTATE PROBLEMS

The prostate gland lies at the base of the bladder. About the size of a walnut, it is a part of the male reproductive system and supplies part of the seminal fluid. Various things can go wrong with it.
- *Prostatitis* is inflammation of the prostate. It causes general malaise, and frequent and uncomfortable urination. The prostate does not become enlarged, but is very tender.
- *Enlarged prostate* is usually a disorder in older men. The prostate grows larger, compressing the urethra which it surrounds and subsequently the bladder itself. It becomes difficult either to start the flow of urine or to stop it. Because the bladder does not empty completely, CYSTITIS may develop. Sometimes the bladder is blocked completely.
- *Cancer of the prostate* is the third commonest CANCER in men after lung and stomach. It can be quite symptomless, and rarely occurs in men under 60.

ORTHODOX TREATMENT
Antibiotics (*prostatitis*); surgery (*enlarged prostate*); hormone therapy, surgery (*cancer of the prostate*).

ACUPUNCTURE
When the kidneys are weak, excesses of damp and heat may accumulate in them and move downward giving the symptoms of chronic prostatitis.
Acupressure The prostate gland can be influenced by pressure on points 44 and any other sensitive points on the midline of the lower abdomen and 34 on the inner side of the lower leg (see pp. 104–5).

HERBAL TREATMENT
Short term inflammation or enlargement of the prostate gland will often respond to herbal teas, but if no improvement takes place or the symptoms recur, consult a herbal practitioner.

A decocotion of equal quantities of gravel root, sea holly and hydrangea root taken in 45–60 ml/3–4 tbsp doses 3 times a day will ease inflammation and reduce the frequency and discomfort of passing urine. Marshmallow leaves could be added for their demulcent properties if burning and heat persist.

Horsetail is astringent and can be used if small amounts of blood are passed and for frequent urination at night. Combine it with hydrangea for greater affect on an enlarged gland.

HOMEOPATHY
- *Sabal serrulata* Where there is an enlarged prostate.
- *Causticum* Where coughing and sneezing cause involuntary urination.

P

NATUROPATHY

Diet: Maintain a wholefood diet. Avoid refined carbohydrates, coffee, strong tea and alcohol. For prostatitis and enlarged prostate, increase fluid intake and eat 25 g/1 oz pumpkin seeds daily. The high zinc content of pumpkin seeds helps to reduce the size of the prostate.

Hydrotherapy: Spray lower abdomen and pelvic area with warm and cold water, alternating 3 minutes hot 1 minute cold; or use sitz baths. Sit in hot water with feet in cold for 3 minutes, then change over to sitting in cold with feet in hot for 1 minute.

Exercise: Maintain regular exercise.

VITAMIN AND MINERAL TREATMENT

Extra zinc (up to 50 mg daily) and polyunsaturated fatty acids such as safflower or wheat germ oil (12 capsules of either daily). Regular intakes of zinc (15 mg daily) and polyunsaturated fatty acids (3–6 capsules daily) in later life may help prevent development of problems.

PSORIASIS

Psoriasis is a skin disease in which the skin grows too rapidly on certain parts of the body, forming thick red inflamed patches covered with a silvery scale. In severe cases the skin may crack and bleed.

It is disfiguring and embarrassing but not infectious. It usually runs in families and is commonest in the 15–25 age group. The cause is unknown, but attacks can be triggered by nervous TENSION and stress, illness, surgery sunburn, or certain prescribed drugs.

SYMPTOMS

The red scaly patches appear most often on the knees and elbows but can erupt anywhere. They are itchy and weepy. Severe attacks cause emotional distress to the sufferer who feels they cannot display their body in public at the beach or the swimming pool. Overall, the disease seems to be better in summer than winter. It may go away on its own, but once you have had psoriasis, it is always possible that it will recur.

ORTHODOX TREATMENT

Coal tar and dithranol ointments; mild steroid creams; PUVA treatment, combining the drug Psoralens with ultraviolet A radiation.

SELF-HELP

Gentle exposure to sunlight is effective, but avoid sunburn at all costs.

ACUPUNCTURE

Acupuncture is often successful in obtaining long remissions by treating those organs whose imbalance is reflected in the skin.

HERBAL TREATMENT

Persistence with blood purifying herbs and herbal lotions or ointment under the supervision of a herbal practitioner has proved successful.

HYPNOTHERAPY

Hypnosis can be effective in helping to control itching.

MASSAGE

Massage the affected area with two drops of calendula oil and one of lavender in 30 ml/2 tbsp almond oil.

NATUROPATHY

Adopt a wholefood diet. Restrict dairy produce, especially milk, meat, refined carbohydrates, coffee, strong tea, and sugar. Increase protein intake with nuts, seeds, grains and pulses.

Seek advice from a naturopath for specific nutritional guidance. Most dermatologists dismiss the idea of diet being implicated in psoriasis, but clinical ecologists have evidence that fundamental changes of diet and digestive enzyme supplements can help some sufferers. Since these changes can do no harm, it is worth trying.

(See *also* ALLERGY, FOOD INTOLERANCE).

RELAXATION TECHNIQUES

Autogenics and **biofeedback** (p. 97).

Psychotherapy may be useful in overcoming the difficulties of interpersonal relationships which are likely to occur if the psoriasis is disfiguring. **Bioenergetics** (*see* p. 95) will appeal to younger people in particular.

VITAMIN AND MINERAL TREATMENT
Can be treated with oral vitamin A and vitamin A applied to the skin, retinoic acid and synthetic vitamin A derivatives. Do not continue for long periods as excessive vitamin A can cause liver problems.

R

RESTLESS LEGS

See *also* CRAMP
This is a very common and frequently misdiagnosed condition.

SYMPTOMS
Within a few minutes of sitting down, the sufferer experiences pins and needles, burning sensations and pain in the legs, sometimes accompanied by a jerking movement. The symptoms can only be relieved by standing up and walking around, but they return as soon as the sufferer sits down again. The condition results in loss of sleep and often interferes severely with social life, making car journeys, dinner parties or theatre visits impossible.

The commonest cause, especially in women is iron deficiency. In fact restless legs can be the first symptom of ANAEMIA due to gradual and chronic blood loss. Sometimes, it may be caused by involuntary muscle spasms, resulting from epilepsy, spinal cord injury or neurological disease, but this is very rare.

ORTHODOX TREATMENT
Iron, folic acid and vitamin E.

NATUROPATHY
Diet: Adopt a diet rich in iron rich foods (green leafy vegetables, liver, whole grains, eggs).
Hydropathy: Contrast bathing of the legs in hot and cold water affords relief.

VITAMIN AND MINERAL TREATMENT
Take vitamin E (200 iu daily) and iron supplements.

RHEUMATISM

A commonly used term for any painful problem in muscles and joints. See FIBROSITIS.

Rheumatoid arthritis *see* ARTHRITIS

RINGWORM

(TINEA)

Ringworm is an infection and inflammation of the outer layer of skin caused by microscopic fungi or moulds. On the body it produces red circular patches with a raised edge that looks like a worm — hence its common name. It is very common and highly contagious, being spread by direct physical contact.

SYMPTOMS
The usual sites affected by ringworm are the scalp, beard, groin ('dhobie itch'), and between the toes (athlete's foot). All of them itch; skin may peel off and leave a raw red area between the toes; small clumps of hair fall out on the scalp.

ORTHODOX TREATMENT
Antifungal powders and cream or benzoic acid preparations; oral drugs.

SELF-HELP
- Keep towels and flannels separate from family linen and boil after use.
- Avoid low temperature washing powders in your machine, as the

fungus may survive and spread to the rest of the wash.

- Athlete's foot sufferers should wear cotton socks and leather shoes (trainers have greatly increased the spread of this version of ringworm). Change socks and wash feet twice a day. Dry thoroughly, patting not rubbing.
- If ringworm affects the groin, wear only cotton underwear and shirts. Shower or bathe frequently, at least once a day, more in hot damp conditions — fungi thrive in warm moist conditions.

Herbal Treatment
Footbath: Take 25 g/1 oz each of red clover, sage, calendula and agrimony and simmer in 3 l/5¼ pts water for 20 minutes. Strain, keeping herbs for a poultice between the toes. Add 10 ml/2 tsp cider vinegar and leave to cool. Bathe feet for half an hour. Dry carefully and powder with arrowroot. Repeat daily.

Homeopathy
Consult a homeopath.

Calendula ointment can be applied locally.

Rubella *see* GERMAN MEASLES

Rupture *see* HERNIA

S

SCARLET FEVER

This is a form of tonsillitis (see TONSILS AND ADENOIDS) caused by bacteria. The infection is spread by droplets in the air from coughing. It occurs mainly in childhood.

Symptoms
A sore throat accompanied by a scarlet rash, FEVER and tender neck glands. Some children are only mildly affected.

Severe cases may have the rash (which resembles sunburn with goose pimples) all over the body, a flushed face with a pale patch around the lips, inflamed tonsils with spots of pus and a red, raw tongue. The skin may peel a week to two after recovery.

Complications may be middle ear infections (see EARACHE), SINUSITIS and infected neck glands.

Orthodox Treatment
Antibiotics.

Self-help
For natural therapies and general care see CHILDREN'S ILLNESSES.

Vitamin and Mineral Treatment
Vitamin C (500 mg 3 times daily) will help strengthen the body's own anti-bacterial defences.

Sciatica *see* BACK PAIN, SLIPPED DISC

Scoliosis *see* POSTURAL PROBLEMS

Sea Sickness *see* TRAVEL SICKNESS

Shingles *see* HERPES

SHOCK

A serious condition in which blood pressure falls rapidly, reducing the amount of blood circulating to the tissues. Reduced flow to the brain can be fatal. Shock can follow major injury, BURNS or acute infectious disease and is frequently the cause of death. It may also follow acute vomiting or DIARRHOEA when there is great fluid loss, or severe allergic reactions to STINGS, drugs (especially antibiotics) or inhaled allergens (see ALLERGY).

Symptoms
Someone in shock feels faint and nauseous with pale, clammy skin and a weak, rapid pulse. Unconsciousness follows as the brain becomes more deoxy-

genated. The symptoms are part of a vicious circle: falling blood pressure deprives the heart of oxygen so it cannot pump at the normal rate, and this in turn makes blood pressure fall further. The declining spiral is fatal unless stopped by treatment.

First Aid
Attend to obvious causes of shock, such as severe BLEEDING, burns or injury where possible; lie the person down with feet raised and clothing loosened. Keep them warm. Get professional help quickly, and do not move the patient unnecessarily.

NEVER apply hot water bottles
give hot drinks
give alcohol.

Orthodox Treatment
With most types of shock, the definitive treatment is to replace lost body fluid, usually with blood transfusions. Pain-relieving and calming drugs may be given, and occasionally ones which raise blood pressure.

Herbal Treatment
Antispasmodic formula.

Homeopathy
- *Aconite 30* Every 15 minutes if fear is marked.
- *Arnica 30* Every 15 minutes after injury or bleeding.
- *Carbo vegetabilis* When cold, short of air, cold breath but wanting to be fanned.
- *Veratrum album* When there are icy cold sweats and cold skin.

SINUSITIS

An inflammation of the mucous membranes lining the sinuses, the air spaces in the bones of the skull above and below the eyes.
- *Acute sinusitis* is frequently caused by COLDS or bacterial and viral infections of the nose, throat and upper respiratory tract.
- *Chronic sinus problems* may be caused by small growths in the nose, injury of the nasal bones, smoking, irritant fumes and smells, common allergies such as HAY FEVER and food allergies, especially to milk and dairy products (see FOOD INTOLERANCE). More children suffer than adults.

Symptoms
HEADACHE, loss of the sense of smell, pain in the teeth, behind and between the eyes and tenderness over the forehead and cheekbones, possible high temperature and general malaise are common. Sometimes sinusitis produces a swollen face followed by a stuffy nose and thick discharge of infected mucus. This in turn can lead to repeated bouts of respiratory infection, ear infections, EARACHE and temporary loss of hearing (*see* HEARING PROBLEMS).

Orthodox Treatment
Antibiotics, nose drops, nasal sprays and decongestants.

Self-help
- Stop smoking; parents of children who suffer should also stop. Children brought up in 'smoking homes' have double the incidence of sinusitis, ear and respiratory problems as children brought up in 'smoke free homes'.
- Never fly when you have sinusitis. Pressure changes can cause severe pain and even damage the eardrum, particularly in children.

Acupuncture
Acupuncture aims to clear any obstruction of the Energy flow of the Lungs which are the 'cleansers' of the respiratory system, including the sinusus. **Acupressure** on points about the nose and eyes—49, 50, 51 and 52 and behind the head, may relieve symptoms (see p. 104–5).

S

Homeopathy

Consult a homeopath as the remedy may vary as the sinusitis progresses. *Allium cepa, kali. bich., pulsatilla* and *sulphur* are often used.

Massage

Manipulation of the neck vertebrae and soft tissue massage to the neck and shoulder muscles encourages sinus drainage. Specific massage to the sinuses helps encourage the passage of mucus and relieves congestion and resulting pain.

Naturopathy

Diet: Keep to a wholefood diet. Exclude dairy products altogether and limit refined carbohydrates. A cleansing regime of raw juice and fresh fruit followed by salads, vegetables and a low starch diet is helpful.
Hydrotherapy: Hot and cold splashing or sponging of the face and sinus areas (2 minutes hot and 1 minute cold) for 10–15 minutes will relieve pain. Steam inhalations alleviate symptoms. Add a few drops of herbal aromatic oils to the water.

Vitamin and Mineral Treatment

Vitamin C (500 mg 3 times daily) may help reduce inflammation and strengthen the body's defences.

Sleep problems *see* INSOMNIA

SLIPPED DISC

(Prolapsed Intervertebral Disc)

See *also* BACK PAIN; PAIN AND PAINKILLERS

The much maligned intervertebral disc is blamed for many symptoms of BACK PAIN in which it is not involved and is ignored in other areas where it is the primary cause of the problem. The myth of the slipped disc has yet to be eradicated: an intervertebral disc *cannot* slip. It can rupture, it can bulge and it can be subject to disease but it cannot slip.

The intervertebral disc is a flexible pad made up of an elastic envelope with a thick jelly-like core in the middle. The pressure in the centre of the disc keeps the vertebrae separate and is responsible for the stability and mobility of the vertebral column.

When a disc ruptures, the wall of the disc tears allowing the gelatinous content to bulge through the wall into the space between the vertebrae, causing pressure on the surrounding tissues especially nerve roots and ligaments.

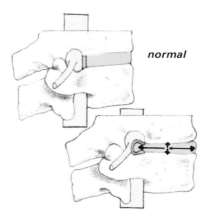

Slipped disc
There is no such thing as a 'slipped disc'. The intervertebral disc is the shock absorber which is found between each pair of vertebrae in the spine. It resembles a plastic bag filled with jelly and in some circumstances the wall of the 'plastic bag' can stretch or break allowing the 'jelly' to squeeze out and press on the spinal cord or the nerve roots coming off it causing excruciating pain.

Why discs 'slip'

Disc problems occur in three ways:
● abnormal stress on a normal disc.
● normal stress on an abnormal disc.
● normal stress of a normal disc when the body is not sufficiently prepared for that stress.

Obesity, occupation or sport can weaken the wall of the disc. Then one final accident, sometimes remarkably slight, causes the rupture of the wall. Few people suffer acute disc pain as a result of a single incident, no matter how severe.

Symptoms
Instant pain in the back, which is the result of muscle spasm and irritation of the spinal nerve. Pain and numbness (sharp, dull intermittent or continuous) radiates into the leg. (Sometimes back and leg pain are simultaneous.)

This pain is *sciatica*. Changing activities or posture may relieve the pain or make it worse. How far down the leg the pain travels and where there are areas of numbness or pins-and-needles depend on the level of the disc injury (higher or lower in the spine). When numbness takes over from pain, it may indicate a much greater and more long standing pressure on the nerve root. Muscle weakness implies an even greater amount of pressure.

Diagnosis and Treatment
Effective treatment depends on correct diagnosis. It is essential to differentiate between back problems caused by joint problems, muscle injury or disc damage. A history of the course and location of the pain will help the practitioner to make an accurate diagnosis and ascertain the exact level at which the disc has ruptured.

Very rarely, surgery is the only suitable treatment. More and more surgeons are reluctant to operate unless all other avenues have been explored. Manipulative therapy is now the first treatment attempted.

Bed rest is always the first step in treatment. The pressure within the disc is 30 per cent less when the sufferer is lying down than when upright.

Self-help
Learning to lift, move and carry objects properly, and the best posture for household tasks will help prevent the likelihood of disc rupture (see **Positive Health/Back Pack** pp. 53–9).

Acupuncture
Local acupuncture techniques relieve acute pain and muscle spasm. Where stimulation treatments are indicated, moxibustion will be used.

Acupressure on point 17 may help relieve pain (see p. 103).

Alexander technique
This technique will help relieve pressure on the disc.

Manipulative Techniques
This is the best treatment for a slipped disc. The disc cannot be put back in place (that would be like trying to squeeze toothpaste back into a tube). An osteopath may say that is what is being done, but this may be an attempt to simplify the complex terms of manipulation.

The enormous relief obtained from manipulative treatment arises from the creation of a better environment for the disc. Relaxation of the muscles, relief of ligament inflammation, separation of the intervertebral spaces to relieve pressure on the disc, mobilization and manipulation to restore proper mechanical function to the joint are all part of the therapeutic armoury of the osteopath and the chiropractor.

Massage
Extremely helpful between manipulative treatments, as it encourages relaxation of the powerful supportive muscles of the spine. This in turn minimizes muscular contortion and distortion of posture.

Psychotherapies
Long-term sufferers are likely to experience DEPRESSION and psychotherapy will be helpful here.

Vitamin and Mineral Treatment
Pain and inflammation may be reduced by high doses of calcium pantothenate (vitamin B$_5$) 2,000 mg daily, calcium orotate (1,600 mg daily) and Bromelain (600 mg daily) until relief is gained; then gradually reduce intake to a level that maintains relief.

Smoking *see* ADDICTIONS

Sore Throat

(Pharyngitis)

Sore throats can be caused by anything that irritates the sensitive mucous membranes at the back of the throat and mouth. This includes viral and bacterial infections; allergic reactions; irritants like dust, smoke, fumes and excessively hot food or drink; tooth or gum infections; abrasions (from fish bones for example); chronic coughing, excessive talking, shouting or screaming, particularly in children and babies. Hoarseness is a common side effect.

Sore throats accompany SCARLET FEVER; TONSILLITIS and rheumatic fever.

Laryngitis is inflammation of the larynx, the section of the wind pipe containing the voice box; it is caused by bacterial or viral infection and often follows a cold. It is particularly common among people who use their voice a lot, such as actors, clergymen and singers. Symptoms are pain on speaking, hoarseness, painful cough and excessive production of mucus.

Any long term changes in the character and pitch of the voice should be investigated without delay.

Orthodox Treatment
Antibiotics; steam inhalations.

Self-help
Stay in a warm atmosphere, rest the voice and inhale olbas oil, Friar's balsam and plain steam occasionally.

Herbal Treatment
Gargles: A weak infusion of sage several times daily (swallow 5 ml/1 tsp every 8 hours); agrimony gargle used 4 or 5 times a day; mullein leaves and flowers (25 g/1 oz to 0.5 l/1 pt water) simmered for 4 minutes, cooled and strained can be used every half hour if necessary for hoarseness and voice loss.
Infusions: Sage and thyme (30 ml/2 tbsp of each) and 2 peeled licorice sticks to 0.5 l/1 pt water boiling, simmered for 2 minutes then cooled and strained can be taken in doses of 15 ml/1 tbsp every 4 hours (add 5 ml/1 tsp of wild indigo to the infusion if available); marshmallow leaf infusion taken several times a day in 45–60 ml/3–4 tbsp doses soothes inflammation and helps hoarseness and voice loss.
Fomentation: Mullein leaves and infusion may be applied as a hot fomentation.

Take garlic oil tablets and echinacea daily (when able to swallow) to help combat the toxins in the body.

Homeopathy
For chronic sore throats consult a homeopath. Specific treatments for sore throat include:
- *Aconite* For laryngitis, sore throat following from exposure to cold dry winds and where there is a numb prickly feeling or croupy cough.
- *Hepar sulph* Where the patient feels chilly and irritable and upset by draughts of cold air; also for a fishbone sensation in the throat.
- *Apis* Where there are stinging pains, depression, and a bright red, shiny throat.
- *Belladonna* Where the throat is very sore, there is spasm on movement, hoarseness and pains spread to the head.
- *Mercurius solubilis* Where throat is dark red, swollen, sore, the breath is offensive and there are hot sweats.
- *Lachesis* Where soreness starts on the left side and the patient cannot bear tightness around the neck.

Specific treatments for laryngitis include:
- *Phosphorus* Where there is hoarseness, irritating dry cough, and a thirst for ice-cold drinks.
- *Causticum* For hoarseness, a raw feeling in throat and chest, and a cough with loss of urine or pain in the hip.
- *Spongia* For a dry barking cough.
- *Kali bichromicum* Where there is stringy sticky sputum, difficult to clear.

Naturopathy
Diet: adopt a fruit and fruit juice only diet for the first 24 hours (not for chil-

dren under 2 years old). Restrict dairy products, which encourage mucus production, until the symptoms have passed, and sugar and starch.
Heat/cold treatment: A cold compress to the throat is helpful for all age groups.

VITAMIN AND MINERAL
Vitamin C (500 mg 3 times daily) will enhance the body's resistance to infection. Sucking vitamin C plus zinc gluconate lozenges can also help by attacking micro-organisms at the site of infection.

Spastic Colon *see* IRRITABLE BOWEL SYNDROME

Spondylolisthesis *see* BACK PAIN

SPRAINS AND STRAINS

Sprains are the result of over-stretching ligaments that attach muscles to bones around a joint. They are painful and cause swelling and bruising.
Strains of muscle fibre are due to over use, excessive weight loading or falls.

SELF-HELP
Treat immediately by applying a cold compress or icepack (a bag of frozen peas works well) to speed recovery and minimize discomfort. An elastic bandage will also help, but it must not be so tight as to impede circulation.

HERBAL TREATMENT
Make an infusion of comfrey leaves (whole) place between sheets of muslin or gauze and wrap around affected area.

Soak a cotton wool pad with tincture of arnica (10 ml/2 tsp to 1 cup of cold water) and keep in place with a bandage until the swelling subsides.

A poultice of pounded ginger is helpful.

HOMEOPATHY
- *Arnica 30* Give at once then every hour.
- *Rhus tox 6* 4 times daily for muscular strain.
- *Ruta grav 6* 4 times daily for ligament strain.

MASSAGE
Massage to alleviate aches.

NATUROPATHY
Exercise: Ensure adequate balance of exercise to rest.
Heat/cold treatment: Apply hot and cold fomentations to specific muscle groups, (3 minutes hot to 1 minute cold for 20 minutes.)

STIFF NECK

See *also* TORTICOLLIS; POSTURAL PROBLEMS

A stiff neck is almost always caused by strain of the muscles and ligaments (see STRAINS AND SPRAINS), although bone, nerve and muscle disease, injury and ANXIETY are other possible causes.

An acute bout of stiffness should be investigated by a practitioner, as a stiff neck is one of the symptoms of meningitis.

ORTHODOX TREATMENT
Liniments, creams and sprays to stimulate the circulation and generate local heat may be prescribed.

SELF-HELP
Good posture (see **Positive Health/ Back Pack** p. 53) and exercise will help a stiff neck. Here is a simple one:
- Clasp hands together and cup over back of the head.
- Drop head forward. Feel the stretch.
- Using one hand, pull head over to one side and let it stretch.
- Then do the same on the diagonal.
- Repeat on the other side.

ACUPUNCTURE
Acupressure on any painful point

S

under the occiput, or on either side of the cervical and upper thoracic vertebrae, or along the muscle that makes up the top of the shoulder. (N.B. not if the stiffness is due to an inflammatory condition.)

ALEXANDER TECHNIQUE
This will be very helpful.

HERBAL TREATMENT
Relaxants such as valerian and compresses of anti-inflammatory herbs such as willow are helpful.

MANIPULATIVE TECHNIQUES
Manipulative therapy will bring instant relief if stiff neck is the result of minor dislocation of the vertebral joints in the neck.

MASSAGE
Massage will relax the muscles and help counteract tendency to spasm; pressure point massage will alleviate pain.

NATUROPATHY
Apply hot and cold fomentations (3 minutes hot, 1 minute cold) to back of neck and shoulders for 20 minutes 2 or 3 times a day.

RELAXATION TECHNIQUES
Relaxation techniques can help, especially **yoga** (*see* p. 99).

PSYCHOTHERAPIES
Recurrent stiff neck may be stress related (*see* ANXIETY, DEPRESSION, TENSION); in these cases psychotherapy will be helpful.

VITAMIN AND MINERAL TREATMENT
See ARTHRITIS

STINGS

Ants, bees, hornets and wasps can all sting. They inject poison into the skin, sometimes leaving their 'sting' in the puncture hole. Stings can be extremely irritating, and some people have severe allergic reactions to them (see ALLERGY) sometimes going into SHOCK.

People in shock must be seen by a medical practitioner at once.

SELF-HELP
If the insect sting is visible, remove with tweezers. Apply vinegar or lemon juice to wasp and ant stings. Dab bicarbonate of soda, washing blue or ammonia onto bee stings.

HERBAL TREATMENT
Antispasmodic formula dabbed onto the sting will relieve irritation.

A cooled infusion of elderflowers and applied on clean lint or cotton wool is soothing.

HOMEOPATHY
- *Ledum 30* Every 15 minutes immediately.
- *Apis Mell 30* Every 15 minutes if the sting produces swelling and a bad reaction.

STOMACH ACHE

See *also* DIGESTIVE DISORDERS; INDIGESTION

Ordinary stomach ache is most commonly caused by abuse of the digestive system, with excessive input of food, alcohol, fat, or inappropriate mixtures of food. A wide range of organisms can produce sickness (see NAUSEA) and DIARRHOEA with severe stomach pain. ANXIETY can cause bouts of acute griping pain.

Occasional episodes for obvious reasons, which soon clear up and have no long term effect on digestion, weight or general health, should be treated as minor discomforts.

Stomach pain associated with drastic weight loss, loss of blood, continual vomiting, prolonged periods of constipation or diarrhoea, or alternate episodes of both, may indicate more serious disorders and medical advice should be sought immediately.

ACUPUNCTURE
By harmonizing the energy of Stomach and Spleen obstructions, and therefore aches, that have been caused by climatic, emotional or nutritional excesses can be dispersed, but the causes have to be analysed and treated and not the symptom itself.

Acupressure on point 23 outside of the lower leg and point 27 in the midline of the abdomen will encourage Energy flow (see p. 102–3).

HERBAL TREATMENT
Adults should drink chamomile tea before meals. Peppermint tea is helpful at all times of day. For children, mix 5 ml/1 tsp powdered slippery elm bark to a paste with a little honey, and add gradually a cup of boiling water. Give this 2–3 times daily.

HOMEOPATHY
Consult a homeopath in cases of chronic inexplicable stomach ache.

NATUROPATHY
Recurrent mild attacks of stomach ache not associated with any underlying disease can be controlled by a sensible diet, including plenty of fibre and a reduction in caffeine and fat intake. You should also stop smoking.

RELAX
Relaxation exercises are helpful in the relief of stress-related stomach aches.

PSYCHOTHERAPY
May be indicated if the pain is a symptom of anxiety.

VITAMIN AND MINERAL TREATMENT
See DIGESTIVE PROBLEMS.

Stress see ANXIETY; BLOOD PRESSURE; TENSION; see also **Stress and how to deal with it** (p. 43) and **Relaxation Therapies** (p. 96).

Stretch marks see PREGNANCY AND CHILDBIRTH

STYES

Styes are BOILS on the margin of the eyelid, usually the lower one, caused by inflammation of a hair follicle. They are most common in people with poor general health.

A stye should come to a head after 4 or 5 days, and the enclosed pus released. Sometimes there is an eyelash in the middle of the stye; it should be taken out to encourage the pus to drain away more quickly. If it becomes infected, a stye may grow to the size of a pea, causing general inflammation of the eyelid and infection in the eye itself.

ORTHODOX TREATMENT
Antibiotic ointments; surgery.

SELF-HELP
- Do not rub the eye; you will spread infection. Children should have the affected eye covered with a pad of sterile gauze.
- Apply compresses of sterile cotton wool soaked in hot water to soothe the pain and help to bring the stye to a head.

HERBAL TREATMENT
Compresses: An infusion of plantain leaves and melilot left for 15 minutes then strained will ease pain and inflammation; finely grated carrot in a muslin bag compress will help bring the stye to a head; pulped raw groundsel in a muslin bag compress is antiseptic.
Eyebath: Use the plantain leaves and melilot infusion warm to bathe the closed eye.

Recurrent styes indicate a low level of vitality and blood cleansing remedies should be used. Consult a herbal practitioner.

HOMEOPATHY
For recurrent styes, consult a homeopath.
- *Aconite* To ease the pain when the stye erupts.

S

● *Pulsatilla* If aconite not effective.

VITAMIN AND MINERAL TREATMENT
Take a multimineral/multivitamin preparation plus extra vitamin C (500 mg 3 times daily) and extra zinc (15 mg daily).

SUNBURN

Sunburn is caused by the ultraviolet rays of the sun, and is more likely when the sun is at its highest. Ultraviolet rays are absorbed by the pigment produced by the skin, and if pigment-producing cells are lacking or have not had time to produce pigment — they need about 48 hours — the rays will burn the skin. This causes, at best, the skin to peel, removing what little tan you have acquired, and at worst, dehydration, blisters, sunstroke and serious illness.

Ultraviolet rays can also produce an allergic reaction (see ALLERGY) in as much as 10 per cent of the population, women rather more than men.

Excessive and prolonged exposure to the sun causes the skin to age quicker and, more importantly, is a major cause of skin cancer.

N.B. Sessions on a sunbed do *not* protect the skin from sunburn.

ORTHODOX TREATMENT
In severe burns, steroid ointments.

HERBAL TREATMENT
A mixture of 2 parts cider vinegar and 1 part olive oil helps moisten the skin and prevent sunburn, and its soothing qualities will relieve sunburn. A cool infusion of elderflowers, nettles or chamomile flowers, applied frequently and liberally, will reduce the heat. St John's wort will relieve the pain quickly.

VITAMIN AND MINERALS
There is no evidence to support the theory that taking vitamins will either protect you from sunburn or promote tanning. However, vitamin E will help

healing and prevent scarring: apply the cream directly and take 200 iu, 3 times daily. Vitamin C (1,000–1,500 mg daily) will help healing and prevent infection. In addition, zinc (15 mg daily) will also be beneficial.

Systemic lupus erythematosus (SLE) *see* ARTHRITIS

T

TEETH GRINDING

(BRUXISM)

Teeth grinding, when the jaws are clenched and the teeth ground together, especially during sleep, is usually a reflection of underlying stress or ANXIETY, but it can also be caused by discomfort in the mouth such as that produced by a badly done filling. Children commonly grind their teeth during sleep, often for no reason, but they usually grow out of it.

Teeth grinders may be completely unaware that they are doing it, but will wake to find the joints at the angle just in front of the ears are sore and painful. If intense teeth grinding persists it can wear away the enamel that covers the back teeth. The uneven wear of the teeth can lead to disturbance of the bite, producing in turn stresses on the joints of the jaw and consequently muscle and nerve tension which may lead to MIGRAINE.

ORTHODOX TREATMENT
The effects of teeth grinding are obviated by the fitting of a small plastic bite guard (made by a dentist) inserted between the back teeth before sleep.

ACUPUNCTURE
If the complaint is associated with stress acupuncture and moxibustion can help.

Acupressure on points 4 and 18 before going to bed may prevent teeth grinding (see pp. 104–5).

HYPNOTHERAPY
If due to underlying tension, hypnosis could help identify the source of it.

MANIPULATIVE THERAPIES
Manipulative treatment to the muscles and joints of the neck and shoulders will relieve habitual patterns of tension.

PSYCHOTHERAPIES
Teeth grinding can occur in sleep when the person is under severe stress and can give rise to pain in the jaw. Anger is often the underlying cause, since repressed anger can result in clenching of the teeth and chronic spasm of the facial muscles. Psychotherapies which allow for the release of anger can therefore be helpful. **Bioenergetics** (see p. 95) and encounter therapy can be helpful.

RELAXATION TECHNIQUES
Biofeedback (see p. 97) is especially helpful in learning to control the tension in the jaw muscles.

TENNIS ELBOW

Pain and stiffness in the elbow caused by local inflammation of the tendons from muscle stress and strain. Most typically this occurs through overuse or poor technique in racquet games, but other activities may spark it off.

Housemaid's Knee is the same pain and stiffness, but in the knee.

ORTHODOX TREATMENT
Anti-inflammatory drugs; injections of steroid and anaesthetic.

ACUPUNCTURE
Stimulating treatments with moxibustion applied direct to the skin or via needles are helpful.

HERBAL TREATMENT
Anti-inflammatory herbs such as willow and primula are extremely effective.

MANIPULATIVE THERAPY
This is often the most successful form of treatment.

MASSAGE
Effleurage (see p. 87) and the use of essential oils such as lavender or rosemary will stimulate circulation.

NATUROPATHY
For the first 24 hours, rest the arm and apply ice packs. Then stimulate circulation in the affected joint by contrast bathing, or apply ice packs followed by a quick hot rub and brisk towel dry.

VITAMIN AND MINERAL TREATMENT
See ARTHRITIS

TENSION

Tension is the contraction of the muscle fibres and the shortening of their ligaments. It is the outer physical sign of inner emotional problems such as ANXIETY, DEPRESSION anger and frustration.

SYMPTOMS
Tension can cause a chronic pain, often in the big muscles of the neck and shoulders (leading to HEADACHE); in the muscle between the shoulder blades (producing pain that radiates around the rib cage into the front of the chest); in the lower back muscles (producing LUMBAGO) and the abdominal muscles. It produces many symptoms such as hyperventilation, MIGRAINE, ASTHMA, DIARRHOEA, CONSTIPATION, NAUSEA, pins and needles in the extremities, raised BLOOD PRESSURE, irritability and considerable personality changes.

Tension and its side effects can become a self-perpetuating cycle. Emotional stress causes muscle tension and physical discomfort which in turn aggravates emotional distress.

ORTHODOX TREATMENT
Behaviour-modifying drugs and tranquillizers.

ACUPUNCTURE

Can be used to treat the Conception meridian (involved in higher thought processes) reducing excessive amounts of Energy and restoring a more harmonious balance.

ALEXANDER TECHNIQUE

This is usually very helpful.

HERBAL TREATMENT

See ANXIETY.

HYPNOTHERAPY

Hypnotherapy can alleviate the symptoms of tension.

MANIPULATIVE THERAPY

This can help dissipate the physical tension in the muscles.

MASSAGE

A full body massage with aromatic oils to enhance the treatment is relaxing. (Use a mixture of jasmine, rose, sandalwood and lavender, 15 drops to 50ml/about 3 tbsp almond oil.)

NATUROPATHY

Avoid excessive use of stimulants such as caffeine, nicotine, alcohol, and cut out junk food and sugar.

PSYCHOTHERAPIES

See ANXIETY.

RELAXATION TECHNIQUES

Yoga (p. 99) and **autogenics** (p. 97).

VITAMIN AND MINERAL TREATMENT

High potency vitamin B complex, preferably the prolonged release variety, plus vitamin E (100 iu with every meal) offer relief. Lack of calcium can lead to tension, nerve irritability and feelings of twitchiness in the limbs. Take a supplement if you have these symptoms.

THRUSH

(CANDIDIASIS)

This is a common infection caused by the yeast-like fungus *candida albicans.* Normally, this fungus lives in healthy balance with the other (benign) bacteria and yeasts that inhabit our mouths, bowels, skin — anywhere there is mucous membrane. When this natural balance is upset, the candida fungus multiplies dramatically and lodges deep into the tissues causing an outbreak of thrush. This may happen in the mouth, the throat, around the anus (especially in babies) in the urinary tract, the vagina or the head of the penis.

CAUSES OF THRUSH

The contraceptive pill, antibiotic drug therapy, immuno-suppressive drugs, diabetes mellitus (see DIABETES), and, in some cases, PREGNANCY can all upset the delicate bacterial balance and precipitate thrush. Debilitating diseases such as leukaemia have the same effect. In this case the infection may become systemic, carried by the bloodstream around the whole body. Thrush is also a common factor in recurring bouts of CYSTITIS.

Babies may contract thrush during their passage down the birth canal, and bottle-fed babies may develop it in their mouths. It can also occur on top of NAPPY RASH, since this provides the perfect environment for fungi to grow.

SYMPTOMS

In the vagina, thrush produces a large amount of unpleasant-smelling yellow/white discharge and intense itching.
In the mouth, small white sore patches form on the lips, tongue, gums and inside the cheeks.
In the penis, the tip may become inflamed (*balanitis*), the penis will be red and sore and there may be discharge from the urethra.
On the hands, the nail cuticles may be damaged; the infection can be painful and may deform the nails.

ORTHODOX TREATMENT

Fungicides used as a cream, lotion, ointment, pessary, tablets or injections.

T

- Thrush is very contagious and easily transmitted by sexual intercourse. If you or your partner suspect you have thrush (and it is much more prevalent among those women who take the contraceptive pill), you must BOTH be treated to avoid constant reinfection.
- Wear cotton pants, and avoid tights, hot bubble baths, excessive washing with strong soap and disinfectants.
- Live yoghurt is very helpful, either eaten, or applied directly to the vagina (use a tampon applicator).

HERBAL TREATMENT
Consult a herbal practitioner. A douche of myrrh and calendula may be recommended.

MYALGIC ENCEPHALOMYELITIS
Recently, some clinical ecologists have come to believe that many of the vague feelings of malaise, and fatigue, depression and symptoms associated with food intolerance may be related directly to thrush. The candida fungus is a highly allergenic organism, and the American ecologist, Dr Orion Truss, was the first to recognize that these allergenic factors could be the cause of various multiple food allergies and other allergic responses in certain people. This malaise has now been given a name — myalgic encephalomyelitis (ME) or Post Viral Fatigue Syndrome (PVFS). The symptoms vary — flu-like aches and pains, memory loss, irritability, depression, sometimes suicidal — but always include extreme muscular fatigue. Some people develop the illness after a bout of a different disease, indicating that the low state of their auto-immune system has allowed candida to take over.

This illness responds very well to natural therapies which help build up the body's own immune system, in tandem with orthodox treatments to control the candida, and the removal of the original cause — antibiotics, contraceptive pill, allergy etc.

HOMEOPATHY
Homeopathic doses of *candida* will help, but you must consult a homeopath.

NATUROPATHY
Naturopathic remedies are particularly helpful for those suffering from ME.
Diet: Cut out all starchy foods that yeasts feed on — sugars, refined carbohydrates, bread — and mushrooms, tea, coffee, chocolate and alcohol while the infection remains. Eat plenty of vegetables, salads, wholegrain cereals and fruit. Garlic (natural or as tablets) and olive oil will attack the yeast, and acidophilus (available as powder, tablets or in certain yoghurts) will help restore the correct bacterial balance. ME sufferers will have to keep this up for longer than those with a short bout. They may also have to try an exclusion diet (see p. 104) to ascertain if they are allergic and if so to what, and cut out any suspect food for life.
Exercise: ME sufferers must *not* over-exercise, and should consult a medical practitioner, preferably a clinical ecologist or naturopath.

VITAMIN AND MINERAL TREATMENT
High potency vitamin B complex, biotin (900 mcg daily) and high potency lactobaccilus acidophilus tablets help suppress excess yeast growth.

Tinea *see* RINGWORM

T

TINNITUS

See *also* HEARING PROBLEMS
A distressing condition in which buzzing, ringing or whistling noises are heard in the ear — usually intermittently, but at its worst, continuously. The noise is usually worse at night.

Common causes are damage to the ear through exposure to continuous noise, diseases of the ear and its nerve (*see* EARACHE), excessive wax in the ear, chronic CATARRH and SINUSITIS, and the use of aspirin-derived drugs and quinine. Deaf people commonly suffer tinnitus.

SELF-HELP
- Make sure ears are free of wax (see EARACHE).
- A personal stereo (at low volume) or a loudly ticking clock will sometimes help to mask out the inner sounds.

ACUPUNCTURE
This may bring partial relief.

NATUROPATHY
Avoid alcohol, nicotine and strong tea.

VITAMIN AND MINERAL TREATMENT
It may respond to high potency vitamin B complex, preferably the prolonged release variety.

TONSILS AND ADENOIDS

Tonsillitis is an acute infection of the tonsils, normally bacterial but occasionally viral.

The tonsils are the body's first line of defence against bacteria, trapping and killing them before they can reach and infect the lungs. During this defensive process, the tonsils may become infected themselves and the adenoids at the back of the nose are nearly always infected with them. When this happens, the adenoids become enlarged, blocking the passage of air through the nose into the Eustachian tubes. Sufferers are forced to breathe through the mouth, may lose the sense of smell and taste, and are prone to ear infections (see EARACHE) and BRONCHITIS.

SYMPTOMS
A SORE THROAT with red, enlarged tonsils, which may be covered in yellow spots of pus. There is pain on swallowing, swollen glands, FEVER and a furry tongue.

Complications are middle ear infections, and, rarely, rheumatic fever.

ORTHODOX TREATMENT
Antibiotics; children who have recurrent bouts may need surgery.

SELF-HELP
For general treatment see under CHILDREN'S ILLNESSES

HERBAL TREATMENT
Gargle with red sage extract (2.5 ml/½ tsp) in a cup of warm water several times daily. Make an infusion of 12 g/½ oz each of agrimony and raspberry leaves in 1 l/1¾ pts boiling water. Leave for 15 minutes then strain. Take 45–60 ml/3–4 tbsp 4 times daily.

Paint eucalyptus oil onto the tonsils, using a good quality soft brush.

HOMEOPATHY
For recurrent attacks, consult a homeopath. For specific remedies:
- *Belladonna* In the first stage, if there is high fever, delirium and a bright red face.
- *Hepar. sulph.* If there is the sensation of a fishbone in the throat, much yellow matter on the tonsils and chilly, irritable feeling.
- *Lachesis* If infection starts on the left side, and throat is extremely sensitive to touch and pressure of clothes.
- *Mercurius solubilis* If there is sweating, bad breath and excessive salivation.

NATUROPATHY
Diet: Check with a naturopath to see if dairy products should be excluded (if adenoids are affected).

Give plenty of fluids, especially pineapple juice, to children. Adults should adopt a cleansing regime or fast of pure unsweetened fruit juices 3–4 times daily for 3 days, followed by fruit, salads and vegetables and grain in a return to a wholefood diet.
Heat/cold treatment: Cold compresses round the neck will be soothing.

T

Children should take extra vitamin A and C. Adults should take 500mg vitamin C daily on top of any other therapy.

TOOTHACHE

Toothache can be caused by caries, an abscess or GINGIVITIS. Caries (tooth decay) is a very common condition, afflicting a quarter of all children under 12 in Britain.

All toothache is excruciating, but the kind of pain and its duration will indicate what is causing the trouble.

- *Short bursts* of pain triggered by sugary foods or hot and cold drinks mean you have caries with slight inflammation of the pulp within the tooth.
- *Long periods* of pain triggered by hot or cold drinks, or severe pain which arrived unheralded and is worse at night means the tooth pulp is very badly inflamed.
- *Intense throbbing* pain, especially associated with a tender patch of gum, is probably caused by an abscess; the abscess may push the tooth up from its socket and there is likely to be obvious inflammation and swelling around the tooth, slight FEVER and a general feeling of malaise.

TREATMENT
Go to your dentist. It is a great mistake to treat toothache with PAINKILLERS for long periods. Eventually the tooth pulp will die, the pain will go away but you will possibly develop an abscess and certainly lose the tooth.

SELF-HELP
Prevention is the best self help.
- Follow the 'Guidelines for Healthy Nutrition' (**Nutrition** pp. 18–19) and see also **Positive Health/ Teeth** pp. 50–1.
- Yearly visits to the dentist for a check-up are essential.

ACUPUNCTURE
Toothache may either be a condition of excess and relate to the energy of the Stomach, or of deficiency, with involvement of the Kidneys.

Treatment would aim to ensure the free flow of Chi energy through those pathways to the offending teeth.

Acupressure on the web of the hand between the thumb and forefinger at A and at either B and C on the foot may give temporary relief.

HERBAL TREATMENT
Oil of cloves provides immediate pain relief. Paint it on the surrounding gum, or if there is a cavity, plug it with cotton wool soaked in the oil.

The juice of a grated raw onion used in the same way is also soothing.

TORTICOLLIS

See *also* TENSION

A distressing condition in which the head is twisted to one side the neck bent, commonly backwards. It is caused by the involuntary spasm of one of the two large sternomastoid muscles, which run from the collar bone to behind the ear on each side of the head.

Babies are sometimes born with torticollis after damage to one of the muscles during birth.

In adults, it is usually caused by injury or may be a result of ANXIETY.

ORTHODOX TREATMENT
Simple exercises, surgery (babies); sedative drugs, physiotherapy, surgery (adults).

ACUPUNCTURE
Local treatment to the affected muscle with needles and moxibustion is used. Where the cause is emotional, the appropriate meridian will be treated.

ALEXANDER TECHNIQUE
This can be beneficial (*see* ANXIETY).

T

241

Manipulative therapy
Stretching of muscles and ligaments, mobilization and rehabilitation exercises can all help.

Massage
Massage may bring relief.

Psychotherapies
This is helpful when the underlying cause is emotional disturbance or anxiety.

Relaxation Techniques
Autogenics (p. 97)

Tranquillizer abuse *see* ADDICTIONS

TRAVEL SICKNESS

Any form of motion — cars, boats, planes, fairground rides — can cause travel sickness. This may range from slight NAUSEA to severe vomiting, DIZZINESS and FAINTING.

Orthodox Treatment
Anti-histamine drugs.

Herbal Treatment
Chew on a few pieces of crystallized ginger from time to time to alleviate sea sickness. Chamomile tea taken as a cool drink at intervals will help.

Homeopathy
- *Coccolus* When sickness associated with vertigo and is worse sitting up; sense of emptiness in head; the smell of food is upsetting.
- *Tabacum* When weak, sweating and trembling.
- *Petroleum* When there is wind in the stomach, water collects in the mouth, and you feel better for eating.

Vitamin and Mineral Treatment
Take vitamin B_6 (adults 25mg, children 10mg) an hour before the journey. Repeat the dose every 2 hours when travelling. The vitamin is more effective if taken with the herb ginger.

Trigeminal neuralgia *see* NEURALGIA

U

ULCERS

See *also* VARICOSE VEINS

Ulcers are eroded, inflamed patches on the surface of the skin or the internal mucous membranes that fail to heal. There are various kinds; the most common of which is MOUTH ULCERS.
- **Skin ulcers** occur in the legs as a result of VARICOSE VEINS. They may also be the result of pressure sores or BEDSORES.
- **Peptic ulcers** is the group name for duodenal and gastric ulcers, which are very similar but have to be distinguished as treatment for each differs.
Duodenal ulcers are distinct breaks in the mucous membrane of the duodenum caused by excessive enzymes and stomach acid. Stress is probably a triggering factor.
Gastric ulcers occur in the stomach, but are basically the same as duodenal ulcers, though less common. They occur mostly in older men.
Peptic ulcers occasionally rupture causing severe haemorrhage.

Orthodox Treatment
Drugs based on a synthetic derivative of licorice; antihistamine drugs; surgery (*peptic ulcers*).

Self-help
- Eat little and often as food is a buffer between your ulcer and your gastric juices.
- Don't rely on a 'bland diet' alone as this may be deficient in vitamin C which reduces the ability of the cells body to heal.

- Avoid smoking (especially if you have gastric ulcers).
- Cut down on alcohol (total abstention is not necessary).
- Rest and relax.
- If you take antacid tablets take them about 2 hours *after* a meal with additional doses as required until you next eat. (The dose of liquid antacid should be about 30 ml.) Food in the stomach is protecting you, so you don't need antacids while eating or digesting.

HERBAL TREATMENT
Consult a herbal practitioner for all ulcers.

External ulcers need the advice of a herbalist, but slippery elm bark powder can be dusted onto the ulcer and calendula ointment smeared round the margin.

Peptic ulcers are not for self treatment, but the following are treatments the herbalist will recommend:

Slippery elm powder will soothe inflamed painful tissue. It is available in tablets, or you could mix 5 ml/1 tsp to a paste with a little honey and a teacupful of boiling water or milk and water. Drink a teacupful 2 or 3 times daily.

A decoction of marshmallow root taken in 45–60 ml/3–4 tbsp doses 2 or 3 times daily is soothing and healing. A decoction of meadowsweet herb will alleviate acidity. Take 45–60 ml/3–4 tbsp before meals. Raw cabbage juice (1 1/2 pts daily taken in 6 doses) is a successful treatment.

HOMEOPATHY
Consult a homeopath for chronic cases.
Skin ulcers:
- *Arsenicum album* Where there are severe burning pains.
- *Kali bich* When ulcer has a clear cut edge, white mucus forms and there is pain in single spots.
Peptic ulcers:
- *Argentum nitricum* Where there is flatulence, butterfly feelings in the stomach, craving for sweet foods and tendency to PHOBIAS.

- *Nux vomica* For irritable pain that starts half an hour after pain; when there is CONSTIPATION.
- *Anacardium* For pain 2 hours after eating that is relieved by food.

HYPNOTHERAPY
Certainly hypnosis can help with pain; maybe also with acid levels.

MANIPULATIVE THERAPIES
By concentrating on the relevant areas of the spine, manipulative therapy can improve the nerve supplies to the stomach area and promote healing of peptic ulcers.

NATUROPATHY
Skin ulcers: Try a wholefood diet supplementing protein intake with nuts, seeds, grains and pulses.
Peptic ulcers: Gradually introduce a diet containing more vegetables and fresh fruit, which should be finely grated or puréed in the early stages. Cooked vegetables will be more easily digested. Increase grains and pulses to provide fibre and strengthen digestive functions. A high fibre diet will halve the likelihood of peptic ulcers recurring.

RELAXATION TECHNIQUES
Meditation (p. 98).

VITAMIN AND MINERAL TREATMENT
Skin ulcers may respond to oral vitamin E (400–600 iu daily) plus direct application of vitamin E cream. Leg ulcers sometimes associated with DIABETES have the same treatment plus folic acid (5 mg 3 times daily) and injections of 20 mg twice weekly in serious cases. *Gastric ulcers* have responded to 150,000 iu vitamin A daily for 4 weeks but only under medical supervision.

Urticaria *see* NETTLE RASH

U

V

Varicose Veins

See *also* PILES

These are distended veins occurring frequently in the rectum wall but most commonly in the legs.

The pumping action of the calf muscles and one-way valves inside the leg veins help blood back upwards to the heart. If the valves stop working efficiently blood collects in the veins, stretching them and producing varicosity. Weakness of the valves is often hereditary, but common causes of varicose veins are prolonged standing, OBESITY, PREGNANCY, CONSTIPATION and lack of exercise.

In severe cases the veins become inflamed producing ECZEMA and skin ULCERS.

ORTHODOX TREATMENT
Injections to divert blood to other blood vessels; surgery.

SELF-HELP
- Improve your diet to eliminate CONSTIPATION and avoid OBESITY (see **Nutrition** pp. 14–15).
- Don't stand or sit without movement for long periods.
- Don't sit with your legs crossed.
- Rest the legs with feet raised at the end of the day.
- Exercise regularly, especially walking.

HERBAL TREATMENT
Apply distilled witch hazel or tincture of calendula to the vein 2 or 3 times daily. Rutin helps strengthen blood vessels; it is available in tablet form and should be taken daily.

HOMEOPATHY
- *Arnica* Where veins feel bruised.
- *Hamamelis* Especially if associated with piles.
- *Carbo vegetablis* When circulation sluggish.
- *Fluoric acid* For simple cases where 'knots' appear in veins.
- *Pulsatilla* Useful during and after pregnancy.

MASSAGE
A very gentle soothing massage up the legs towards the heart is beneficial. Essential oils of calendula, lavender and rosemary will help. Use 15 drops to 50 ml/about 3 tbsp almond oil.

NATUROPATHY
Diet: Adopt a wholefood diet to avoid constipation and obesity.
Hydrotherapy: Contrast bathing with hot and cold water will ease the pain in the legs.

VITAMIN AND MINERAL TREATMENT
Bioflavonoids (100 mg daily) plus vitamin C (500 mg daily) can help reduce the condition. Vitamin E (400–600iu) daily can reduce swelling, pain, and prevent phlebitis. Lecithin (5–15 mg daily) complements the action of vitamin E.

Verruca *see* WARTS

Vertigo *see* DIZZINESS

Vitamin and Mineral Deficiency

See *also* **Nutrition** pp. 25–8

It is a sad fact that we can no longer rely on our food to deliver all our vitamins and minerals to us intact.

By the time we get to our food, many of the micronutrients have been stripped from it by the refining process. Then there is further despoliation in the kitchen: unnecessary peeling and chopping and over-long cooking can take away the little that is left. Try to make sure you get as much as you can out of your food:

- buy it whole as much as possible — brown rice, wholemeal bread etc.
- buy fresh vegetables every day.
- never peel vegetables unless the skin is extremely thick and horny; all the nutrients are found just under the skin; scrub them instead.
- never soak vegetables in water for long periods; all the vitamins leach out.
- never cut vegetables up very small — the longer they are on the chopping board and exposed to air, the more you are losing. Prepare vegetables quickly just before you need them.
- cook them in as little water as possible and do not throw the water away; save it for the stock pot — that way you get the minerals back.
- avoid frozen fruit and vegetables if possible — all the minerals lovingly locked in leach away when the vegetables defrost.

WHO NEEDS SUPPLEMENTS?

If you follow the tips above and eat a healthy diet you should be taking in the minimum recommended requirement (see chart). However, people who have no control over the buying and preparation of their food will need a daily multivitamin and mineral supplement. These are supplied in the minimum daily intake doses.

If you are young, old, pregnant, a heavy drinker or smoker, take the contraceptive pill or are on any other drugs, you will definitely be deficient.

Growing children need an assured daily intake of vitamins A, C and D; pregnant women will need supplements of the B complex and folic acid; elderly people may need extra calcium, vitamins B and C, or (if they don't nourish themselves properly because they live alone) the whole range. A daily multivitamin supplement with extra vitamin C (250–500 mg) will benefit most elderly people. Women taking the contraceptive pill need extra B_6.

The chart below indicates the minimum recommended daily requirement of the major vitamins and minerals, and the symptoms experienced if there is a deficiency. Symptoms only are listed, not specific deficiency diseases such as scurvy (vitamin C) pellagra (vitamin B_3) or beri beri (vitamin B_1) as these are extremely rare and caused by chronic vitamin deficiency rather than a temporary shortfall.

See also the Vitamin and Mineral charts on pp. 26–8, 245–7 for further information.

Vitamin and mineral deficiency chart

Vitamin	Daily need	Deficiency symptoms/effects	Other factors
A (retinol)	750 μg/2500 iu	night blindness, catarrhal and bronchial infections, dry flaky skin, general fatigue	deficiency may be caused by certain drugs, liquid paraffin and malabsorption of fats.
B_1 (thiamine)	1.5 mg	nervous disorders, anorexia, fatigue, anxiety states, heart problems, depression, skin and hair problems	alcohol, tobacco and high carbohydrate diets may cause deficiency
B_2 (riboflavin)	1.7 mg	anaemia, mouth and tongue ulcers, poor vision; very rare in man	contraceptive pill may induce deficiency
B_3 (niacin, nicotinic acid)	19 mg (21 mg during lactation)	dermatitis, diarrhoea, dementia, skin goes dark and scaly when exposed to sunlight	an excessive intake of refined foods can cause deficiency

V

Vitamin	Daily need	Deficiency symptoms/effects	Other factors
B_5 (pantothenic acid)	10 mg	insomnia, fatigue, 'burning feet' syndrome; deficiency is unlikely	excessive intake of refined foods might cause deficiency
B_6 (pyridoxine)	2 mg 10 mg for pregnant women 25 g for women for 10 days before menstruation 25–30 mg for women taking contraceptive pill	mild depression, insomnia, nerve problems, irritability, certain anaemias	pregnancy, contraceptive pill, smoking, alcohol, anti TB drugs and antibiotics can all cause deficiency
B_{12}	3 μg 5 μg for pregnant women + women taking contraceptive pill 4 μg during lactation	pernicious anaemia, nervous disorders, burning sensation of tongue	vegan diet, contraceptive pill, heavy smoking and many antibiotics and other drugs all cause deficiency
folic acid	400 μg 600 μg for pregnant women 500 μg during lactation	anaemia	pregnancy, contraceptive pill, alcohol and many drugs can cause deficiency
biotin	300 μg	depression, loss of appetite, nausea, muscular pain, dermatitis	eating raw eggs can cause deficiency
C (ascorbic acid)	60 mg 80 mg for pregnant women	slow wound healing, sore gums, scaly skin, easy bruising, pains in joints, lack of resistance to infection	aspirin, contraceptive pill, alcohol, smoking, corticosteroids and other drugs can all cause deficiency
D	10 μg/400 iu	bone deformities and degeneration, tooth decay	lack of sunshine and dairy products or fish oils, malabsorption of fat and liquid paraffin can all cause deficiency
E (tocepherol)	30 mg	anaemia in infants, muscle wastage	contraceptive pill, excessive intake of refined vegetable oil and liquid paraffin can all cause deficiency
K	500–1000 μg	blood fails to clot in normal time; haemorrhage, deficiency unlikely as vitamin made by body in intestines	antibiotics, liquid paraffin and malabsorption of fats may cause deficiency

V

Mineral	Daily need	Deficiency symptoms/effects	Other factors
Calcium (Ca)	1,000 mg	stunted growth in children, rickets, osteoporosis, loss of muscle control	vitamin D deficiency will hinder absorption
Phosphorous (P)	1,000 mg	loss of appetite, weakness, but very rare in man	excessive use of antacids may cause deficiency
Sodium (Na)	1,200 mg	muscle cramp, dehydration, mental apathy, low blood pressure	heavy work/exercise, heavy sweating can cause deficiency. NB excess sodium can cause high blood pressure
Potassium (K)	3,000 mg	muscle weakness, cramps, irregular heartbeat, mental deficiency	purgatives and diuretics cause deficiency
Magnesium (Mg)	400 mg	apathy, muscle weakness, convulsions, trembling	excessive diarrhoea and heavy drinking causes deficiency
Iron (Fe)	18 mg	anaemia	vitamin C deficiency hinders absorption
Zinc (Zn)	15 mg	failure to grow, poor appetite, poor wound healing, infertility, mental apathy, loss of taste, skin diseases, anorexia, acne, behavioural disorders in children	a diet of refined food, drugs such as corticosteroids, pregnancy, contraceptive pill, heavy drinking can all cause deficiency
Iodine (I)	200 μg	enlarged thyroid gland, drowsiness, coarse skin and hair, weight gain, apathy, muscle weakness	lack of iodine in the soil in which the food grows causes deficiency
Copper (Cu)	4 mg	anaemia, greying hair, lowered resistance to infection	a diet of exclusively refined food may cause deficiency
Manganese (Mg)	5 mg	no established deficiency symptoms	
Chromium (Cr)	200 μg	diabetes in pregnancy and elderly people	eating only refined food can cause deficiency
Selenium (Se)	200 μg	some types of anaemia	excessive intake of refined foods and deficiency in the soil can cause deficiency or loss
Cobalt (Co)	1 μg	see vitamin B_{12} (cobalt occurs with this vitamin)	see vitamin B_{12}
Sulphur (S)	800 mg	no known symptoms	
Molybdenum (Mo)	500 μg	dental caries, male impotence, irritability, irregular heartbeat, lack of uric acid production	high intakes of refined, processed food and deficiency in the soil may cause deficiency

● iu stands for international units; this is an old fashioned method of measuring vitamins, and only three are still measured this way: A, D and E. In the chart, measurement are given both in ius (where relevant) and in milligrams (mg) or micrograms (μg).

V

Heavy drinkers and smokers, who may well be taking in the minimum requirement recommended will need supplements because their habits inhibit the action of the vitamins and minerals they do consume. People taking medicinal drugs also need supplements: antibiotics mean extra vitamins B and K; corticosteroids need extra vitamin B_6, C, calcium and zinc; diuretics need extra potassium; aspirin and anti-inflammatory drugs need extra vitamin C. The supplements may need to be up to 5 times the minimum recommended requirement.

Undiagnosed mineral deficiencies can cause a wide range of problems. One of the most important is zinc deficiency which can be detected by a simple zinc taste test. Adolescents, pregnant and nursing mothers have increased needs for zinc and should take a zinc supplement.

If you think you are in need of a vitamin supplement because of suspected deficiency, always consult a naturopath or medical practitioner first: it is easy to overdo the dose, especially important with vitamin A.

The recommended daily requirements for the average healthy person are given in the chart.

> When wholemeal flour is refined into white flour, this is what you lose:
> 60 per cent calcium
> 77 per cent potassium
> 78 per cent sodium
> 71 per cent phosphorous
> 32 per cent sulphur
> 89 per cent cobalt
> 98 per cent chromium
> 68 per cent copper
> 76 per cent iron
> 85 per cent magnesium
> 86 per cent manganese
> 48 per cent selenium
> 78 per cent zinc
> Calcium and iron are replaced, albeit not entirely, but the other minerals are not.

Vomiting see NAUSEA; see also ANOREXIA NERVOSA; PREGNANCY AND CHILDBIRTH

W–Z

WARTS

Warts are caused by a virus and are highly infectious. There are several strains of wart virus, giving rise to warts on different parts of the body: thick, hard, painful warts on the soles of the feet (verrucae), flat warts on the face, rough, horny cauliflower like warts on the knees and on the knuckles and nail folds of the hands, and ano-genital warts are all common.

Warts incubate for several months before breaking out. The body's own immune system will eventually kill them off, but this can take a long time, up to two years. When the warts do go, they drop off very quickly, giving rise to legends of 'miracle cures' if the miracle remedy has been applied just before the body has cured the wart by itself.

Verrucae in children should always be treated by a chiropodist as they are painful and spread easily in schools and swimming pools.

Genital warts are transmitted by sexual contact. They must be treated quickly by a medical practitioner as they spread like wildfire. There is some evidence that links genital warts with cervical cancer, so it is important to follow up treatment with regular cervical smear tests.

ORTHODOX TREATMENT
Freezing or burning.

FIRST-AID
Left alone, most warts go away of their own accord, but if they are distressing, a proprietary wart remover may be useful. Patent treatments do not kill the wart virus, only remove the hard horny layers of skin that the virus produces. Most of them are based on salicylic acid, so be careful not to spill them onto healthy skin.

Soak the affected area in warm soapy water for a few minutes, then gently rub the horny layer of the wart with a fine pumice stone. Apply a corn plaster with a hole in the middle over the wart to protect the surrounding skin and paint the wart with the remover.

Do not treat facial or genital warts in this way as scarring and irritation will result.

HERBAL TREATMENT
Verrucae and warts can be treated in the same way. Rub the wart with a crushed garlic clove or garlic juice, lemon juice, castor oil, dandelion stalk juice or the juice from the stalks of the greater celandine (do not let this spill onto normal skin). Wash your hands thoroughly afterwards to prevent the spread of infection.

WHIPLASH

Whiplash is an injury to the vertebrae, muscles and ligaments of the neck caused by sudden and violent backward jerk of the neck. It is commonly caused by rear-impact car accidents. Muscles fibres and ligaments can be torn and the spine damaged—at worst, there may be injury to the spinal cord and paralysis.

The pain from whiplash is often longstanding and may become chronic and disabling in itself. Natural therapies can help here. (See *also* PAIN AND PAIN-KILLERS.)

ORTHODOX TREATMENT
Painkillers; supportive cervical collar.

SELF-HELP
Fit properly adjusted head rests to front and rear seats of your car. The adjustment should be easy to suit all your different passengers. DO NOT USE THEM AS NECK RESTS, as this increases the risk of serious injury.

ACUPUNCTURE
Acupuncture can help combat the pain.

ALEXANDER TECHNIQUE
This is very helpful during recovery.

HERBAL TREATMENT
Consult a herbal practitioner who will prescribe anti-inflammatory herbs such as willow.

MANIPULATIVE THERAPIES
Manipulative treatment is particularly effective in correcting sprains and dislocations; it cannot be used if there is injury to the spinal cord or fracture of the vertebrae.

MASSAGE
Massage and remedial exercises will help restore normal movement as soon as possible and to alleviate the chronic pain.

VITAMIN AND MINERAL TREATMENT
Stiffness may be relieved by high-dose calcium pantothenate (vitamin B_5). Start with 2,000 mg daily (preferably in prolonged release form); once relief is obtained, reduce dose gradually to the level which maintains relief.

WHOOPING COUGH

(PERTUSSIS)

This is a highly infectious bacterial illness of childhood, affecting the respiratory system. It is most infectious in the early stages and spread by coughs and sneezes. The illness can last up to three months; most children recover completely, but it is dangerous in very young babies, who may have to go into hospital.

Whooping cough occurs epidemically every four years or so.

SYMPTOMS
Normal cold symptoms of a cold, (runny eyes, nose, cough and slight temperature) followed after two weeks,

by the main symptom of violent and uncontrollable bouts of coughing often followed by vomiting. The child cannot breathe during the coughing spasms and may appear to be suffocating. Bouts are followed by the typical 'whoop' sound as the child gasps to breathe in again. Small babies can become short of oxygen and find it difficult to breathe in again after coughing spasm.

Complications are encephalitis, brain damage from lack of oxygen or the rupturing of blood vessels in the brain, secondary chest infection and sometimes PNEUMONIA.

ORTHODOX TREATMENT
Antibiotics; immunization.

SELF-HELP
For general guidelines see CHILDREN'S ILLNESSES.

HERBAL TREATMENT
For the cough: Add one large clove of garlic, finely sliced to 100 g/4 oz runny honey. Cover and leave overnight. Add 5 ml/1 tsp to a cup of warm water and sip (4 times daily). Simmer 15 ml/1 tbsp crushed linseed and 25 g/1 oz peeled licorice sticks with water in a covered pan for half an hour. Pour 0.5 l/1 pt over 25 g/1 oz each of white horehound and coltsfoot, and 15 ml/1 tsp thyme. Cover, cool and strain through a coffee filter or fine cloth. Take every 4 hours (5 ml/1 tsp under 2 years, 10 ml/2 tsps for 2 to 5 years and 12 ml/1 dessertsp over 5 years.)
For breathing: Rub the chest with olbas oil to improve breathing.
As antibiotic: Rub the soles of the feet with cut cloves of garlic or garlic salve. Research has proved this to have good results; it reaches the lungs in half an hour.

HOMEOPATHY
Consult a homeopath.

NATUROPATHY
Maintain a high liquid intake especially if child is vomiting after coughing. Give small quantities of light food between coughing bouts, rather than 3 meals a day. Avoid all dairy products and give fruit and vegetable juice and easily digested food such as brown rice, wholemeal toast, wholemeal pasta, porridge made with water, yeast extracts and clear soups until the appetite returns.

VITAMIN AND MINERAL TREATMENT
Vitamin C (500 mg 3 times daily) may be given to strengthen the body's defences (This is in addition to any other therapy.)

Whooping Cough and Vaccination
The adverse publicity of the side-effects of whooping cough vaccine has generated increased interest in the use of homeopathic vaccinations for this disease. Many homeopaths believe that homeopathic vaccination is effective but there is no clinical evidence to support this claim, so the Faculty of Homeopathy at The Royal London Homeopathic Hospital has stated that all children should receive the conventional immunization against whooping cough unless there is a definite medical contraindication.
The most important contraindications for the vaccine are as follows:
- children who have ever suffered from convulsions.
- children who suffered neurological damage at birth, however slight.
- children whose parents or brothers and sisters suffer from convulsions or brain damage.

Furthermore, pharmacists have been advised by the Council of the Pharmaceutical Society of Great Britain only to supply homeopathic whooping cough vaccine against a prescription, and to advise people trying to buy them to see their GP.

The statistics apparently show that there is more risk of severe illness arising from whooping cough than there is from using the orthodox immunization. Parents must make their own judgement in this area but should take sound objective advice.

Wry neck *see* TORTICOLLIS

Yeast Infections *see* THRUSH

RESOURCES

Below are some useful addresses and further reading

General
British Holistic Medical Association
179 Gloucester Place
London NW1 6DX
01 262 5299
01 402 2768

College of Health
18 Victoria Park Square
London E2 9PF
01 980 6263

Institute for Complementary Medicine
21 Portland Place
London W1N 3AF
01 636 9543

Research Council for Complementary Medicine
Suite 1
19a Cavendish Square
London W1M 9AD
01 493 6930

Acupuncture
British Acupuncture Association and Register
34 Alderney Street
London SW1 4EV
01 834 1012

British College of Acupuncture
44 New Market Square
Basingstoke,
Hants

Addictions
Alcoholics Anonymous
PO Box 514
11 Redcliffe Gardens
London SW10 9BQ
01 352 9779

153 Lisburn Road,
Belfast BT9 6AJ
0232 681084

Al Anon Family Groups
61 Great Dover Street
London SE1 4YF
01 403 0888

Alcohol Concern
305 Grays Inn Road
London WC1X 8QF
01 833 3471

The Accept Clinic
200 Seagrave Road
London SW6
01 381 2112

Alexander Technique
Society of Teachers of the Alexander Technique
10 London House
226 Fulham Road
London SW10 9EL
01 351 0828

2 Royal Terrace
Glasgow G3 7NT
Scotland

90 Ninian Road
Roath
Cardiff
Wales

7 Dun An oir
The Old Bawn
Tallaght
Co. Dublin
Eire

SATA
64 Alfred Street
Milson's Point
New South Wales 2061
Australia
929–8910

Allergy
Allergy Foundation of America,
801 2nd Avenue
New York
NY 10017
USA

Arthritis
Arthritis Care
6 Grosvenor Crescent
London SW1X 7ER
01 235 0902

Meall Ruidh
Carie
by Rannoch Station
Perthshire PH17 2QJ
Scotland
08822 357

19 Tathan Crescent
St Athan
Barry
Glamorgan CF6 9PE
Wales
0446 750456

31 New Forge Lane
Belfast B19 5NW
N. Ireland
0232 669882

Arthritis and Rheumatism Council
41 Eagle Street
London WC1
01 405 8572

Autogenics
Centre for Autogenic Training
15 Fitzroy Square
London W1
01 388 1007

Back Pain
Back Pain Association
31–33 Park Road
Teddington
Middlesex TW11 0AB
01 977 5474

The Back Store
324a King Street
Hammersmith
London W6 0RF
01 741 5022

Chiropractic
Anglo-European College of Chiropractic
13–15 Parkwood Road
Bournemouth
Hants BH5 2DF
0202 431028

British Chiropractors Association
5 First Avenue
Chelmsford
Essex CM1 1RX
0245 358487

Australian Chiropractors Association
1 Martin Place
Linden
NSW 2778
Australia

Chiropractors Registration Board
McKell Building
Rawson Place
Sydney
NSW Australia

Chiropractors and Osteopaths Registration Board of Victoria
PO Box 4790
GPO
Melbourne
Victoria 3001

Herbalism
British Herb Growers Association
17 Hooker Street
London SW3

The British Herbal Medicine Association
The Old Coach House
Southborough Road
Surbiton
Surrey

The National Institute of Herbal Medicine
148 Forest Road
Tunbridge Wells
Kent
0892 30400

The General Council and Register of Consultant Herbalists and The British Herbalists Union Ltd
93 East Avenue
Bournemouth
Hants

The Herb Society of America
300 Massachusetts Avenue
Boston
Massachusetts 02115
USA

The Herb Society of South Australia Inc
PO Box 140
Parkside
South Australia 5063

The Queensland Herb Society
23 Greenmount Avenue
Holland Park
Brisbane
Queensland
Australia

The National Institute of Medical Herbalists Ltd
20 Osborne Avenue
Jesmond
Newcastle on Tyne

Herbal suppliers
Potter's Ltd
Douglas Works
Leyland Mill Lane
Wigan
Lancs WN1 2SB

Weleda UK Ltd
Heanor Road
Ilkeston
Derbyshire DE7 8DR

The Bach Centre
Mount Vernon
Sotwell
Wallingford
Oxon OX10 0PZ

Abbotts's Physio Laboratories Ltd
56 Railway Road
Leigh
Lancs

Homeopathy
The Homeopathic Development Foundation Ltd
19a Cavendish Square
London W1M 9AD
01 629 3204

The Royal London Homeopathic Hospital
Great Ormond Street
London WC1N 3HR
01 837 3091

Homeopathic Suppliers
A Nelson & Co Ltd
73 Duke Street
London W1M 6BY
01 629 3118

Ainsworths' Homeopathic Pharmacy
38 New Cavendish Street
London W1M 7LH
01 935 5330

Hyperactivity
Hyperactive Children Support Group
59 Meadowside
Angmering
Sussex BN16 4BW

Hypnotherapy
Association of Hypnotists and Psychotherapists
Blythe Tutorial College
25 Market Square
Nelson
Lancs
0282 699378

British Hypnotherapy Association
67 Upper Berkeley Street
London W1H 7DH

Migraine
The British Migraine Association
178a High Road
Byfleet
Weybridge
Surrey KT14 7ED
09323 52468

The Migraine Trust
45 Great Ormond Street
London WC1N 3HD
01 359 3563

Myalgic Encephalomyelitis (ME)
The ME Association
PO Box 8
Stanford-le-Hope
Essex

Naturopathy
Incorporated Society of Registered Naturopaths
1 Albemarle Road
The Mount
York YO2 1EN

British College of Naturopathy and Osteopathy and British Naturopathic and Osteopathic Association
Frazer House
Netherall Gardens
London NW3 5RR
01 435 8728

Chiropractic and Osteopathy
The British Naturopathic and Osteopathic Association
Frazer House
Netherhall Gardens
London NW3 5RR
01 435 8728

The British College of Naturopathy & Osteopathy
Frazer House
Netherhall Gardens
London NW3 5RR

The British School of Osteopathy
1–4 Suffolk Street
London SW1Y 4HG
01 839 2060

European School of Osteopathy
104 Tonbridge Road
Maidstone
Kent ME16 8SL

Australian Osteopathy Association
252 Packington Street
Geelong West 3218
Victoria
Australia

Chiropractors and Osteopaths Registration Board of Victoria
PO Box 4790
GPO
Melbourne
Victoria 3001

Psychotherapy
The Albany Trust
24 Chester Square
London SW1
01 730 5871

Association for Humanistic Psychology
62 Southwark Bridge Road
London SE1
01 928 8253/4

Boyesen Centre
Acacia House
Centre Avenue
The Vale
London W3
01 793 2437

Co-Counselling Phoenix
5 Victoria Road
Sheffield
Yorks S10 2DJ
0742 686371

Family Welfare Association
501–5 Kingsland Road
London E8
01 254 6251

Holwell Centre for Psychodrama
East Down
Barnstaple.
Devon
027 1822681

North Street Counselling Centre
23 Grove Road
Leighton Buzzard
Beds LU7 8SF
0525 379574

Philadelphia Association
14 Peto Place
London NW1
01 486 9012

The Psychotherapy Centre
1 Wythburn Place
London W1H 5WL
01 723 6173

British Association of Psychotherapists
121 Hendon Lane
London N3 3PR
01 346 1747

Vegetarianism
The Vegetarian Society
53 Marloes Road
London W8 6LA
01 937 7739

Vegan Society
47 Highlands Road
Leatherhead
Surrey
0372 372089

Yoga
The British Wheel of Yoga
80 Lechampton Road
Cheltenham
Gloucestershire

FURTHER READING

General
Herbert Benson
The Relaxation Response
Fountain Press, Surbiton, Surrey 1971

Boston Women's Health Collective
Our Bodies, Our Selves
Penguin 1978

Fritjof Capra
The Turning Point
Fontana 1983

Ivan Illich
Limits to Medicine
Boyars 1976

Brian Inglis and Ruth West
The Alternative Health Guide
Mermaid/Michael Joseph

Thomas Mckeown
The Role of Medicine: Dream, Mirage or Nemesis?
Blackwell 1979

Kenneth Pelletier
Mind as Healer, Mind as Slayer: a holistic approach to preventing stress disorders
Allen & Unwin 1979

Patrick C Pietroni
Holistic Medicine: new map, old territory
British Journal of Holistic Medicine vol 1, 3–13 1984

Mike Samuels and Hal Bennett
The Well Body Book
to overcoming cancer for patients and their families
Bantam 1980
Wildwood House 1974

Carl O. Simonton *et al*
Getting Well Again: a
step-by-step self-help guide

Back pain
Dr David Imrie with Colleen Dimson
Goodbye Backache
Sheldon Press

Dr Alan Stoddard
The Back: Relief from Pain
Martin Dunitz

Bates Training
W H Bates MD
Better Eyesight without Glasses
Panther Books

Herbalism
Philip M Chancellor, ed
Handbook of the Bach Flower Remedies
CW Daniel & Co Ltd

Nalda Gosling
Successful Herbal Remedies
Thorsons

Barbara Griggs
Green Pharmacy
Jill Norman Publishers

Loewenfeld and Back
Herbs for Health and Cookery
Pan Books

Schauenberg & Paris
A Guide to Medicinal Plants
Lutterworth Press

Richard le Strange
A History of Herbal Plants
Angus & Robertson

Malcolm Stuart
An Encyclopedia of Herbs and Herbalism
Orbis

William A R Thomson
Healing Plants
Macmillan

Robert Tisserand
Aromatherapy
Mayflower Granada Publishing

Doris Grant and Jean Joice
Food Combining for Health: a new look at the Hay system
Thorsons

Maurice Hanssen
E for Additives and E for Additives Supermarket Shopping Guide
Thorsons

Leonard Mervyn
Thorsons Complete Guide to Vitamins and Minerals
Thorsons

Thorson's Diet to Help series Including *Hay Fever and Asthma, Heart Disease, Cystitis, Diabetes* and *Control Cholesterol.*

Massage
Claire Maxwell-Hudson *et al*
The Book of Massage
Ebury Press

Naturopathy
Roger Newman Turner
Naturopathic Medicine
Thorsons

Psychotherapy
Lewith and Kenyon
Clinical Ecology
Thorsons

Anthony Clare and Sally Thompson
Let's Talk about Me
BBC Publication

J Kovel
A Complete Guide to Therapy from Psychoanalysis to Behaviour Modification
Pelican

A Lowen
Bioenergetics
Penguin

F Perls
The Gestalt Approach
Bantam

C R Rogers
On Becoming a Person
Constable

INDEX

PHOTOGRAPHIC CREDITS

Pages 70 and 71: Rex Features/P H Hutchings; page 81: Daily Telegraph Colour Library/Geg Germany; page 85: British Chiropractic Association, Alan F Raymond.